ANESTHESIA IN COSMETIC SURGERY

One major by-product of the aging baby-boom generation has been a surging interest in cosmetic surgery. Outpatient cosmetic surgery clinics have sprouted up in droves all over the United States, and the number of cosmetic procedures performed in 2005 increased by more than 95% from the previous year. Although procedures like facelifts and abdominoplasties are considered minimally invasive, the anesthetic protocols and regimens involved are often overly complex and unnecessarily toxic. Major complications involving anesthesia in this (and any other) surgical milieu can range from severe postoperative nausea and vomiting (PONV) to postoperative pain to mortality. Although mortality may be rare, there have been many cases in which perfectly healthy cosmetic surgery patients require emergency intervention due to a severe complication involving anesthesia. In recent years, many new anesthetic protocols have been developed to reduce the incidence of PONV and other complications, while ensuring that effective pain management and level of "un-awareness" during surgery are always maintained.

Barry L. Friedberg, M.D., is a volunteer assistant professor at the Keck School of Medicine, University of Southern California. Since 1992, he has practiced exclusively in the subspecialty of office-based anesthesia for elective cosmetic surgery. He founded the Society for Office Anesthesiologists (SOFA) in 1996 that he merged in 1998 with the Society for Office Based Anesthesia (SOBA), another non-profit, international society dedicated to improving patient safety through education. Dr. Friedberg is the developer of propofol ketamine (PK) technique designed to maximize patient safety by minimizing the degree to which patients need to be medicated to create the illusion of general anesthesia, that is, "no hear, no feel, no recall."

Anesthesia in Cosmetic Surgery

BARRY L. FRIEDBERG, M.D.

Assistant Professor in Clinical Anesthesia
Volunteer Faculty
Keck School of Medicine
University of Southern California
Los Angeles, CA

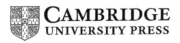

CAMBRIDGE UNIVERSITY PRESS
Cambridge, New York, Melbourne, Madrid, Cape Town, Singapore, São Paulo

Cambridge University Press
32 Avenue of the Americas, New York, NY 10013-2473, USA

www.cambridge.org
Information on this title: www.cambridge.org/9780521870900

First published 2007

Printed in the United States of America

A catalog record for this publication is available from the British Library.

Library of Congress Cataloging in Publication Data

Anesthesia in cosmetic surgery / [edited by] Barry L. Friedberg.
    p. ; cm.
Includes bibliographical references and index.
ISBN 978-0-521-87090-0 (hardcover)
1. Anesthesia.   2. Surgery, Plastic.   I. Friedberg, Barry L., 1948—
[DNLM: 1. Anesthesia—methods.   2. Cosmetic Techniques.   3. Surgical Procedures, Elective.
WO 200 A579543 2007]
RD81.A5445   2007
617.9′6–dc22   2007001311

ISBN 978-0-521-87090-0 hardback

Come mothers and fathers
Throughout the land
And don't criticize
What you can't understand
Your sons and your daughters
Are beyond your command
Your old road is
Rapidly agin'
Please get out of the new one
If you can't lend your hand
For the times they are a-changin.'

– Robert "Bob Dylan" Zimmerman
"The Times They Are A-Changin," 1963

To my parents, my first teachers, who taught me it was acceptable to not be like everyone else as long as I aspired to be the best I could be.

To Willy S. Dam, M.D., of Bispebjerg Hospital, Copenhagen, my first anesthesia teacher, who encouraged me to become an anesthesiologist.

To all the patients who have suffered from previous anesthetics and who may now be relieved of their PONV, postoperative pain, and prolonged emergences.

Contents

Foreword

Physicians, like all people, live in a world that is proscribed more by what we do in rote fashion every day than by what we understand in any meaningful way. Our modern lives have become so harried that most of us barely have enough time to pause and reflect on what we have done and where we are going.

Dr. Barry L. Friedberg, at great personal effort and time, has put forth this pearl of a book: ideas, methods of practice, and salient knowledge on the cutting edge of modern medical practice as they apply to the world of minimally invasive anesthesia for cosmetic surgery. As many of our practices prove every day in operating rooms across the United States and beyond, the information and anecdotes provided here apply equally well to a whole host of different anesthetic and surgical settings.

Modern science is replete with heroic strides in improving patient care and decreasing perioperative morbidity and mortality—and yet, today, we still do not understand the underlying mechanisms of general anesthesia on the brain, *much less the construct of consciousness itself!*

The field of anesthesiology and perioperative medicine achieved unprecedented gains in patient outcomes through the advent of pulse oximetry decades ago. Since then, we have refined our techniques, implemented new airway devices, decreased postoperative nausea and vomiting, improved our times to "street readiness," and done a better job of managing pain. Now is the time to move to the next level of patient care.

Dr. Friedberg, through unrelenting drive and perseverance, has brought to light the benefits of the age-old concept that "less is more." Through the use of minimally invasive anesthetic techniques, a resurgence in the prudent use of ketamine via the propofol-ketamine (PK) technique, and the application of brain wave (level-of-consciousness) monitoring, Dr. Friedberg has brought anesthesia care to a higher plane.

When Albert Einstein died, curious scientists autopsied his brain in the futile quest to glean some insight into one of humanity's greatest minds. They were desperately seeking answers to how this one man transformed Newtonian physics into an advanced understanding of the universe itself. Today, physicists struggle with String Theory and other abstract mathematical concepts to solve the ultimate riddle of bridging relativity theory with quantum mechanics in one grand unifying equation. But back in 1905, when Einstein's first papers were reaching the scientific print, he was greeted as a heretic. At one point, a group of one hundred of the world's most renowned scientists signed a document stating that Mr. Einstein was not correct in his radical departure from conventional theory. Albert Einstein is reported to have replied, in paraphrase, "if they were so sure that they were right and I was wrong, then why does this letter contain one hundred signatures—in that case, they should need only one signature!"

In this same vein, there have been those detractors who espouse opposition to some of the elegant medical practices and insights put forth by Dr. Friedberg. To those voices, hiding in the shadow of inexperience, I say with a loud and confident voice—come join us, read on, and enjoy this journey along the road to greater insight and knowledge. Some have suggested that Dr. Friedberg is "redefining anesthesia"—and, in some contexts and practice paradigms, this may be true. I like to think of his work, and this book, as a stepping-stone to the next level of patient care.

Adam Frederic Dorin, M.D., M.B.A.
Medical Director
Grossmont Plaza Surgery Center
San Diego, CA

Acknowledgments

I wish to express my appreciation to the following individuals for their help during the creation of this book.

Raymond Hasel, M.D., an early propofol ketamine adopter, for his valuable suggestions regarding my chapters.

The librarians at Hoag Hospital Medical Library, especially Cathy Drake, Michele Gordaon, and Barbara Garside for their generous support.

Marc Strauss, my editor and friend, who displayed extraordinary sagacity and forebearance in making this book a reality.

Ken Karpinski, my project manager, who guided me through the production processes.

Brian Bowles for his help with the copyediting and Constance Burt for her assistance with the final proofing and corrections to the manuscript.

Introduction

Anesthesiology has undergone remarkable changes in recent years. Among them is the development of anesthesia subspecialties and of anesthesiologists who focus most or all of their time in one area of anesthesia practice. This change has several advantages for patients, surgeons, and anesthesiologists. For one, the anesthesiologist learns the needs and expectations of the surgeon, which optimizes surgical outcome for patients. Furthermore, knowing what to expect, the anesthesiologist is better able to adjust both the doses and timing of drugs so that patients are adequately anesthetized for surgery but then emerge from anesthesia in a timely and comfortable manner. Nowhere are these issues more important than when surgery is performed in the ambulatory or office-based setting. Expectations are that patients undergoing surgery in these settings will go home the same day. Resources for extended care are usually nonexistent, as they should be.

Providing anesthesia for office- or clinic-based cosmetic surgery has emerged as one subspecialty area for anesthesiologists. For patients, convenience is greatly enhanced and costs are greatly decreased in office- or clinic-based cosmetic surgery. To provide the best anesthetic care in this specialized setting requires certain skills that are not emphasized in most anesthesia training programs. Fortunately, we are blessed with a resource prepared by a highly skilled and experienced anesthesiologist.

In this book, Dr. Barry L. Friedberg has assembled a compendium of his fifteen years of providing anesthesia care in the office setting. Where scientific documentation is available, Dr. Friedberg provides it. Where it is lacking, he guides the reader with recommendations that represent both reasoned judgment and innovative, effective results. He knows what works and what doesn't and explains his views in text and illustrations that are concise and informative.

Any anesthesiologist contemplating providing anesthesia care for cosmetic surgery, regardless of the surgical setting, needs to read this book. For those providing care in the office or clinic setting, it is virtually mandatory. By reviewing this text, anesthesiologists will avoid the pitfalls that exist in this practice and conclude their days with grateful patients and happy surgeons.

C. Philip Larson, Jr., M.D., C.M., M.A.
Professor Emeritus
Anesthesiology & Neurosurgery, Stanford University
Professor of Clinical Anesthesiology
David Geffen School of Medicine at UCLA

Preface

The very essence of leadership is that you have a vision.
—Theodore Hesburgh

Caesar's *Gallic Wars* begins with the observation that "All Gaul is divided into three parts." *Anesthesia in Cosmetic Surgery* is also divided into three parts.

Part I, Chapters 1–10, is devoted to minimally invasive anesthesia (MIA)® for minimally invasive surgery. (The United States Patent and Trademark Office [USPTO] granted trademark serial number 76/619,460, file number 067202-0312946 to minimally invasive anesthesia [MIA] to Dr. Friedberg in 2005.)

Part I advances the premise of a unitary anesthetic technique for *all* elective cosmetic surgery. Part I challenges the belief that only some types of elective cosmetic surgery are suitable for intravenous sedation. Many readers may be similarly challenged by the description of abdominoplasty, an extraperitoneal procedure, as a minimally invasive surgery.

Inasmuch as the MIA™ technique is not universally applicable for every surgical personality, Part II, Chapters 11–13, is dedicated to providing a comprehensive view of other anesthetic techniques administered by dedicated anesthesia professionals. Deliberately omitted are those approaches of oral and intravenous sedation directed by the surgeon in the absence of a dedicated anesthesia provider.

There is much about the practice of anesthesia in cosmetic surgery that is not specifically related to anesthetic technique. Part III, Chapters 14–18, and Appendices A and B illustrate the chasm between the medically indicated (third-party reimbursed) anesthesia practice and that particular to anesthesia for elective cosmetic surgery.

The reader who demands Level 1 study to accept new solutions to clinical problems is reminded that neither aspirin nor penicillin ever had a Level 1 study to validate their efficacy. Nonetheless, both are well-accepted therapeutic agents. The efficacy of the MIA™ technique will eventually make it a widely accepted practice.

"Insanity" is sometimes defined as performing the same act in the same way, over and over, yet expecting a different outcome. Only by changing the "script" can outcomes be improved. MIA™ for minimally invasive surgery represents a paradigm shift or change in the "script" for the anesthetic management of the patient intraoperative experience. **MIA™ technique is not only different from anesthetic techniques described in Part II but also safer.** Superior postoperative outcomes for postoperative nausea and vomiting (PONV) and pain management with MIA™ technique are described in Part I.

In 2007, American soldiers are dying in Afghanistan and Iraq. HIV/AIDS is still causing deaths throughout the world. Deaths from malnutrition, starvation, and natural disasters still plague the third world. A nuclear disaster from weapons of the former Soviet Union in the hands of rogue nations or terrorists remains a threat. According to the National Highway Transportation and Safety Administration (NHTSA), on American highways in 2004, there were 105 daily deaths (or 38,253 for the year) from motor vehicle accidents. Whereas death is a constant in life, the public has grown somewhat able to accept these kinds of deaths. Death surrounding elective cosmetic surgery, surgery without medical indication, is never an acceptable outcome for the patient, the patient's family, the anesthesiologist, the surgeon, or the lay public.

There is a "perfect storm" of forces that have made this book not only possible but necessary. The baby-boom or "me generation," born 1946 to 1964, is beginning to age. Social forces creating the "sandwich" effect of simultaneously caring for parents and children have created economic forces dictating that this generation will postpone retirement. The work force is a competitive environment with a heavy emphasis on a youthful appearance. The combination of narcissism and the need to remain competitive at work has created a huge impetus for "boomers" to seek cosmetic relief of the aging process.

In the course of seeking cosmetic surgery, many patients receive general anesthesia, opioid-based IV sedation, or regional anesthetics in hospital surgicenter (ASC) and office-based settings (see Part II). When death occurs in the office-based setting, the public and media find it unacceptable. "Dying to be beautiful," read the headlines. States like Florida, California, New York, and others have rushed to regulate the office surgical suite because it is frequently the site for elective cosmetic surgery.

Sadly, what remains is the absurd situation that it is acceptable to have a death from a pulmonary embolism following an abdominoplasty in a hospital or ASC setting but not the exact same outcome in an office-based setting. The emerging hypocrisy is that the hospital and ASC lobbies in Florida (and others to follow) have persuaded the legislatures to mandate reporting of all mortalities from office-based cosmetic surgery while remaining exempt from the same requirement. This is clearly not in the interest of public safety. *All* deaths from elective cosmetic surgery should be subject to the same reporting and scrutiny as those in the office-based setting.

The old maxim that "while the surgeon can only maim, the anesthesiologist can kill" rings true in the effort to affect the ultimate negative anesthesia outcome. How can tragic deaths in cosmetic surgery be avoided? Is the answer somewhere in the future with better drugs or better monitors? *It is not possible to get the right answer by asking the wrong question.* "Have we overlooked existing drugs, techniques, and/or monitors that can provide for a safer anesthetic with better outcomes?" is, perhaps, the more insightful question. The answer to this question is at the heart of the MIA™ technique.

Barry L. Friedberg, M.D.
Corona del Mar
California

List of Contributors

David Barinholtz, M.D.
President and CEO
Mobile Anesthesiologists, LLC
Chicago, IL

Meena Desai, M.D.
Managing Partner
Nova Anesthesia Professsionals
Villanova, PA

Adam Frederic Dorin, M.D., M.B.A.
Medical Director
Grossmont Plaza Surgery Center
San Diego, CA

Norig Ellison, M.D.
Professor of Anesthesia
University of Pennsylvania
Philadelphia, PA

Holly Evans, M.D., F.R.C.P.
Associate Professor
Department of Anesthesiology
Division of Ambulatory Anesthesiology
Duke University Medical Center
Durham, NC

Barry L. Friedberg, M.D.
Assistant Professor in Clinical Anesthesia
Volunteer Faculty
Keck School of Medicine
University of Southern California
Los Angeles, CA

Scott D. Kelley, M.D.
Medical Director
Aspect Medical Systems, Inc.
Norwood, MA

Marc E. Koch, M.D., M.B.A.
Founder and CEO
Somnia Anesthesia Services, Inc.
New Rochelle, NY

C. Philip Larson, Jr., M.D., C.M., M.A.
Professor Emeritus
Anesthesiology & Neurosurgery
Stanford University
Palo Alto, CA
Professor of Clinical Anesthesiology
David Geffen School of Medicine at UCLA
Los Angeles, CA

Norman Levin, M.D.
Chief, Department of Anesthesiology
Century City Hospital
Los Angeles, CA

Ann Lofsky, M.D.
Staff Anesthesiologist
Saint John's Hospital
Santa Monica, CA
Anesthesia Consultant and Governor Emeritus
The Doctors' Company
Napa, CA

Joel McMasters, M.D., M.A.J., M.C., U.S.A.
Assistant Chief of Anesthesia
Director of Total Intravenous Anesthesia
Brooke Army Medical Center
San Antonio, TX

Joseph Niamtu III, D.M.D.
Private Practice
Cosmetic Facial Surgery
Richmond, VA

Rodger Wade Pielet, M.D.
Clinical Associate
Department of Surgery
University of Chicago
Chicago, IL

Chris Pollock, M.B.
Consultant in Pain Management and
    Anaesthesia
Hull and East Yorkshire Hospital Trust
Hull, England

David Rahm, M.D.
President and CEO
Vitamedica
Manhattan Beach, CA

David B. Sarwer, Ph.D.
Departments of Psychiatry and Surgery
The Edwin and Fannie Gray Hall Center for
    Human Appearance and the Weight
    and Eating Disorders Program
University of Pennsylvania School of Medicine
Philadelphia, PA

James A. Snyder, D.D.S.
Founder and CEO
Center for Dental Anesthesiology
Alexandria, VA

Susan M. Steele, M.D.
Professor
Department of Anesthesiology
Division of Ambulatory Anesthesiology
Duke University Medical Center
Durham, NC

1 | Propofol Ketamine with Bispectral Index (BIS) Monitoring

Barry L. Friedberg, M.D.

INTRODUCTION

Anesthesiologists are trained to administer anesthesia for surgery. Elective cosmetic surgery is commonly performed in an office-based facility with patients discharged to home. However, elective cosmetic surgery differs from elective or emergency surgery in many substantial aspects (see Tables 1-1 and 1-2).

"Cosmetic surgery is almost always elective, and patients are almost always in good health. The patient, however, is willing to risk this good health (at least to a limited extent) in order to experience improvements in physical appearance, and perhaps more importantly, self-esteem, body image, and quality of life."[1]

There is *no medical indication* for elective cosmetic procedures, excluding breast reconstruction post-mastectomy. One may consider risk-benefit ratios of differing anesthetic regimens in *medically* indicated surgery. However, surgery *without* medical indication should not accept *any* avoidable risk. Halogenated inhalation anesthetics are triggering agents for malignant hyperthermia (MH),[2] carry an increased risk of deep venous thrombosis with potential pulmonary embolism,[3] and are emetogenic.[4] If the patient is interested and the surgeon is willing, **all** cosmetic procedures *can* be performed under local *only* anesthesia. Therefore, *any* additional anesthetic agents should be subject to the highest justification.

Most patients desire *some* alteration of their level of consciousness from fully awake through completely asleep. Given that all known risks *should* be avoided, when possible, then which agents are best suited to the task, what monitors should be employed, and to what level

Table 1-1. Elective cosmetic procedures

Commonly performed cosmetic surgical procedures. All procedures have successfully been anesthetized with PK MAC/MIA™ technique in the office-based setting.

1. Rhinoplasty (closed or open)
2. Liposuction or suction assisted lipoplasty (SAL)
3. Blepharoplasty (open, transconjuctival, or endoscopic)
4. Rhytidectomy (open or endoscopic)
5. Breast augmentation, subglandular, subpectoral (via areaolar, inframammary, transaxilllary, or transumbilical approach)
6. Hair transplantation with or without scalp reduction
7. Facial resurfacing (laser, chemical peel, or mechanical dermabrasion)
8. Brow lift (coronoplasty or endoscopic)
9. Abdominoplasty (classical or simple skin)
10. Otoplasty
11. Genioplasty (mandibular advancement or recession)
12. Facial implants (malar and mandibular with silicone or autologous fat)
13. Lip enlargement (autologous fat transfer, radiated cadaver material [Alloderm®], Gortex® extrusions, Restylane,® Juvaderm,® etc.)
14. Platsyma band plication
15. Composite procedures; i.e., (a) endoscopic brow lift and endoscopic rhytidectomy, with open platysma band plication, (b) blepharoplasty, rhinoplasty, and rhytidectomy, or (c) breast augmentation with abdominoplasty

Table 1-2. Cosmetic procedures by type from PK MAC/MIA™ technique case log March 26, 1992 – March 26, 2002 [12]

	N	%
Liposuction	663	(25)
Breast augmentation	489	(18)
Facial resurfacing mechanical abrasion, chemical peel, or laser resurfacing	389	(14)
Rhytidectomy	305	(11)
Blepharoplasty	198	(7)
Rhinoplasty	81	(3)
Fat transfer	57	(2)
Abdominoplasty	54	(2)
Composite or misc. procedures	447	(18)
Total	2,683	(100)

"We hold the basic premise that the less the involvement of the patient's critical organs and systems (i.e., the lower the concentration of the agent, or the less 'deep' the anesthesia), the less will be the damage to the patient, whether this be temporary or permanent."[6]

"For the anesthetic itself, overall experiences indicate that the least amount of anesthetic that can be used is the best dose. Local and monitored anesthesia care (MAC) is preferable to regional. Regional techniques are preferable to general anesthesia."[7]

Table 1-3. Minimally invasive surgeries appropriate for BIS-monitored PK MAC, the MIA™ technique

1. *All* cosmetic procedures (see Table 1-1)
2. Gyn: laparoscopy (tubal ligation, fulgeration endometriosis)
3. Ortho: arthoscopy
4. Urology: lithotripsy
5. Gen. surg.: herniorraphy & breast cancer surgery
6. Neuro: microdiscectomy, microlaminectomy, carpal tunnel release
7. sedation for morbidly obese
8. peripheral injuries in U.S. Army field hospitals in Iraq, Afghanistan

Cases being performed with PKR[a] TIVA
1. U.S. Army neurosurgery in Iraq.
[a] Propofol-Ketamine-Remifentanil

of anesthesia should be administered (i.e., minimal sedation ["anxiolyis"], moderate ["conscious"] sedation, deep sedation, or general anesthesia [GA])? (See Appendix 1-1, Defining Anesthesia Levels). If better outcomes are the goal, doesn't minimally invasive anesthesia for minimally invasive surgery make sense?[5] (See Table 1-3.)

WHY IS MINIMALLY INVASIVE ANESTHESIA® IMPORTANT?

"Less is more" is a Mies Vanderohe principle applied to the Bauhaus school of minimalist architecture. "Doing more with less" is a Buckminster Fuller concept of housing applied to his geodesic domes.

"When possible, procedures longer than three or four hours should be performed with local anesthesia and intravenous sedation because general anesthesia is associated with deep venous thrombosis at much higher rates under prolonged operative conditions."[3]

"Newer techniques for intravenous sedation that include the use of propofol, often in combination with other drugs, have made it possible to perform lengthy or extensive procedures without general anesthesia and *without the loss of the patient's airway protective reflexes.*"[9]

"When you can measure what you are speaking about, and express it in numbers, you know something about it; but when you cannot measure it, when you cannot express it in numbers, your knowledge is of a meager and unsatisfactory kind; it may be the beginning of knowledge, but you have scarcely, in your thoughts, advanced to the stage of science." (William Thompson, knighted Lord Kelvin. Popular lectures and addresses [*1891–1894*])

The bispectral index (BIS) monitor facilitates a numerical expression of the *hypnotic* component (anesthesia = hypnosis + analgesia) of the anesthetic state and may permit a reasonable inference about the analgesic state. Heart rate, blood pressure, and other clinical signs are notoriously unreliable indicators of anesthetic depth.[10] BIS provides new information about patients that is simply unavailable from any other vital or clinical sign.[11] BIS, as an index, has no units. The scale is 0–100, with 100 representing awake and zero representing isoelectric (or zero) brain activity. Hypnosis compatible with general anesthesia (GA) occurs between BIS 45–60. BIS 45–60 with *systemic* analgesia defines general anesthesia. BIS 60–75 with adequate *local* analgesia is a major part of the MIA™ technique. Patients who received MIA™ neither hear, nor feel, nor remember their surgical experience.[12]

Monk et al. published an associated 20% increase in the one-year mortality risk *associated* with every hour of BIS <45.[13] Therefore, BIS <45 for cumulative periods greater than one hour must be considered as overmedicating.

The routine practice of overmedicating for fear of undermedicating is no longer a desirable or acceptable practice (see Table 1-4).

Monk et al. postulated that the increase in one-year anesthetic mortality might be related to an inflammatory response from excessively deep anesthesia.[13] A more recent prospective, randomized controlled study demonstrated

Table 1-4. BIS levels and levels of sedation/anesthesia

BIS	Sedation/Anesthesia Level
98–100	Awake
78–85	Minimal Sedation ("Anxiolysis")
70–78	Moderate ("Conscious") Sedation[a]
60–70	Deep Sedation[b]
45–60 + systemic analgesia	General Anesthesia[c]
<45, >1 hr.	Overanesthetized![13]

[a]With moderate sedation, *passive* maneuvers like extension and rotation of the head or shoulder pillow may be all that are necessary to maintain the airway.
[b]With deep sedation, *active* maneuvers, like nasal airway or LMA, may be required to maintain airway patency.
[c]See Appendix 1-1.

increased C-reactive protein levels with BIS <45 for more than 50% of the cases.[14]

The BIS monitor does not replace traditional vital-sign monitoring, that is, EKG, NIABP, SpO_2, (or $EtCO_2$ when indicated). When measured, the $EtCO_2$ typically runs between 38–42 with the MIA™ technique. The $EtCO_2$ offers the display of the waveform of the patient's respiration. Many experienced anesthesiologists are capable of assessing adequate respiratory movement without this information. Over 3,000 PK MAC cases have been safely anesthetized without $EtCO_2$ monitoring.

Titrating anesthesia with BIS trend is limited by the fact that the processing required for the BIS algorithm is delayed 15–30 seconds behind real time. This delay has given rise to the legitimate criticism that BIS does not predict patient movement. BIS, a measure of the hypnotic state, was not designed to predict patient movement (see Chapter 3).

EMG is the instantaneous display of the frontalis muscle activity if the XP software version of the BIS A2000, or later, is used. Inadequate analgesia leading to patient movement is predictable if the EMG is selected from the advanced screen menu to trend as a secondary trace. A spike in EMG (when BIS is 60–75, in spontaneously breathing patients) nearly always predicts inadequate analgesia, preceding patient movement (see Fig. 1-1). The anesthesiologist should utilize the 15–30 second delay in the change of the BIS value to simultaneously bolus propofol while encouraging the surgeon to supplement the local analgesia.

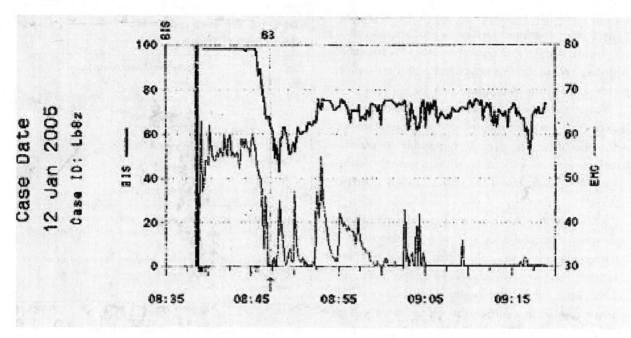

Figure 1-1. Incremental propofol induction began 08:45. Ketamine 50 mg IV administered 08:47, BIS = 63. In this particular case, BIS increases post-ketamine dose. However, the increase does **not** defeat the ability to titrate propofol to BIS 60–75!

Postoperative Nausea and Vomiting (PONV)

Macario et al. conducted a statistically validated survey of a panel of expert anesthesiologists on what postoperative anesthetic outcome *they* believed patients most wanted to avoid.[15] The anesthesiologists concluded that **pain** was the number one anesthesia outcome patients most desired to avoid. A follow-up, similarly statistically validated survey of patients' anesthesia outcomes they most desired to avoid was **emesis**![16] Clearly, a disconnect exists between what anesthesiologists believe about their patients and what the patients actually want most to avoid. A potential explanation could be that patients who consent for elective surgery *expect* to have some postoperative discomfort but do not want their pain to be compounded by emesis.

How are PONV, preemptive analgesia, and postoperative pain management related?

There is a consensus among PONV authorities like Apfel, Chung, Gan, Scuderi, and White, that both inhalational anesthetics and opioids are emetogenic agents. "In the *context* of [emetogenic] anesthesia, postoperative pain management and opioid related PONV remain problems."[17] In the context of emetogenic anesthesia, experts advise "multimodal" prophylaxis in the highest risk group.[18]

Apfel's recent NEJM article identifies the highest PONV risk group of patients as nonsmoking females, with a history of previous PONV and/or motion sickness, having emetogenic (i.e., elective cosmetic) surgery of two or more hours.[4] Apfel's criterion of high risk applies *exceptionally* well to Friedberg's previously referenced series of 2,683 patients.[12]

Elective cosmetic surgery anesthesia for the "rich and famous" of Beverly Hills and Newport Beach is the highest risk PONV population! This conclusion reflects the southern California geographic bias of the author. There are many other such communities worldwide.

The MIA™ technique is not perfect but *contextually* nonemetogenic. Without *any* antiemetic prophylaxis, this highest risk group of patients experienced a total of thirteen PONV events for an unprecedented 0.5% PONV rate![12] A 50 mg dissociative dose of ketamine at BIS <75 propofol levels eliminates the noxious input of the injection of local analgesia while avoiding emetogenic agents like the halogenated inhalational vapors and intravenous opioids.

Lidocaine provides intraoperative analgesia with bupivicaine providing postoperative analgesia. In this *context*, it has been extremely rare for patients to require (emetogenic) opioid relief of their postoperative discomfort.

Elimination of all emetogenic triggers defines nonopioid, preemptive analgesia (NOPA). NOPA is the hallmark of the MIA™ technique. In Friedberg's fifteen-year experience, no patients have been admitted to the hospital following PK MAC/MIA™ technique for either PONV or unmanageable pain.

Beware Laryngospasm

No technique is perfect. Classical laryngospasm can be diagnosed by the characteristic "crowing" sound generated by a small gap in the vocal cords owing to their incomplete closure. With ketamine-associated laryngospasm, the vocal cords most commonly close completely. Hence, only rarely will crowing noise alert the anesthesiologist to impending desaturation. Additionally, the usual remedy of positive pressure ventilation combined with anterior jaw thrust is *completely* ineffective. The anesthesiologist must pay particular attention to *sneezing* or *coughing* as the only prodrome warning him of impending laryngospasm.

The treatment of choice is a rapid IV bolus of lidocaine 1 mg · lb^{-1} or 2 mg · kg^{-1}.

Concern about adding more lidocaine in patients receiving relatively large amounts of lidocaine local analgesia has led other anesthesiologists to prefer to deepen the propofol level by adding a 50 mg propofol bolus to break the laryngospasm. However, when IV lidocaine *has* been administered for laryngospasm, no stigmata of lidocaine toxicity have been observed. The BIS showed no decrease in response to the IV lidocaine bolus. There was no transient hypotension or widening of the EKG complex during the case. No patient complained of tinnitus, tremulousness, or metallic taste on the tongue after emergence.

Administering succinylcholine (SCH) to break the spasm is suboptimal because SCH adds unnecessary (and avoidable) risk as an MH triggering agent. (Neither propofol nor ketamine are MH triggering agents.) Further, the myalgias associated with SCH make the agent totally unacceptable in the elective cosmetic surgery patient.

Waiting until desaturation occurs after the prodrome will add a substantial amount of time until the lidocaine can circulate to anesthetize (and open) the vocal cords. Desaturation increases the physiologic stress to the patient. The alarm of the pulse oximeter, accompanied by the bluish discoloration of the patient, increases the psychological stress to the anesthesiologist, surgeon, and operating room nursing staff. This disturbing scenario is best minimized by promptly giving IV lidocaine when the patient coughs or sneezes.

WHAT IS CLONIDINE-PREMEDICATED, BIS-MONITORED PK MAC, OR THE MIA™ TECHNIQUE?

Something old (ketamine), something new (BIS-monitored propofol hypnosis), something borrowed (diazepam ketamine technique[19]), no one blue (SpO$_2$ >90% on room air).

Why Ketamine?

The brain cannot respond to stimuli it does not receive. *Critical concept*: GA does not reliably block all incoming noxious stimuli! The "wind-up" phenomenon,[20] mediated by the NMDA receptors, is often invoked to explain acute postoperative pain after general anesthesia, as well as the formation of chronic pain states.

"Dissociation" refers to a patient who, under the influence of ketamine, remains motionless in response to noxious stimuli.

Based on clinical observation, the NMDA receptor block from a 50 mg dissociative dose of ketamine reliably blocks all incoming noxious stimuli to the cortex (the so-called mid-brain spinal) for a period of 10–20 minutes. After obtaining an equal dissociative effect with a 50 mg ketamine dose in both 90-pound female and 250-pound male patients, the author concluded that *the number of NMDA receptors does not vary with patient body weight in adults.*

Preemptive analgesia is most consistently observed when the NMDA receptors are saturated *prior* to noxious stimulation. Acetaminophen 1,000 mg po is adequate for postoperative pain management (for the few patients who request it) in the context of clonidine-premedicated, BIS-monitored PK MAC patients.[12] (See Table 1-5.)

Making Ketamine Predictable

In *other* contexts, ketamine has a well-deserved reputation for causing hypertension, tachycardia, and an unpredictable 20% of patients experiencing hallucinations or dsyphorias.[21] Hypnotic doses of propofol block ketamine-induced hallucinations as well as undesirable hemodynamic sequellae.[22] Being able to assign a numerical value

Table 1-5. Ketamine tips

1. 80% patients achieve dissociative effect with 25 mg ketamine, 98% with 50 mg ketamine. No "down side" to 50 mg dose as long as BIS <75. Wait 2–3 min. before injecting local. Wait an additional min. if patient is reactive before administering more ketamine.
2. Preemptive analgesia effect is variable when inadequate dissociative effect is obtained. Saturate NMDA receptors!
3. *All adult patients, independent of body weight, require 50 mg ketamine initial dose to saturate NMDA receptors.*
4. Reinjection of previously injected field does NOT require more ketamine.
5. Consider injecting both sides with initial ketamine dose.
6. If prep. is cold, consider injecting 25 mg ketamine 2–3 min. before prep. or consider warming prep. solution!
7. With experience, less ketamine is administered. Friedberg's case log of the last 500 cases (of 2,683 patients) showed 80% performed with either one or two 50 mg doses of ketamine.[12]
8. Mixing propofol with ketamine is TIVA[23] not MAC.
9. Do not exceed an aggregate total of 200 mg ketamine.
10. Do not give ketamine in the last 20–30 minutes of a case.

Table 1-6. Clinical pathway for MIA™ technique

1. Clonidine 0.2 mg PO 30–60 min preop (Systolic >100, body weight >100 pounds).
2. Glycopyrrolate 0.2 mg IV with 2 ccs 1% lidocaine plain.
3. Incrementally *titrate propofol to BIS <75* with multiple, sequential $150 ug \cdot kg^{-1} \cdot 20 sec.$ mini-boluses. *N.B.* If pump does not have a bolus feature, set initial rate to $450 ug \cdot kg^{-1} \cdot min^{-1}$ and reduce the rate toward 50 as soon as the EMG begins to decrease.
4. Basal propofol infusion rate $50 ug \cdot kg^{-1} \cdot min^{-1}$.
5. Ketamine 50 mg IVP @ *BIS <75* 2–3 minutes *prior* to injection local anesthesia.
6. Adjust basal propofol rate upward to maintain BIS 60–75 if ketamine causes an increase.
7. Inject adequate local analgesia.
8. Administer more ketamine only after two reinjections of the field fail to eliminate patient movement.
9. Maintain propofol at BIS 60–75, EMG 0 on BIS scale, 30 on EMG scale.
10. Bupivicaine in field before closure, especially for browlift, subpectoral breast augmentation, and abdominoplasty.

with BIS to the level of propofol hypnosis, *prior* to administering the ketamine, was an enormous breakthrough in making ketamine a predictable agent. Not only could the initial ketamine dose be administered without problems, but also subsequent doses, when needed, could be given with assurance.

First, create a *stable* level of propofol in the brain by performing an incremental, not bolus, induction. The incremental induction maintains spontaneous ventilation, commonly maintains masseter tone, avoids propofol waste, and is less apt to produce induction hypotension. Incremental propofol induction provides hypnosis with a minimal physiologic and pharmacologic trespass to the patient. *Lesser trespass increases patient safety.*

Lesser trespass increases the probability of maintaining the SpO_2 >90% on room air (i.e., room air, spontaneous ventilation, or RASV). *Key concept*: Titrate propofol to BIS <75 *before* giving the ketamine! Do NOT give ketamine at BIS >75.

Because the elective cosmetic surgical patient tends to be healthy, cardiac output and redistribution from the brain tend not to be significant factors in altering established brain levels of propofol. However, the nineteenfold interpatient variation in propofol hydroxylation may play a significant role in the ability to maintain a stable level of propofol in the brain.[23] Measuring an individual patient's *brain* response to propofol with BIS would appear to be a more effective strategy than employing target controlled infusions (TCI) to achieve specific *blood* levels of propofol (see Table 1-6).

Premedication

PK MAC was derived from diazepam ketamine MAC technique, which was first published in 1981.[19] Vinnik clearly enumerated that only *after* the patient was soundly asleep from the diazepam was the ketamine to be administered.[19] Diazepam hypnosis, followed by ketamine dissociation, followed by local anesthetic injection was Vinnik's clinical pathway. Although Guit was the first to publish the combination of propofol and ketamine, the technique was described as a total intravenous anesthetic (TIVA).[24] TIVA strongly implies that the local analgesia injected by the surgeon is not essential for the success of the TIVA technique. In contradistinction, the surgeon's local analgesia *is* essential for the success of PK MAC.

Guit's TIVA technique was unknown to Friedberg in 1992 when Friedberg embarked on *replacing* Vinnik's diazepam with propofol. The surgeons quickly complained about the cost of the propofol and pleaded for relief. Friedberg added midazolam in an effort to reduce the amount of propofol. From March 26, 1992 through March 26, 1997, the case log Friedberg maintained contained patient's names, dates, surgeons, patient age, gender, weight, surgical procedure(s) (see Table 1-2), midazolam, propofol, ketamine, and anesthesia times.[8] Propofol rates, $mg \cdot min^{-1}$ and $ug \cdot kg^{-1} \cdot min^{-1}$, were calculated *retrospectively*.

If 2 mg midazolam was good, perhaps 4 mg midazolam could be better for propofol-sparing purposes. In the aforementioned case log, a total of 354 patients received 0 mg midazolam, 316 patients received 2 mg, and another 303 patients received 4 mg midazolam premedication from 1992–97. No consistent, incremental relationship could be established in propofol savings between the 0, 2, and 4 mg midazolam groups.[8] In June 1997, Friedberg eliminated the midazolam from PK MAC.

In September 1997, Oxorn published a very elegant Level I study confirming Friedberg's uncontrolled, clinical experience in 973 patients.[25] Oxorn reported that there was no statistical difference in either induction or maintenance doses of propofol between those patients who received 2 mg midazolam premedication and those who received none.[25] *However, the unexpected finding was that a statistically significant threefold number of patients who received midazolam required pain medication in the PACU.*[25]

From July 7, 1997, through December 21, 1998, 268 patients received BIS-monitored PK MAC *without* premedication, midazolam, or other benzodiazepine. During BIS-monitored propofol hypnosis, there were no patients who suffered from hallucinations or a lack of amnesia. This experience led Friedberg to conclude that benzodiazepine premedication was superfluous to provide amnesia or to prevent hallucinations *in the presence of BIS monitoring.* Some of these patients were included in a subsequent publication.[26]

Patients continued to request premedication to calm them. After attending the New York Postgraduate Assembly (PGA) in December 1998, Friedberg returned with the renewed notion of adding po clonidine as a premedication. Like Vinnik's concept of administering sleep doses of diazepam to block ketamine hallucinations, clonidine for premedication had also been previously reported in the plastic surgery literature.[27,28]

Inconsistent propofol sparing results were observed with 0.1 mg po clonidine. A therapeutic clonidine dose should be in a range between 2.5–5.0 $ug \cdot kg^{-1}$.[29] Clonidine 0.2 mg mg po achieves that range in patients weighing between 95–175 pounds. The higher dose of clonidine provided consistent propofol sparing results and further refinement of BIS-monitored PK MAC.[30]

From January 26, 2001 to September 2002, rofecoxib 50 mg po was added to the clonidine. When the drug was voluntarily withdrawn from the market, rofecoxib was deleted from the premedication. While the *addition* of the rofecoxib appeared to benefit the patient, the *deletion* of the agent did not appear to increase (the already few) postoperative patient complaints of discomfort.

At the present time, only clonidine 0.2 mg po (30–60 minutes preoperatively) and glycopyrrolate 0.2 mg with 2 cc 1% lidocaine IV are given as premedication (see Table 1-6).

Fluid Management

The long-standing teaching that patients who are NPO after midnight are at least 500–1,000 ccs behind on their fluids is not especially relevant for elective cosmetic surgery patients. As stated earlier, these are by and large essentially healthy patients who are far different from the debilitated ward patients on whom most anesthesia trainees learn about anesthesia. Elective cosmetic surgical patients are not "dry." Vasodilating anesthetics are no longer being administered. Lastly, large fluid shifts and blood loss are atypical experiences in most elective cosmetic surgery.

Other authors have analogized the insult produced by liposuction to that of a burn injury. However, burn patients do not have compression garments applied to obliterate the "third space" created by the aspiration of subcutaneous fat.

Fluid replacement regimens based on experience in burn patients are inappropriate for liposuction patients.

Especially for cases up to 5,000 ccs of liposuction, fluid replacement should remain modest, that is, not more than 1,000 ccs. Otherwise, one may risk fluid overload,

---

Table 1-7. MIA™ airway algorithm (assumes incremental propofol induction)

1. Extend and laterally rotate head, one side may have better gas exchange than the other.
2. Insert shoulder (not neck) pillow to increase force of extension.
3. Insert lubricated nasal airway (#28 FR most commonly).
4. Insert lubricated LMA (#4 most commonly).
5. No ET required: >15 yrs, >3,000 patients; no opioids, benzodiazepines, or muscle relaxants.

Table 1-8. Local anesthesia tips

1. PDR limit of 500 mg lidocaine with epinephrine (7 mg · kg^{-1}) is outdated and overly conservative. Neither the 2005, 2006 nor the 2007 (print or electronic) editions of PDR have *any* entry for injectable lidocaine!
2. 200 ccs of 0.5% lidocaine (1,000 mg) with epinephrine is well tolerated and without sequellae of toxicity
3. Tumescent or "wetting" solution = 500 mg lidocaine, 1 mg epinephrine in 1,000 ccs NSS (Klein) or LR (Hunstead)
4. 5,000 ccs of tumescent solution = 2,500 mg lidocaine
5. 5,000 ccs of tumescent solution in a 60 kg female patient = 42 mg · kg^{-1}
6. Avoid >50 cc 0.25% (125 mg) bupivicaine for postoperative analgesia.

---

pulmonary edema, and dilution of platelets and other coagulation factors.

Another unaesthetic consequence of 2,000–4,000 ccs fluid replacement in this patient population is enuresis on the operating room table. This will embarrass the patient and annoy the nurse who had to clean it up. Catheterizing the patient to compensate for inappropriate fluid administration exposes the patient to the risk of an unnecessary bladder infection.

Patients who experience caffeine withdrawal headache without their morning caffeine are encouraged to drink their cup of coffee black or with non-dairy creamer, if necessary. Apple juice or water is permitted up until an hour before surgery. Patients who are hungry upon awakening are encouraged to have toast and jam. Simple carbohydrates and sugars are rapidly absorbed by the stomach and pose no real threat to patient safety. It is far better to have the patient arrive without hypoglycemia. Patients are encouraged to void before getting on the operating table. (See Table 1-7.)

Major Confounding Principle

A blanched surgical field does *not* guarantee adequate surgical analgesia. More local analgesia resolves the patient movement 99% of the time. Administer more ketamine only after two reinjections of the field fail to eliminate patient movement.

BIS becomes much more than a simple tool with which to titrate propofol. BIS becomes a case management tool. By being able to demonstrate adequate propofol levels (i.e., BIS 60–75) *during* patient movement, the surgeon

can be educated to inject more analgesia. In addition to the *initial* injection of the local analgesia, the patient is spared noxious, painful input during the surgery. The brain cannot respond to stimuli it does not receive. *Postoperative pain management begins intraoperatively!* Reproducible preemptive analgesia occurs under conditions of adequate dissociation secondary to the saturation of the NMDA receptors. (See Table 1-5.)

BIS as Fianchetto

From Italian, *fianchetto* is a chess term meaning a "double move." In a "binary" system of anesthesia (hypnosis + analgesia = anesthesia), being able to measure hypnosis permits an inference about the adequacy of analgesia. Adequate analgesia produces de facto muscle relaxation for minimally invasive surgery. BIS 60–75 with EMG = 0 (on the BIS scale, 30 on the EMG scale) defines adequate hypnosis for the MIA™ technique. Therefore, *adequate* hypnosis in the presence of patient movement (usually preceded by a spike in EMG) infers *inadequate* analgesia!

Postoperative Pain Management

In the context of clonidine-premedicated, BIS-monitored PK MAC, now formally known as the MIA™ technique, postoperative pain is minimal to nonexistent. Part of this phenomenon may be explained by having patients emerge from propofol with the clonidine still in effect. Patients who have lower anxiety levels, secondary to lowered catecholamines from the clonidine, tend to have less pain complaints. In the diethyl ether era, "stormy induction, stormy emergence" was the common rationale for premedicating surgical patients. Preoperatively, a clonidine-premedicated patient may not appear drowsy but, upon questioning, usually admits to feeling "calmer." A further explanation for the remainder of the observation of minimal-to-no postoperative pain appears to be the phenomenon of preemptive analgesia.

With the dissociative effect of ketamine, no noxious signals reach the cortex during the injection of local anesthesia. *GA does NOT reliably block all incoming noxious stimuli.* Use the BIS to not only maintain hypnosis at 60–75 but also to assure inadequate local analgesia is dealt with appropriately (i.e., more local) and not by subterfuge (i.e., more ketamine, propofol, or opioids). Lastly, bupivicaine, especially for browlift, breast augmentation, and abdominoplasty, provides long-lasting nonopioid relief. Do not exceed a total of 125 mg bupivicaine (or 50 ccs 0.25%) for postoperative analgesia. Because the bupivicaine quickly binds to tissue, it is necessary only to splash it into the operative field. Some surgeons prefer to close the wound and inject the bupivicaine retrograde up the suction drainage tube(s). Both approaches with bupivicaine are effective.

All of the anesthesiologists' efforts to prevent PONV and effect adequate pain management may be for naught if the surgeon discharges the patient home with an opioid-containing analgesic (i.e., Vicodin® or Tylenol #3®). Darvocet® or other similar nonopioid analgesics may provide an increment of relief greater than 1,000 mg acetaminophen every six hours. Oral diazepam is especially effective for decreasing the muscle spasm associated in subpectoral breast implant patients. *N.B. This is also a useful strategy for any other submuscular implants; i.e., gluteal.*

The few patients who do complain of pain present a differential diagnosis of "central" (or supratentorial) versus "peripheral" (infratentorial) pain. *Both complaints are real.* Some patients may complain of pain when they had been predominantly immobile for the surgery. This pain is more likely to be "central" in origin. This type of patient may respond better if 50 mg po diphenhydramine (Benadryl®)

Table 1-9. Errors to avoid

1. Ketamine before propofol: NO
2. Ketamine at BIS >75: NO
3. Bolus propofol induction: NO
4. Inadequate local analgesia: NO
   BIS as *fianchetto* for adequate propofol *and* lidocaine
5. Opioids instead of more lidocaine: NO
6. Ketamine instead of more lidocaine: NO
7. >200 mg *total* ketamine or any in last 20 min. of case: NO
8. Tracheostomize patient for laryngospasm instead of IV lidocaine: NO
9. SCH instead of lidocaine for laryngospasm: NO

is added to the 1,000 mg acetaminophen (Tylenol P. M.®). More experience with the MIA™ technique will eliminate most of the patient movement seen with inadequate local analgesia. These patients may require ketorolac 30–60 mg IV to deal with "peripheral" pain issues. As the surgeon becomes more willing to inject additional local analgesia *during* the case when patient movement occurs at BIS 60–75, fewer issues of "peripheral" pain will be manifest. None of the more than 3,000 PK MAC patients has ever required hospital admission for intractable pain. (See Table 1-9.)

CONCLUSION

One must empathize with those who, understandably, have difficulty believing that a subpectoral breast augmentation in combination with a classical abdominoplasty can be performed as an office-based or day surgery without PONV or postoperative pain management issues. "Cognitive dissonance" is the psychological principle that precludes individuals from believing what they observe when it sharply contradicts what they have been taught to believe.

The On-Q® pump may have some additional value; but in the context described in this chapter, it offers little pain management benefit to offset the additional $280 cost (in 2005 dollars). While dexmedetomidine may possess 8 times the alpha$_2$ agonist potency of clonidine, it is 400 times more expensive (2005 dollars) and more tedious to administer. There are no current plans to replace clonidine with dexmedetomidine in the MIA™ technique.

The MIA™ technique reproducibly provides preemptive analgesia and is not technically difficult to execute. It does, however, require the active cooperation of the surgeon. Surgeons have become more interested in the use of local anesthesia to diminish PONV and postoperative pain management problems they perceive to be produced by the emetogenic agents the anesthesiologist chooses to administer.

Although initially developed for office-based, elective cosmetic surgery, the MIA™ technique is by no means limited to these types of cases (see Table 1-3). The MIA™ technique offers superior outcomes to alternative forms of anesthesia (see Part II) for cosmetic surgery (i.e., essentially **zero** PONV *without* the use of anti-emetics and minimal postoperative pain management).

In the final analysis, the MIA™ technique provides safety, simplicity, and satisfaction for all parties involved in the surgical experience: patients, their at-home caregivers, surgeons, nurses, and anesthesiologists.

REFERENCES

1. Goldwyn RM: Psychological aspects of plastic surgery: A surgeon's observations and reflections, in Sarwer DB, Pruzinsky T, Cash TF, et al. (eds.), *Psychological aspects of reconstructive and cosmetic plastic surgery.* Philadelphia, Lippincott, Williams & Wilkins, 2006; p13.
2. www.mhaus.org
3. McDevitt NB: Deep venous thrombosis prophylaxis. *Plast Reconstr Surg* 104:1923,1999.
4. Apfel CC, Korttila K, Abdalla M, et al.: A factorial trial of six interventions for the prevention of PONV. *N Engl J Med* 350:2441,2004.
5. Friedberg BL: Minimally invasive anesthesia for minimally invasive surgery. *Outpatient Surgery Magazine.* Herrin Publishing Partners LP, Paoli, PA. 2:57,2004.
6. Cullen SC, Larson CP: *Essentials of Anesthetic Practice.* Chicago, Year Book Medical Publishers, 1974; p82.
7. Laurito CE: Anesthesia provided at alternative sites, in Barasch PG, Cullen BF, Stoelting RK (eds.), *Clinical Anesthesia,* 4th ed., Philadelphia, Lippincott, Williams & Wilkins, 2001; p1343.
8. Friedberg BL: Propofol-ketamine technique, dissociative anesthesia for office surgery: A five-year review of 1,264 cases. *Aesth Plast Surg* 23:70,1999.
9. Lofsky AS: Deep venous thrombosis and pulmonary embolism in plastic surgery office procedures. *The Doctors' Company Newsletter.* Napa, CA, 2005. www.thedoctors.com/risk/specialty/anesthesiology/J4254.asp
10. Flaishon R, Windsor A, Sigl J, et al.: Recovery of consciousness after thiopental or propofol. *Anesthesiol* 86:613, 1997.
11. www.aspectms.com/resources/bibliographies
12. Friedberg BL: Propofol ketamine anesthesia for cosmetic surgery in the office suite, chapter in Osborne I (ed.), *Anesthesia for Outside the Operating Room. International Anesthesiology Clinics.* Baltimore, Lippincott, Williams & Wilkins, 41(2):39,2003.
13. Monk TG, Saini V, Weldon BC, et al.: Anesthetic management and one-year mortality after non-cardiac surgery. *Anesth Analg* 100:4,2005.
14. Kersssens C, Sebel P: Relationship between hypnotic depth and post-operative C-reactive protein levels. *Anesthesiol* 105:A578,2006.
15. Macario A, Weinger M, Truong P, et al.: Which clinical outcomes are both common and important to avoid? The perspective of a panel of expert anesthesiologists. *Anesth Analg* 88:1085,1999.
16. Macario A, Weinger M, Carney K, et al.: Which clinical anesthesia outcomes are important to avoid? The perspective of patients. *Anesth Analg* 89:652,1999.
17. White PF: Prevention of postoperative nausea and vomiting—A multimodal solution to a persistent problem. *N Engl J Med* 350:2511,2004.
18. Scuderi PE, James RL, Harris L, et al.: Multimodal antiemetic management prevents early postoperative vomiting after outpatient laparoscopy. *Anesth Analg* 91:1408, 2000.
19. Vinnik CA: An intravenous dissociation technique for outpatient plastic surgery: Tranquility in the office surgical facility. *Plast Reconstr Surg* 67:199,1981.
20. Thompson SWN, King AE, Woolf CJ: Activity-dependent changes in rat ventral horn neurons in vitro, summation of prolonged afferent evoked depolarizations produce a D-2-amino-5-phosphonovaleric acid sensitive windup. *Eur J Neurosci* 2:638,1990.
21. Corssen G, Domino EF: Dissociative anesthesia: further pharmacologic studies and first clinical experience with the phencylcidine derivative CI-581. *Anesth Analg* 45:29, 1968.
22. Friedberg BL: Hypnotic doses of propofol block ketamine induced hallucinations. *Plast Reconstr Surg* 91:196,1993.
23. Court MH, Duan SX, Hesse LM, et al.: Cytochrome P-450 2B6 is responsible for interindividual variability of propofol hydroxylation by human liver microsomes. *Anesthesiol* 94:110,2001.
24. Guit JBM, Koning HM, Coster ML, et al.: Ketamine as analgesic with propofol for total intravenous anesthetic (TIVA). *Anaesthesia* 46:24,1991.
25. Oxorn DC, Ferris LE, Harrington E: The effects of midazolam on propofol-induced anesthesia: propofol dose requirements, mood profiles and perioperative dreams. *Anesth Analg* 85:553,1997.
26. Friedberg BL, Sigl JC: Bispectral (BIS) index monitoring decreases propofol usage in propofol-ketamine office based anesthesia. *Anesth Analg* 88:S54,1999.

27. Man D: Premedication with oral clonidine for facial rhytidectomy. *Plast Reconstr Surg* 94:214,1994.
28. Baker TM, Stuzin JM, Baker TJ, et al.: What's new in aesthetic surgery? *Clin Plast Surg* 23:16,1996.
29. Goyagi T, Tanaka M, Nishikawa T: Oral clonidine premedication reduces awakening concentrations of isoflurane. *Anesth Analg* 86:410,1998.
30. Friedberg BL, Sigl JC: Clonidine premedication decreases propofol consumption during bispectral (BIS) index monitored propofol-ketamine technique for office based surgery. *Dermatol Surg* 26:848,2000.

APPENDIX 1-1 DEFINING ANESTHESIA LEVELS: THE TERMINOLOGY

Monitored anesthesia care (MAC) is a term created to include all anesthesia services except general or regional anesthesia. MAC is not especially useful to describe a particular anesthetic state or spectrum of states. MAC remains a term of exclusion in that it specifically is NOT general or regional anesthesia.

PK MAC connotes separately administering ketamine *after* inducing the patient with a continuous infusion of propofol.[1] The MIA™ technique adds the layer of BIS monitoring along with *po* clonidine premedication and infusion pump administered propofol.[2]

BIS-monitored PK MAC or the MIA™ technique falls well within the scope of the definition of IV sedation for an AAAASF Class B facility, except in the (current) regulations of the AAAASF and the state of Florida. The MIA™ technique provides a *measure* of the level of hypnosis achieved. The MIA™ technique *intensifies* but does not *depress* the laryngeal or "life-preserving" reflexes.

MINIMAL, MODERATE, DEEP SEDATION & GENERAL ANESTHESIA*

Minimal sedation (Anxiolysis)

Minimal sedation is a drug-induced state during which patients respond normally to verbal commands. Although cognitive function and coordination may be impaired, ventilatory and cardiovascular functions are unaffected.

* Excerpted from ASA position on Monitored Anesthesia Care in ASA manual for Anesthesia Departmental Organization and Management, 2003–4. Reprinted with written permission of the American Society of Anesthesiologists. A copy of the full text can be obtained from ASA, 520 N. Northwest Highway, Park Ridge, Illinois 60068-2573.

Moderate Sedation/Analgesia ("Conscious Sedation")

Moderate sedation/analgesia is a drug-induced depression of consciousness during which patients respond purposefully to verbal commands, either alone or accompanied by light tactile stimulation. No interventions (*Editor's note*: "*intervention*" *is undefined.—BLF*) are required to maintain a patent airway, and spontaneous ventilation is adequate. Cardiovascular function is usually maintained.

N.B. A *second* physician is involved in: Deep sedation analgesia.

Deep Sedation/Analgesia

Deep sedation/analgesia is a drug-induced depression of consciousness during which patients cannot be easily aroused but respond purposefully following repeated or painful stimulation. The ability to independently maintain ventilatory function may be impaired. Patients may require assistance (*Editor's note*: "*assistance*" *is undefined. -BLF*) in maintaining a patent airway, and spontaneous ventilation may be inadequate. Cardiovascular function is usually maintained. Reflex withdrawal from a painful stimulus is NOT considered a purposeful response.

General Anesthesia (GA)

General anesthesia is a drug-induced loss of consciousness during which patients are not arousable, even by painful stimulation. The ability to independently maintain ventilatory function is often impaired. Patients often require assistance in maintaining a patent airway, and positive pressure ventilation may be required because of depressed spontaneous ventilation or drug-induced depression of neuromuscular function. Cardiovascular function may be impaired.

Because sedation is a continuum, it is not always possible to *predict* how an individual patient will respond. Hence, practitioners intending to produce a given level of sedation should be able to rescue patients whose level of sedation becomes deeper than initially intended. Individuals administering moderate ("conscious") sedation/analgesia should be able to rescue patients who enter a state of deep sedation/analgesia, while those administering deep sedation/analgesia should be able to rescue patients who enter a state of general anesthesia.

COMMENT ON THE FOUR CLASSES OF SEDATION/ANESTHESIA

Neither the term "intervention" (for "conscious" or moderate sedation) nor "assistance" (for deep sedation) to maintain an airway is defined in the preceding ASA position paper.

"Intervention" for "conscious" or moderate sedation may be any passive maneuver to maintain airway patency. "Interventions" include, but are not limited to, extending the head with or without lateral rotation, and placement of a one liter bag (or similar device) under the patient's shoulders. "Interventions" are designed to exert more force on the genioglossus muscle, elevating the tongue off the back of the oropharynx, and opening the airway. *(The genioglossus muscle is so named because it connects the "genu," or "knee," of the mandible to the "glossus," or tongue.)*

An intermediate maneuver between "intervention" and "assistance" is sometimes referred to as a "chinner" in the dental and oral surgical community. A "chinner" is the manual support of the chin to open the airway long enough for drug levels to decrease enough to allow the patient to regain an adequate SpO_2. By definition, a "chinner" is a *transient* maneuver as opposed to either a continuous passive "intervention" or an active "assistance."

"Assistance" for deep sedation may be any supraglottic mechanical device actively inserted into the nose or mouth to maintain airway patency. Examples of such devices are nasal airways, oral airways, cuffed oropharyngeal airways

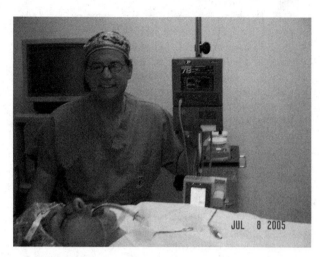

Figure 1-1. The patient is prepared for a rhinoplasty, is asleep at BIS 78, spontaneously breathing room air through an LMA. $SpO_2 > 96\%$.

(COPA®), laryngeal mask airways (LMA®), and even Combitube.®

Propofol administered at an infusion rate sufficient to produce a BIS 60–75 (moderate to deep sedation) will depress the *pharyngeal* reflexes and inhibit swallowing (see Table 4-2). The pharyngeal reflexes are not "life preserving" because they do not protect the glottic chink.

If the patient maintains a preinsertion BIS value of 60–75 after the insertion of a supraglottic device (meaning that a deeper level of anesthesia was neither required for the insertion nor maintenance), then the insertion of a

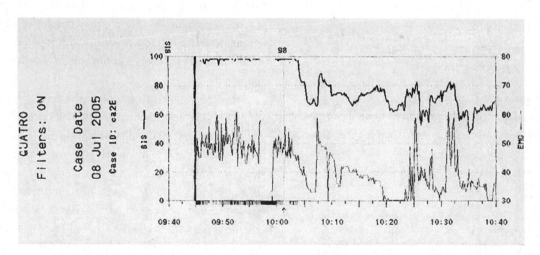

Figure 1-2. The BIS trace for the entire case. Note that at no time during the LMA insertion or the majority of the case does the patient require BIS 45–60 (hypnosis compatible with GA) to tolerate her LMA. Clearly, the insertion of an LMA *per se* does not transform PK MC/MIA™ technique from a sedation to general anesthesia!

supraglottic device, per se, does not transform a deep sedation case into a general anesthetic! LMA does not equal GA![3]
See Figures 1-1 and 1-2.

Modification of the AAAASF classification to include either a separate level or subsection of Level C should be created to account for nontriggering anesthesia.

A Class C facility typically must have an anesthesia machine, scavenging, and dantrolene to safely provide general anesthesia. The MIA™ technique is a nontriggering technique. Therefore, *no* increment in patient safety (i.e., substantial cost-zero benefit) will be achieved by requirements that ignore the value of measuring the patient's level of consciousness. Intravenous sedation can be minimal, moderate, or deep sedation as well as general anesthesia (*vide supra*).

In an attempt to bring a semblance of order into the chaotic nomenclature of levels of sedation/anesthesia, the ASA has defined four specific clinical levels. The attempt to differentiate "conscious sedation" as being performed by a *single* physician would appear to preclude the possibility of "conscious sedation" being provided by a second physician (i.e., an anesthesiologist or nurse anesthetist). This is incompatible with current clinical practice.

All of the first three levels of sedation may be described MAC because they are neither general nor regional anesthesia. One of the most cogent points contained in the ASA position on MAC was the statement that it is not always possible to *predict* how an individual patient will respond!

CORRELATING DEFINITIONS WITH CLINICAL PRACTICE

Benzodiazepines may be used to provide minimal, moderate, and deep states of sedation. Propofol can produce *all* four levels of hypnosis for sedation/anesthesia. However, benzodiazepines are not well measured by the BIS or other currently commercially available level-of-consciousness monitors. Propofol *is* well measured by BIS[17,18] (see Table 1-4). Propofol alone can provide minimal sedation "anxiolysis" (BIS 78–85). Propofol in conjunction

with *intermittent* ketamine may be either moderate or "conscious" sedation (BIS 70-78) or deep sedation (BIS 60–70) depending on whether passive "intervention" or active "assistance" for airway maintenance is required (*vide supra*).

The MIA™ technique may be classified as minimal (BIS 78–85), moderate "conscious" sedation (BIS 70–78), or deep sedation (BIS 60–70), depending on whether a *passive* intervention (moderate sedation) or an *active* assistance (deep sedation) is required to maintain the airway. The insertion of an LMA without increasing the depth of anesthesia below BIS 60–75 does not transform a sedation case into a general anesthesia. *The MIA™ technique is MAC, not GA or TIVA.* The MIA™ technique does not require an anesthesia machine,[21] scavenging, or dantrolene to be safe, simple reproducible, and effective for patients having *ill* elective office-based cosmetic surgeries.

Numerical terminology is more precise than verbal terminology to describe levels of sedation and anesthesia. Numerical terminology permits more precise and effective communication of the level of hypnosis and analgesia between the anesthesiologist and his surgeons as well as his fellow anesthesiologists.

REFERENCES

1. Friedberg BL: Propofol-ketamine technique. *Aesth Plast Surg* 17:297,1993.
2. Friedberg BL: Minimally invasive anesthesia for minimally invasive surgery. *Outpatient Surgery Magazine.* Paoli, PA, Herrin Publishing Partners LP 2:57,2004.
3. Friedberg BL: Does LMA equal GA? (letter). *Outpatient Surgery Magazine.* Paoli, PA, Herrin Publishing Partners LP 6:15,2003.
4. Friedberg BL: Brain is target organ for anesthesia. *Anesthesia Patient Safety Foundation Newsletter* (www.apsf.org) 20(3),Fall 2005.
5. Kearse LA, Rosow C, Zaslavsky A, et al.: Bispectral analysis of the electroencephalogram predicts conscious processing of information during propofol hypnosis and sedation. *Anesthesiol* 88:25,1998.
6. Twersky RS: Office-based anesthesia: Considerations for anesthesiologists in setting up and maintaining a safe office anesthesia environment. Park Ridge, IL, American Society of Anesthesiologists. 2000.

Preoperative Instructions and Intraoperative Environment

Barry L. Friedberg, M.D.

PREOPERATIVE INSTRUCTIONS
  Adjusting Surgeon Expectations
  Adjusting Patient Expectations
CONCLUSION

PREOPERATIVE INSTRUCTIONS

Nothing *per os* (NPO), or nothing by mouth, after midnight is the most commonly given preoperative instruction to *all* surgical patients. This is not unreasonable given the fact that the majority of surgical patients are exposed to emetogenic inhalational vapors and/or emetogenic intravenous opioids. Both inhalational vapors and intravenous opioids depress the laryngeal or "life-protecting" reflexes.

California Assembly Bill (AB)595 specifically mandated office accreditation when sedatives and analgesics are used in a manner that has the probability to depress the "life-preserving" reflexes. The "Catch-22" is that neither the legislature nor the anesthesia community ever defined what the "life-preserving" reflexes are. In both the peer-reviewed literature[1] and in unrebutted public testimony before the CA Medical Board when Dr. Thomas Joas, a prominent anesthesiologist, was its presiding chairman, Friedberg has unequivocally defined the laryngeal reflexes as the "life-preserving" reflexes.

Emetogenic inhalational vapors and/or emetogenic intravenous opioids expose the surgical patient to an increased likelihood of aspiration and death. **If surgical patients cannot reflexly protect their trachea, they cannot preserve their lives.** The lack of pharyngeal reflexes or swallowing seen with propofol sedation/anesthesia does not necessarily mean that the laryngeal reflexes are similarly depressed. In fact, when ketamine is added to the regimen of propofol sedation and opioids are *scrupulously avoided* (i.e., *PK MAC/*MIA™ technique), laryngospasm has been

observed in about 1–2% of patients. Laryngospasm is the *antithesis* of depressed laryngeal reflexes. *Laryngospasm has been observed as long as several hours after a single 50-mg dose of ketamine!* Laryngospasm is the ultimate in *heightened* laryngeal reflex activity. Because it does not depress the "life-preserving" reflexes, *PK MAC/*MIA™ technique is exempted from AB595 mandating office accreditation. Notwithstanding the AB595 exemption, the medical liability carriers will still require that the ASA monitoring standards (i.e., NIABP, SpO_2, EKG) be followed in any anesthetizing situation.

Temperature measurement is not especially relevant with a nontriggering anesthetic technique. $EtCO_2$ tends 38–42 with PK MAC or the MIA™ technique, when measured. Being able to observe the waveform of the exhaled CO_2 may give additional reassurance to the anesthesiologist that the patient is, in fact, breathing. This is potentially significant if the patient is draped in a manner that precludes observation of the rise and fall of the chest wall (Barinholtz D, personal communication. 2005). $EtCO_2$ monitoring, per se, does little to enhance patient safety with an opioid avoidance technique like the PK MAC/MIA™ technique.

Additionally, there must be a source of oxygen (i.e., an E tank), a means of positive pressure ventilation (i.e., an Ambu® bag), and suction readily available in any anesthetizing situation. Lastly, insurers will defer to the state authorities for any requirement for a crash cart and a defibrillator (see Chapter 18). Friedberg has never discouraged offices from seeking accreditation despite the fact that *PK MAC/MIA™ technique is exempted from AB595. However, he has safely administered PK MAC/MIA™ technique for offices either in the process of accreditation or unaccredited ones that have met the prerequisites for the safe administration of PK MAC/MIA™ technique.*

In every state except Florida, PK MAC/MIA™ technique is recognized as IV sedation. Florida Medical Board regulations follow those of the American Association for the Accreditation of Surgical Facilities (AAAASF). The Medical Board of Florida has arbitrarily classified PK MAC/MIA™ technique as GA. The net effect of this ruling is to require every office-based surgery suite in Florida desiring to have the safer, superior outcomes of PK MAC/MIA™ technique to be required to increase their classification from a "B" to a "C" facility. All "C" facilities must have (1) an anesthesia machine, (2) scavenging, (3) dantrolene. PK MAC/MIA™ technique is a nontriggering IV technique. Florida's requirements add substantial costs without adding a scintilla of patient safety. Both the AAAASF and the Florida Medical Board have rebuffed numerous phone calls and e-mail entreaties to calendar this item on their meeting agenda to even permit a discussion of the factual definition of sedation versus general anesthesia (see Chapter 1, Appendix 1-1).

Friedberg's preoperative instructions have evolved after lengthy experience with a nonemetogenic anesthetic regimen (see Table 2-1). In general, patients who are *stable*

Table 2-1. Preoperative instructions

1. Patients taking antihypertensives, antidepressants, beta-blockers, asthma medications, or oral hypoglycemic agents should maintain their usual morning dosage with enough water to comfortably get their medications down. Asthmatics should bring their inhalers with them to surgery.
2. Patients who regularly consume caffeinated beverages and who experience headache without the usual morning caffeine dose are encouraged to have their usual morning dose of caffeine WITHOUT any dairy product. Nondairy creamers are acceptable, if needed.
3. Patients who are very hungry upon awakening may have toast and jam and/or apple juice if so desired.
4. Patients who are scheduled for afternoon surgery may have a light breakfast not closer than four hours prior to their surgery. Again, "light" means **NO DAIRY PRODUCTS** (i.e., milk, cream, butter, yogurt, or cheese).

---

on their preoperative regimen of medications should continue taking those medications with the following exceptions. Hypertensive patients on diuretics like furosemide or hydrochlorothiazide are instructed **not** to take their a.m. dose as this will tend to cause their bladder to become full under anesthesia. A full bladder can cause patients to squirm about the OR table, elevate their blood pressures, or void spontaneously (enuresis). Owing to the higher probability of blood loss and fluid replacement, a three-to-four–hour hospital-type noncosmetic surgery case is often begun with a Foley bladder catheter. *PK MAC/MIA™ technique does not routinely require bladder catheterization. The exception to this caveat is for a case scheduled for at least five to six hours.* For many patients, eliminating the catheterization eliminates the risk of an iatrogenic bladder infection, a decidedly undesirable outcome in an office-based, elective cosmetic surgical patient.

Elective cosmetic surgical patients fasted overnight are **not** generally 500–1,000 ccs "behind" on fluid volume, as is traditionally taught. Blood loss and replacement are **not** contemplated. Fluid shifts do **not** occur. The physiologic insult of liposuction is **not** analogous to burn cases! Even with a tumescent or "super wet" liposuction procedure, the "third space" created by the aspiration of fat is functionally obliterated by the use of compression garments! A recent article in the plastic surgery literature was disingenuous when the authors suggested that liposuction was not for the treatment of obesity.[2] The article subsequently described the means to safely extract more than 5,000 ccs per operative visit! Rebuttal to the liposuction advisory panel was subsequently published.[3] Liposuction is clearly safer when 5,000 ccs or less are aspirated. Friedberg supports both the Florida and California medical boards' limitations (4,000 and 5,000 ccs of fat, respectively) on the amount of liposuction that may be safely performed in a single office-based surgery.

Florida's board mandates the reporting of hospital admissions and deaths from office-based cosmetic surgery. Public safety also demands the **same** mandatory reporting requirements for elective cosmetic surgery deaths in hospital and ASC settings! An eight-hour limitation in Florida on office-based surgical procedures is reasonable and likely to improve patient safety. Both mandatory reporting and surgery time limitations are supported by Friedberg.

Patients who are very hungry upon awakening may have toast and jam and/or apple juice if so desired. Simple sugars and carbohydrates are readily absorbed from the stomach. The stomach will be empty without having the patient present hypoglycemic (or, at the least, unhappily hungry) before surgery. Management of the patients' blood sugar has been greatly facilitated by the advent of the battery-operated glucose meter, that is, Accu-Check® or One Touch.® Nonetheless, it is still incumbent on the anesthesiologist to assure that hypoglycemia under anesthesia does not occur. Juvenile, Type I, or insulin-dependent diabetic patients should avoid their full a.m. dose of insulin. However, they should have *some* insulin! One half to one third of their usual morning insulin dose should be satisfactory for control without substantially risking hypoglycemia for two-to-four–hour morning cases. For these patients, an hourly check of their blood sugars *during* anesthesia is strongly recommended.

*Insulin-dependent diabetics should **not** be scheduled as afternoon elective cosmetic surgery cases!*

Diabetics brittle enough to require an insulin infusion are not suitable candidates for office-based cosmetic surgery. Postoperative nausea may sometimes be an expression of hypoglycemia. Nausea of this etiology is more appropriately treated with oral or IV glucose, not antiemetic medication. Whether or not the patient is diabetic, it is useful for patient comfort to offer apple juice or a glucose-containing sports drink like Gatorade® at the conclusion of any case, especially those that run longer than two hours. By eliminating the root causes of PONV (i.e., inhalational anesthetics and opioids), patients rapidly emerge PONV free and able to resume PO fluid intake after the propofol is discontinued. Therefore, resumption of PO fluids is an irrelevant discharge criterion for patients anesthetized with *PK MAC*/MIA™ technique.

Given the enormous commercial success of the Starbucks® coffee company, no account of preoperative instructions would be complete without some discussion of the issue of PO intake of caffeinated beverages in the morning of surgery. From 1992 to 1994, Friedberg noted a number of patients complaining of postoperative headache after PK MAC. He asked the patients with headache complaints if they were regular consumers of caffeinated beverages, coffee, tea, or so-called "energy" drinks like Red Bull.® Most patients experiencing headaches answered in the affirmative. Patients who regularly consume caffeinated beverages should be asked preoperatively if they experience headache if they miss their morning drink. For those who answered affirmatively (not all caffeine drinkers will answer so), allowing them to have some caffeine preoperatively will avoid the postoperative complaint of headache.

Taken without dairy products, a cup of caffeinated coffee or tea will have no greater effect on gastric content than water in this author's clinical experience.

For patients who desire some whitening of their coffee, a nondairy "creamer" is acceptable. For anesthesiologists who have difficulty allowing patients to have their coffee, one tablet of No Doze,® an over-the-counter caffeine tablet, with sips of water may be a suitable alternative. Caffeine maintenance has the same logic as does maintenance of preexisting prescription drug therapy.

Patients who are stable on their preoperative prescription medications are best left stable.

Do not abruptly withdraw these agents (caffeine or prescription drugs) unless there is a pressing reason to do so. If any doubt exists, consult with the prescribing physician. Lastly, patients who are scheduled for afternoon surgery may have a light breakfast not closer than four hours prior to their surgery. "Light" means NO DAIRY PRODUCTS, that is, milk, cream, butter, yogurt, or cheese. Water or apple juice may be consumed up to one hour preoperatively if so desired.

Table 2-2 summarizes the elements of the preoperative information routinely elicited from patients (see Chapter 14 for an in-depth discussion of preoperative assessment). Middle-aged (i.e., 35–60), sedentary adults, both men *and* women, *may* have significant coronary artery disease (CAD) without symptoms or taking medications like

---

Table 2-2. Preoperative patient information

1. Age and weight
2. Current medications, including herbal supplements like Ginko Biloba, garlic, or St. John's Wort
3. Smoking status, pack-year history, time from last cigarette
4. Pregnancy status, "Do you believe that you may be pregnant at this time?"
5. Allergies to medication and the specific reaction, i.e., urticaria (hives), problem breathing
6. History of asthma or hepatitis
7. Previous anesthetic experience, i.e., prolonged emergence or PONV
8. History of motion sickness

nitroglycerin to alert the anesthesiologist. These patients are particularly at risk for destabilization of their asymptomatic, underlying CAD. The stress of the injection of epinephrine-containing local anesthetic at the beginning of all cosmetic surgical procedures can potentially produce a "chemical" stress treadmill.

Much confusion continues over whether ketamine produces tachycardia and hypertension. *The answer is both "yes" and "no" depending on the context in which ketamine is administered!*

Ketamine is often given in close temporal sequence to the injection of local anesthesia by the surgeon. When a tachycardia occurs in this *context*, it is clearly impossible to differentiate a ketamine effect from an epinephrine effect. When given as a single anesthetic agent (i.e., $1-2$ mg $\cdot$ kg^{-1}), ketamine will produce hypertension and tachycardia, just as the original investigators described. (Using doses of $2.0-4.0$ mg $\cdot$ kg^{-1} in 1968, Corssen reported an 8.1% incidence of hypertension [25% above resting baseline] and a 4.1% incidence of tachycardia.)[4]

However, the *context* in which ketamine is given in *PK MAC/MIA*™ technique is entirely different. The **incremental** induction technique with propofol is designed to create a stable level of propofol in the brain. By titrating the propofol to a quantitative level with the BIS (i.e., $70-75$), the *context* in which the ketamine interacts with the brain is precisely and *reproducibly* defined. Friedberg has administered the ketamine on many occasions in the course of administering *PK MAC/MIA*™ technique with ten to twenty minutes elapsing before the surgeon was ready to inject the local. In none of those "ketamine-without-local-anesthetic-injection" contexts did tachycardia or hypertension occur.

Fifty mg ketamine, in the *context* of a stable brain level of propofol, produces **neither** tachycardia nor hypertension.

The epinephrine in the surgeon's local anesthetic may cause the heart rate to increase. Diastolic filling time shortens as heart rate increases. Normal coronary arteries dilate to compensate for the shortened filling time. Plaque-filled or atherosclerotic coronaries are *unable to dilate* in response to the demand for increased oxygen with tachycardia. When oxygen demand exceeds the diseased coronaries' ability to supply it to the myocardium, the patient's heart will most likely become destabilized.

Those anesthesiologists unwilling to prevent tachycardia may find the ACLS algorithm for ventricular tachycardia/fibrillation useful.

Cardiac destabilization does not require a full thickness myocardial infarction. Destabilization with a low probability of resuscitation may occur just as easily with a subendocardial infarction.

To anticipate destabilization, it may be useful to routinely monitor a modified V5 (MV5) EKG. This may be accomplished by first selecting lead I on the monitor. Then, place the left arm (black) lead over the point of maximum impulse or apex of the left ventricle, and use the third lead (green or red) on the left shoulder to observe the ST-T waves as an indicator of coronary ischemia. Obviously, monitoring an MV5 during a breast augmentation or mastoplexy case will not be practical.

Even more useful than monitoring MV5 is **preventing tachycardia** in **all** patients over the age of 35 with the judicious use of beta-blockers. Friedberg advocates 10 mg labetolol (Trandate® or Normodyne®) IV push but recognizes propranolol (Inderal®) or esmolol (Brevibloc®) may be acceptable alternatives. In the **context** of opioid administration, it may be unwise to administer more than 5 mg labetolol at a time. However, dividing the labetolol doses may be ineffective in preventing the "chemical" stress treadmill in a timely fashion.

Another advantage of opioid avoidance PK MAC/MIA™ *technique is that one may administer labetolol as a 10 mg bolus without creating a severe bradycardia.*

Elicitation of the patient's body weight will facilitate using any syringe-pump-type device for the administration of propofol. The utility of body weight based dosing of propofol is limited by the fact that there may be as great as a nineteenfold variability in propofol hydroxylation.[5] This variability was most closely correlated with cytochrome P450 P2B6.[5] This interindividual variability confounds the best pharmacokinetic or pharmacodynamic modeling. Interindividual variability is another foundation for using a level-of-consciousness monitor, like BIS, to titrate propofol to produce *PK MAC/ MIA*™ technique (see Chapter 3).

See Chapter 14 and Appendix A for a discussion of the potential impact current medications and herbal supplements may have on anesthetic management. Patient's smoking status is a concern because smokers often do not tolerate oral airways as well as nasal airways.

Table 2-3. Airway management algorithm for the MIA® technique (assumes incremental propofol induction)

---

1. Head extended, rotated laterally (facelift position)
2. 1,000 cc IV bag (or shoulder roll) under shoulders
3. Nasal airway (#28, most commonly), lubricated
4. LMA (#4, most commonly), lubricated. *Patients will breath spontaneously throughout the case. Supplemental oxygen will be applied to maintain SpO2 > 90% and the following sequence of airway interventions will be started until saturation is satisfactory.*

Coughing is more likely to result if the anesthesiologist tries to maintain a patent airway with an oral device instead of the recommended PK MAC/MIA™ airway management algorithm.

All MIA™ patients are managed with the same airway algorithm, namely, whatever level of intervention is required to maintain a patent airway (see Table 2-3).

In Friedberg's experience, smokers tend to have heightened sensitivity of their glottic chink. They are more susceptible to laryngospasm, especially if there is a history of a recent upper respiratory infection (URI).

Wide variability among cosmetic surgery practices exists on how to deal with the sensitive issue of the patient's pregnancy status. At one end of the spectrum of contemporary practice is a patient disclosure: "I do not believe that I am pregnant at this time." An intermediate position would be to use an over-the-counter pregnancy urine spot test to rule out pregnancy. At the other extreme of practice is demanding a human chorionic gonadrotropin (HCG) assay on every female patient prior to giving potentially teratogenic anesthetic agents. In many private practice settings, an HCG test imposes an additional financial burden on the cash-paying cosmetic surgery patient. An HCG test is not as relevant in the menopausal rhytidectomy patient, despite reproductive technology having pushed the typical age boundaries for pregnancy. The HCG test is more relevant to the younger and more fertile breast augmentation or liposuction patient who tends to be more cost-conscious. Increasing the financial burden exacted on these patients preoperatively may increase their motivation to find a different cosmetic surgeon who may be willing to forego this testing. The issue is further compounded

by considerations raised by the new federal privacy statute (HIPAA). HIPAA is principally applicable for medically indicated, third-party, or insurance cases. Elective cosmetic patients are not covered by this statute. A binding arbitration agreement is currently being utilized, placing one more step in the patient's process of filing a lawsuit.

Most allergy histories, if carefully taken, involve known side effects from drugs rather than true allergic reactions. Examples are, "my heart races every time my dentist injects my teeth," or "I vomit every time I take codeine." One must take cognizance of true allergic phenomenon like urticaria, rash, and anaphylaxis. By avoiding neuromuscular blocking agents, especially succinylcholine, PK MAC/MIA™ technique eliminates many of the offending agents. Avoiding morphine will eliminate histamine-type reactions. Avoiding meperidine adds more safety to PK MAC/MIA™ technique, especially if patients are taking the monamine oxidase inhibitors (MAOI) like phenelzine (Nardil®) or tranylcypromine (Parnate®). The hypertensive crisis precipitated by the administration of meperidine to patients on MAOI, although not an allergic reaction, will nevertheless cause considerable but avoidable stress in the office-based surgical suite along with the significant potential of the loss of patient life.

When one elicits a history of asthma, inquire about the most recent attack and what measures were taken to break it. A common response to the question about asthma has been, "I had it as a child but haven't had any problems in years." For the patient who has an active asthmatic history, it is imperative that they bring whatever inhalers they typically use to the office prior to having anesthesia for cosmetic surgery. It is also important to inquire about how well the patient feels they are breathing on admission to the office surgery suite. It is not unreasonable to ask the patient to take a few puffs of their inhaler of choice before inducing anesthesia. Avoiding both inhalational agents as well as endotracheal intubation with PK MAC/MIA™ technique are significant advantages for the asthmatic patient. Ketamine has some bronchodilating properties that may also be advantageous for the asthmatic patient. An asthmatic attack may be triggered by administering beta-blocking drugs to treat tachycardia. Fortunately, actively asthmatic patients tend to be more tolerant of tachycardia than nonasthmatics. Be judicious when deciding to treat tachycardia with beta-blocking agents in this group of patients.

Eliciting a history of hepatitis will not change the dosing of propofol or ketamine but should alert the anesthesiologist to take greater care with blood and bodily fluid exposure. *In the era of HIV/AIDS, anesthesiologists are obliged to use "universal precautions" for all patients.* Nonetheless, one tends to exercise even more caution when dealing with a patient whose lifestyle suggests a greater likelihood of being positive (i.e., intravenous drug using, homosexual males).

Acutely jaundiced patients are not suitable candidates for office-based elective cosmetic surgery.

Patients with previous hepatic injury would probably be better served by avoidance of halogenated inhalational anesthetic agents for elective cosmetic surgery, especially since a suitable alternative in PK MAC/MIA™ technique exists.

During the ten years Friedberg logged his PK MAC/MIA™ technique cases, approximately 35% of all patients admitted to having PONV with previous anesthetic experiences. Few patients answered positively to the open-ended question "Have you had any problems with previous anesthesia?" Only by asking the close-ended question "Did you throw up after your previous anesthesia?" will one discover the surprisingly high levels of previous PONV in the cosmetic surgical patient population. So many patients have experienced PONV that they believe it is a *normal* part of the anesthetic experience! Both Gan[6] and Apfel[7] agree that a positive history of previous PONV is only one marker to determine high risk of repeat PONV. Other risk markers include female gender, nonsmoking status, history of motion sickness and plastic surgery. By all standards, Friedberg's practice would qualify as high risk for PONV. Despite the risk of PONV, antiemetics are not used preemptively for patients receiving the MIA™ technique, *even those with a positive history of PONV.* Only 13 patients experienced PONV out of a total 2,680 patients, an astounding and unprecedented **0.5% PONV rate**, anesthetized with PK MAC/MIA™ technique from March 26, 1992 through March 26, 2002.[8] *All* thirteen patients who experienced PONV stated they would still prefer PK MAC/MIA™ technique to their previous anesthetic. The patients stated that their emesis was a "once-and-done" experience compared to the hours and, sometimes, even *days* of PONV.

Patients repeatedly confirmed Macario's scientifically validated survey[9] that it was preferable to avoid vomiting before avoiding pain. Essentially, all patients who sign up for elective surgery know, at some level (consciously or subconsciously), that they are going to experience some level of discomfort or pain on emergence. **What they are trying to ask of their anesthesiologist is not to "rub salt in their wounds" by making them throw up in addition to their pain!** For many reasons, not the least of which is production pressure, anesthesiologists tend not to take cognizance of their patients' concerns on this issue. It is easier to give ondansetron, et cetera, than to modify one's anesthetic "game plan" of nearly always administering opioids.

Once the hospital or ASC patient is deposited in the PAR, PONV is often no longer the problem of the anesthesiologist. Small wonder why some surgeons regard their anesthesia colleagues as indifferent to the surgeon's problems. Many surgeons (and patients) rightly perceive the anesthesia as the cause. The hostility generated by the anesthesiologists' apparent indifference to PONV is a significant impediment to securing the cooperation of the surgeon to implement the paradigm shift involved in performing PK MAC/MIA™ technique.

The office-based anesthesiologist, in comparison to his institutionally based colleague, does not require a Level I study to learn if his patient is experiencing PONV on emergence. The office-based anesthesiologist is typically *physically present* with the patient during emergence and can readily observe with his own eyes the results of his anesthetic regimen. There is no hiding from the outcomes. They may be quite literally in his face!

Adjusting Surgeon Expectations

There is little likelihood of successfully implementing PK MAC/MIA™ technique without eliciting the active cooperation of the surgeon. It is incumbent on the anesthesiologist attempting to introduce the MIA™ technique to seek to educate his surgeons about the need for *adequate* local analgesia. *A blanched field does not always mean adequate analgesia.* Patient movement in the presence of BIS 60–75 is an indication for the reinjection of the field on which the surgeon is working.

Specifically, the advantages of the MIA™ technique are nonopioid, preemptive analgesia (NOPA), the subsequent elimination of PONV and the overwhelming majority of postoperative pain. One cannot hope to effect this education in the heat of an incipient surgery. Specifically, do not attempt to introduce the MIA™ technique while looking over the ether screen or in the surgical lounge immediately preceding the case. The surgeon is typically distracted by the anticipation of the operation and is rarely receptive to instituting profound changes on the spot. Much preferable to the lounge or the OR is to schedule an outside meeting (i.e., the hospital cafeteria or medical library) to begin a dialogue with the surgeon. Even better, a meeting outside the hospital, ASC, or surgical office is much more likely to produce a more receptive audience and the desired effect of cooperation.

The greater the distance is from the stressor environment (i.e., the OR), the greater the likelihood is of gaining the surgeon's undivided attention.

In this unfettered setting, try to explain to the surgeon that the BIS monitor helps to tell the difference between patient movement that originates from the spinal cord (meaning no issue of awareness or recall) from that originating from the brain. If he appears not to understand, consider using the example of the chicken moving after its head has been severed. Still, no guarantee of success can be offered, even under these circumstances. All people resist change: lay people, surgeons, and even anesthesiologists.

Having the anesthesiologist express his genuine desire to eliminate PONV for his patients and their surgeons is an enormous act of kindness. "A single act of kindness throws out roots in all directions, and the roots spring up and make new trees. The greatest work that kindness does to others is that it makes them kind themselves" (Amelia Earhart, missing pioneering female aviatrix).

The MIA™ technique is not universally acceptable because not all surgeons take their own postoperative patient calls. Therefore, the advantage of decreasing the number of those calls for PONV and pain management is not offset by the minor inconvenience of having to stop operating for ten to fifteen seconds to reinject a field. Most surgeons' eyebrows arch upward when approached with the question, "Are you interested in working with me to eliminate PONV and postoperative pain in our patients?"

Many surgeons have unpleasant memories of performing surgery on patients under IV sedation. (The modern practice of TIVA has helped to erase many of those memories. See Chapter 11.) Those memories usually consist of *intolerable* patient movement, patients being too asleep and then too awake, generally distracting and annoying

Table 2-4. The surgeon's "golden" rules for the MIA™ technique

1. BIS 60–75 means the patient is adequately asleep.
2. A blanched surgical field does not guarantee complete analgesia.
3. Reinject the field if the patient moves at BS 60–75.

the surgeon from his work. In the context of the MIA™ technique, it is almost always difficult to discern from the conduct of a smooth general anesthetic. It is so if the surgeon can learn to follow the "golden" rules of the MIA™ technique (see Table 2-4).

Adjusting Patient Expectations

Elective cosmetic surgery patients complain after anesthesia for cosmetic surgery for a variety of reasons. Sometimes the anesthesiologist wasn't nice to them, didn't appear to take their concerns to heart, or was too busy to listen. This type of complaint illustrates why many otherwise competent anesthesiologists may be unsuited for office-based cosmetic surgery anesthesia. Some anesthesiologists may feel that "frivolous" cosmetic surgery patients are wasting the anesthesiologist's time when there are medically indicated surgeries that need his expertise. Worse still, some anesthesiologists may offer their unsolicited and unwelcome opinion that they do not see anything wrong with the cosmetic surgery patients' appearance. Sometimes the complaint is *only* that the anesthesiologist was rough or hurt them starting the IV.

Other complaints that can be avoided are those necessary to disclose because they are known outcomes or side effects. If patients know what to expect, then it is less likely that they will complain.

Glycopyrrolate causes dry mouth. Complaints about dry mouth can usually be circumvented by explaining that dryness is *expected* for six to eight hours after surgery. It is also useful to apologize, in advance, for the inconvenience of the dry mouth in front of a witness (when available) who will be with the patient after surgery. That the patient may drink and eat freely but their mouth will remain dry until the medicine wears off satisfies most patients. For those still unsatisfied, it may be helpful to explain that the *alternative* to the dry mouth could be a sore throat from suctioning the excess secretions caused by the ketamine.

Table 2-5. Preoperative admonitions

1. Dry mouth for six to eight hours postoperatively
2. Blurry vision
3. Slight discomfort on application of BIS sensor
4. One out of twenty, or 5%, experience pleasant, colorful dreams

To date, given a choice, no cosmetic surgery patient has preferred the pain of a sore throat to the annoyance of a dry mouth. All inconveniences are relative.

Some patients will complain about blurry vision upon emergence unless they are told that ointment intended to protect their corneas (or eyes) will be put in after they are asleep. To date, no cosmetic surgery patient has chosen dry, burning eyes to transient blurry vision. see Table 2-5

If a level-of-consciousness monitor like the BIS is used, it may be helpful to permit patients to touch the back of the sensor where it will meet their skin. The anesthesiologist can reassure the patient that the sensor will not puncture

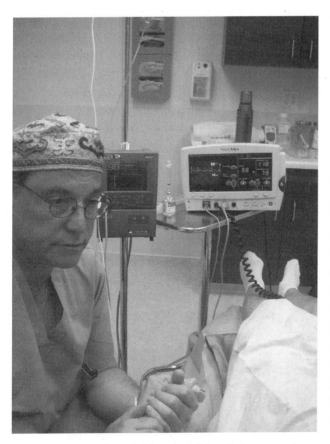

Figure 2-1. Dr. Friedberg holding the left hand of a consenting patient prior to induction. Witnesses are in the OR but out of the picture field.

the skin, even though it is slightly uncomfortable when applied. Many patients have stated that the sensor feels like Velcro® being stuck to their head. Explaining that BIS empowers patients to be in "control" while they are asleep is very comforting for some anxious patients. During the preoperative patient interview, Friedberg writes a series of four numbers with accompanying phrases on the BIS sensor package: 0–100 (range), 98–100 (awake), 60–75 (MIA), and 45–60 (GA). The explanation goes as follows: "For the first twenty years of my practice, I, like most anesthesiologists, would *guess* how asleep you were based on your heart rate and blood pressure. We anesthesiologists formerly believed that any changes in your level of anesthesia in your brain would be reflected by changes in your heart rate and blood pressure. For fear of giving you too little medicine, I would routinely *overmedicate* by a factor of 20–30% for fear of administering too little. By giving me a number by which I may help judge how asleep you are, BIS has revolutionized the delivery of anesthesia care for you, the patient.

BIS is an index with no units like pounds or inches. The range is from 0–100. Right now, all of us in the preoperative room are between 98–100. The deeper your anesthetic becomes, the lower your BIS value will become. By gradually getting you off to sleep with a series of minidoses of propofol, I am able to carefully custom fit your anesthetic to you, the individual, at this moment in time, rather than relying on an off-the-rack, one-size-fits-most approach. By medicating you only to the level of 60–75, we are able to give you the illusion of general anesthesia in that you neither hear, nor feel, nor remember the surgery. I refer to this state as the minimally invasive anesthesia (MIA)™ technique. Giving still more medication will take you down to the level recognized as 'general anesthesia' at 45–60. Using this numerical scale helps to avoid the unnecessary medication we were formerly obliged to administer for fear of giving you too little medication. Why would I not want to know how asleep you are? Isn't measuring better than guessing? The medication I am giving you is not designed to medicate your heart rate or blood pressure. I am trying to medicate your brain! Hopefully, my presentation was simple and easy to understand. Do you have any questions for me?"

If one was initially seated for the interview, try to remain seated when asking if the patients have any questions. Remaining seated conveys a more sincere interest on the part of the anesthesiologist than standing up and beginning to exit the room.

As long as the patient is asked for permission in advance, it is a very supportive gesture to hold the patient's hand during induction see Fig 2-1. *Never induce the patient without another person present in the room.* "No administrator of an anesthetic is safe from having such a charge preferred against him, and if he and his supposed victim are alone, it is simply a case of word against word."[10] Liability suits have been filed when the patient has fantasized and subsequently alleged inappropriate, unprofessional behavior on the part of the anesthesiologist.[11] The anesthesiologist is defenseless without a witness.

CONCLUSION

The office-based nurses who are full-time employees (as opposed to leased solely for the surgical schedule) are more likely to have personal contact with the patients on preoperative as well as postoperative visits in addition to the surgical experience. In contradistinction to the nursing staff in the hospital or ASC (who are more like the leased office employee), the office-based nurses tend to take their work more personally and "bond" with the patients because of the extended contact. This continuity of care promotes the personalization of medical care that is a reason, beyond the welcome financial advantage, that growing numbers of patients prefer to have cosmetic surgery in the office setting. There is a greater perception of "caring" in their care!

REFERENCES

1. Friedberg BL: Propofol-ketamine technique, dissociative anesthesia for office surgery: A five-year review of 1,264 cases. *Aesth Plast Surg* 23:70,1999.
2. Iverson, R. E., Lynch, D. J., and the ASPS Committee on Patient Safety: Practice advisory on liposuction. *Plast Reconstr Surg* 100:1478,2004.
3. Friedberg BL: Inaccuracies and omissions with the report of the ASPS Committee on Patient Safety Practice Advisory on Liposuction. *Plast Reconstr Surg* 117:2142,2005.
4. Corssen G, Miyasaka M, Domino EF: Changing concepts in pain control during surgery: Dissociative anesthesia with CI-581. *Anesth Analg Curr Res* 47:746,1968.
5. Court MH, Duan SX, Hesse LM, et al.: Cytochrome P-450 2B6 is responsible for interindividual variability of propofol hydroxylation by human liver microsomes. *Anesthesiol* 94:110,2001.
6. Gan TJ, Meyer T, Apfel CC, et. al.: Consensus guidelines for managing postoperative nausea and vomiting. *Anesth Analg* 97:62,2003.
7. Apfel CC, Korttila K, Abdalla M, et al.: A factorial trial of six interventions for the prevention of PONV. *N Engl J Med* 350:2441,2004.
8. Friedberg BL: Propofol ketamine anesthesia for cosmetic surgery in the office suite, in Osborne I (ed.), *Anesthesia for Outside the Operating Room. International Anesthesiology Clinics.* Baltimore, Lippincott, Williams & Wilkins, 41:39,2003.
9. Macario A, Weinger M, Carney K, et al.: Which clinical anesthesia outcomes are important to avoid ? The perspective of patients. *Anesth Analg* 89:652,1999.
10. Buxton D: Anaesthetics. London, H.K. Lewis, 1888; p 145.
11. Balasubramaniam B, Park GR: Sexual hallucinations during and after sedation and anaesthesia. *Anaesthesia* 58:1149, 2003.

3 | Level-of-Consciousness Monitoring

Scott D. Kelley, M.D.

INTRODUCTION

Level-of-consciousness monitoring allows anesthesia clinicians to measure the effects of anesthesia and sedation on the brain, allowing them to deliver anesthesia with more precision. With the variety of anesthetic techniques, agents, and approaches utilized during anesthesia for cosmetic surgery, a consciousness monitor is one of the important tools that aid in the goal of improving patient care and achieving excellent outcomes.

EVOLUTION OF PATIENT MONITORING

Patient assessment and intraoperative monitoring during anesthesia has undergone gradual change and refinement. Observations of clinical signs such as pupil response, patterns of respiration, quality of the pulse, and movement were first augmented by direct measurement of physiologic endpoints including blood pressure, heart rate, and respiratory rate and volume. With the development of pulse oximetry and capnography, precise assessments of ventilatory management could be made. The use of end-tidal agent analysis and peripheral nerve stimulation provided anesthesia clinicians the ability to measure pharmacologic agent concentration and effect, respectively. Although not used during cosmetic surgery, cardiac function can be evaluated using technologies that range from pulmonary artery catheters and transesophageal echocardiography to new methods of continuous blood pressure and cardiac output monitoring.

Despite the remarkable improvements in assessment of the cardiovascular and pulmonary function during anesthesia, direct determination of the effect of the anesthetic and sedative agents on the central nervous system has remained limited. Careful clinical investigations demonstrated that hemodynamic responses do not necessarily provide an accurate representation of the central nervous system responsiveness to anesthetic agents. *Therefore, hemodynamic responses were unreliable indicators of brain status.*[1]

In contrast, technologies that permit independent neurophysiological monitoring of the central nervous system provide a direct measure of brain response during anesthesia and sedation, allowing clinicians to fine-tune the perioperative management of each patient. Accurate monitoring and targeting of brain effect, in combination with assessment of clinical signs and traditional monitoring, permit a more complete approach to adjusting the dosing and mixture of anesthetic, sedative, and analgesic agents.

LEVEL-OF-CONSCIOUSNESS MONITORING

Consciousness-monitoring technologies provide measurement of the *hypnotic effect* of anesthesia. They have proven to be accurate and reliable in nearly all patients and clinical settings and are robust in the presence of the most commonly used anesthetic and sedative agents. At the core of most consciousness-monitoring technologies is the surface electroencephalogram (EEG). This complex physiologic signal is a waveform that represents the sum of all brain activity produced by the cerebral cortex. The EEG changes in response to the effects of anesthetic and sedative/hypnotic agents.[2] Although individual drugs can induce some unique effects on the EEG, the overall pattern of changes is quite similar for many of these agents. During general anesthesia, typical EEG-changes responses include an increase in average amplitude (power) and a decrease in average frequency. These changes become more evident as the EEG waveform frequency patterns move from beta to delta—the pattern consistent with deep anesthesia.

The complex EEG waveform can be broken down into its individual components, analyzed using a mathematical technique called *power spectral analysis* and displayed as power per frequency component in a "power spectrum." Power spectral analysis results in one or more numeric descriptors known as processed EEG parameters.[3]

Many attempts have been made to utilize power spectral analysis and processed EEG parameters to gauge the effect of anesthesia on the brain. Processed EEG parameters that have been investigated as indicators of anesthetic effects include the 95% spectral edge frequency as well as the median frequency. These parameters are various characteristics that describe the EEG power spectrum. Median frequency and 95% spectral edge frequency indicate the spectral frequency below that contains either 50% or 95% of the power in the EEG.

Unfortunately, for most anesthetic drugs, the relationship between dosage and changes in EEG power and frequency is not straightforward, so it has been difficult to use traditional processed EEG parameters in a clinically reliable way. A clear challenge for further adoption of the EEG as a reliable indicator of anesthetic effect was to overcome the lack of adequate correlation between anesthetic dose and processed EEG parameters derived from power spectral analysis. New waveform analysis techniques have been developed. Algorithms have been introduced to translate EEG waveform analysis into clinical monitoring platforms. The challenge of using processed EEG parameters to successfully monitor hypnotic level during anesthesia and sedation has been met.

BISPECTRAL INDEX: THE PROTOTYPE LEVEL-OF-CONSCIOUSNESS MONITOR

The Bispectral Index (BIS Index) is the most widely utilized level-of-consciousness monitor. Because of its wide availability and extensive investigation, BIS provides the best method to examine this class of anesthesia-effect monitors. BIS monitoring provides a direct and accurate method for continuous level-of-consciousness monitoring throughout the course of anesthetic or sedative administration in the setting of cosmetic surgery.

The BIS Index is a numerically processed, clinically validated EEG parameter. Unlike traditional processed EEG parameters derived from power spectral analysis, the BIS Index is derived utilizing a composite of multiple advanced EEG signal-processing techniques—including bispectral analysis, power spectral analysis, and time domain analysis.[4] As seen in Figure 3-1, these components are combined to optimize the correlation between the EEG and the clinical effects of anesthesia.

The U.S. Food and Drug Administration cleared the BIS Index (Aspect Medical Systems) as an aid in monitoring

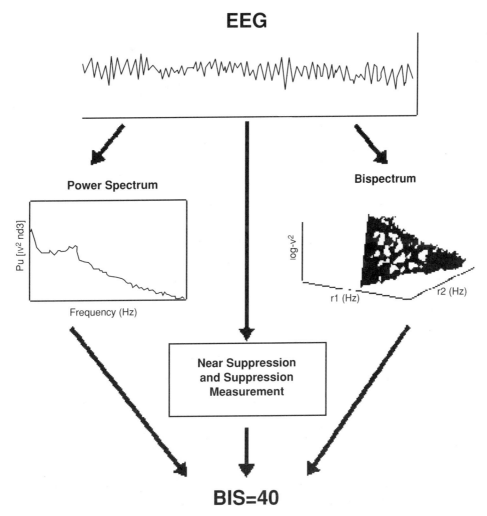

Figure 3-1. Components of Bispectral (BIS) Index.

the hypnotic effect of anesthetics and sedatives in 1996, allowing its introduction into routine clinical practice. Subsequent to BIS, other level-of-consciousness monitors now cleared to measure anesthetic effect in surgical patients include Patient State Index (Physiometrix); Entropy (GE Healthcare), SNAP II (Everest Biomedical), Cerebral State Monitor (Danmeter), and Narcotrend (Schiller Medical).

Focusing on the BIS technology as the prototype consciousness monitor, there are three key elements integral to the system as it functions as a consciousness monitor during anesthesia:

1. EEG Signal Analysis: Bispectral Analysis
2. BIS Algorithm
3. BIS Index

Bispectral Analysis

A portion of the cortical EEG reflects changes attributable to harmonic and phase relationships between cortical and subcortical neural generators. These relationships are altered during hypnosis, producing characteristic patterns in the EEG. Bispectral analysis—and its mathematical results, for example, bicoherence, bispectrum, real triple product—is a sophisticated signal-processing methodology that assesses relationships among signal components and captures synchronization within signals like the EEG. By quantifying the correlation between all the frequencies within the signal, bispectral analysis (together with power spectral and cortical EEG analysis) yields an additional EEG descriptor of brain activity during hypnosis.[4]

BIS Algorithm

A key milestone in the development of a consciousness monitor was to identify EEG features or "descriptors"—bispectral or otherwise—that were highly correlated with sedation/hypnosis induced by the most commonly used anesthetic agents. During development of the BIS Index, several EEG features were identified by analyzing a database of EEGs from more than 5,000 subjects who had received one or more of the most commonly used hypnotic agents and who had been evaluated with simultaneous sedation assessment.[5] Multivariate statistical models were used to derive the optimum combination of EEG features to correlate with clinical endpoints of sedation. From this iterative process, the BIS algorithm that would yield

a clinically tuned, validly processed EEG parameter was developed.

BIS Index

The BIS Index is a number between 0 and 100 scaled to correlate with important clinical endpoints during administration of anesthetic agent (see Fig. 3-2). BIS values near 100 represent an "awake" clinical state while 0 denotes the maximal EEG effect possible (i.e., an isoelectric EEG).

As the BIS Index value decreases <70, the probability of explicit recall decreases dramatically. At a BIS Index value of <60, a patient has an extremely low probability of consciousness.

BIS Index values <40 signify a greater effect of the anesthetic on the EEG. At low BIS values, the degree of EEG suppression is the primary determinant of the BIS value.[6] Prospective clinical trials have demonstrated that maintaining BIS Index values in the range of 40–60 improves the perioperative period following general anesthesia and reduces the risk of intraoperative awareness.[7] During sedation care, BIS Index values >70 may be observed during adequate levels of sedation, but patients may have a greater probability of consciousness and potential for recall.

VALIDATION OF THE BIS INDEX

A number of studies have validated the accuracy of the BIS Index in assessing hypnotic drug effect on level of consciousness. In one investigation utilizing common anesthetic agents and combinations (propofol, midazolam, isoflurane, midazolam-alfentanil, propofol-alfentanil, and propofol-nitrous oxide), simultaneous measurements of the BIS Index and sedation state were obtained.[8] In Figure 3-3, logistic regression curves display the probability of response to voice and the probability of free recall as a function of BIS Index for all agents tested. The overall sigmoid shape of the curve indicates that the BIS Index proved to be a good indicator of hypnotic state. The BIS Index performed as well as (or better than) measured or targeted drug concentration as an indicator of the hypnotic state. Free recall of word or picture cues is lost when the BIS Index decreases to the 70–75 range, indicating that *memory impairment occurs at higher BIS Index values than loss of consciousness.*

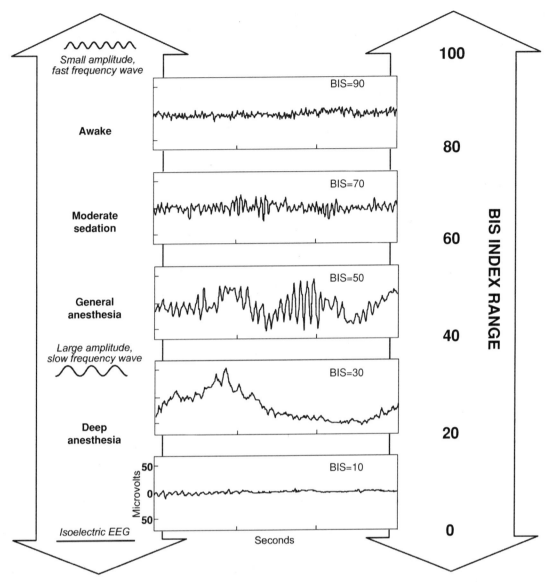

Figure 3-2. BIS index range.

Further investigation has suggested that some memory function—that is, "learning" memory formation without conscious recall—may occur at lower BIS Index values.[9]

This early data has been supported by subsequent investigations that tested the ability of the BIS Index to accurately predict the state of consciousness. In one study, the BIS Index had significantly higher prediction probability for level of consciousness when compared to the traditional hemodynamic variables (blood pressure and heart rate).[10] More importantly, in this study of volunteers during propofol anesthesia, a BIS Index threshold value of 60 achieved a sensitivity of 99% and a specificity of 81% to predict responsiveness to verbal command, indicative of the accuracy of the BIS Index in the assessment of unconsciousness.

ASSESSING THE BIS INDEX IN RECOVERY OF CONSCIOUSNESS

Taken together, these studies support the accuracy of the BIS Index as a measure of hypnotic state. In particular, they validate the ability of the BIS Index to determine the transition into unconsciousness. During general anesthesia care, a key imperative is the maintenance of unconsciousness. Using the isolated forearm technique, accuracy of BIS

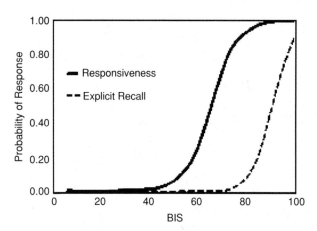

Figure 3-3. Probability of response at differing BIS levels.

Index monitoring to predict the return to consciousness following induction of anesthesia was investigated.[1] After a single bolus dose of propofol or thiopental, patients were assessed for consciousness at intervals by asking them to squeeze the investigator's fingers while the BIS Index was monitored continuously. Although the intensity and duration of hypnotic effect varied considerably among patients, the recovery of consciousness occurred consistently at a BIS Index value above 60. A BIS Index value <65 indicated a probability of <5% that consciousness would return within fifty seconds. Changes in blood pressure and heart rate, in contrast, were poor predictors for the recovery of consciousness.

ASSESSING CONSISTENCY OF BIS INDEX PERFORMANCE

Crucial to the value of level-of-consciousness monitoring is consistency of performance with different anesthetic agents and different patient populations. This consistency is extremely important to anesthesia providers because of the broad range of agents utilized and intrinsic patient variability.

The consistency of the relationship between the BIS Index value and brain status has been tested across different hypnotic agents (intravenous and inhalation anesthetics) as well as different patient types. In the validation studies mentioned earlier, the relationship between the BIS Index and level of clinical response was nearly identical for all hypnotic agents tested or when two anesthetic drugs are combined.[8] Furthermore, during steady-state conditions

of anesthesia or sedation, the BIS Index is a stable measurement of hypnotic effect and does not vary significantly over time.

Patient age is a strong determinant of the anesthetic dose required to produce a clinical effect. For example, the MAC values for inhalation agents decrease as patient age increases. In a study of the influence of age on hypnotic dose requirements, the dose of sevoflurane required to achieve hypnotic effect differed markedly among different age groups and showed the expected decrease in dose required with increasing age. The BIS Index value displayed a consistent relationship to the sedative effects of sevoflurane across this wide range of age groups – unrelated to dosage.[11] Thus, the BIS Index offers a distinct advantage over anesthetic-dose monitoring as a tool to measure and manage depth of sedation.

FACTORS AFFECTING THE CONSCIOUSNESS-MONITOR VALUES

Displayed values on consciousness monitors, such at the BIS monitor, are derived from the preceding ten to thirty seconds of EEG data. As such, the displayed value of a brain monitor is a measure of the state immediately prior to the calculation. A similar analogy would be the data provided by pulse oximetry during management of a difficult airway. There is an expected delay in oxygen saturation that results from physiologic processes, and airway difficulty may be clearly evident prior to any changes in saturation. Similarly, increases in saturation will lag behind the restitution of adequate ventilation and oxygenation of the lungs.

Under steady-state conditions (e.g., in a controlled research trial), most consciousness monitors predict subsequent responses to voice command or memory for words. However, the clinical situation during surgery is notably different because of the lack of steady-state conditions. Intraoperative consciousness-monitor values will be influenced by a number of variables including brain concentration of anesthetic, level of analgesia (via infiltrated local anesthetic or systemic analgesic administration), and degree of surgical stimulation.

It must be recognized that the net brain state, as measured by the BIS Index or another consciousness-monitor parameter, changes as a result of these dynamic variables. Nevertheless, consciousness monitors provide an accurate measure of the net effect and responses of the brain to new conditions. They are unable, however, to predict future changes.

USING CONSCIOUSNESS MONITORS IN ANESTHESIA PRACTICE

The addition of BIS or other forms of level-of-consciousness monitoring adds a new dimension to patient management during anesthesia and sedation. These monitors complement other forms of monitoring and potentially impact all phases of anesthesia care.

Despite significant advances in patient monitoring techniques, most clinicians would agree that patient responses to anesthesia are frequently unpredictable and precise dosing of anesthetics and sedatives remains a challenge. Much of the uncertainty in anesthesia centers on the fundamental concern of "adequacy of anesthesia." Traditionally, this concern is justified since the **hemodynamic parameters used to infer adequacy of anesthetic effect have been shown to be unreliable indicators of brain status.** Clinical judgment and experience remain the cornerstones for managing uncertainty, and consciousness monitoring provides valuable additional data that *enhances* such judgment. Direct measurement of the hypnotic effect of the agent, through continuous consciousness monitoring, substantially facilitates intraoperative patient assessment, titrated dosing and balance of anesthetic agents, and patient recovery process.

Some of the challenges and clinical considerations associated with hemodynamic monitoring are outlined in Table 3-1. *Because heart rate and blood pressure are not exquisitely sensitive to changing levels of consciousness, the patient's hypnotic state cannot be accurately inferred from changes in these vital signs.*[12] For example, administration of cardiovascular agents will change blood pressure and/or heart rate, typically without affecting anesthetic depth. A variety of anesthetic adjuvants, such as neuromuscular blocking agents, reversal agents, and local anesthetic solutions with vasoconstrictors, may have an effect on both cardiovascular reactivity and the anesthetic state but without a direct correlation between the two. Finally, changing levels of surgical stimulation may impact hemodynamics or level of consciousness independently.

Table 3-1. Considerations in hemodynamic monitoring

Average hours at work monitoring traditional vital signs provide a measure of cardiovascular responses to anesthesia administration and surgical stimulation. Although changes in blood pressure and heart rate may correlate with the anesthetic effect in some instances, many factors can interfere with this relationship, including the following:
1. Vasoconstrictor additives to local anesthetic solutions
2. Interaction of multiple anesthetic agents
3. Unexpected synergistic drug effects
4. Patient cardiovascular status
5. Medications that attenuate cardiovascular responses (e.g., clonidine premedication or other antihypertensives)

Anesthetic dosing that ensures adequacy of anesthesia may produce hemodynamic changes close to acceptable limits of cardiovascular response. This approach is further complicated by the difficulty of measuring the therapeutic window in some patients. In these cases, the anesthesia provider may be unable to discriminate between the dose required to achieve the therapeutic effect (i.e., unconsciousness) and the dose producing undesired cardiovascular effects.

Anesthetic agent monitoring (e.g., end-tidal agent analysis), although common in hospital and surgery center locations, is not routinely available in many of the locations where cosmetic anesthesia is provided. Some of the clinical considerations important in utilizing anesthetic agent analysis are highlighted in Table 3-2. End-tidal agent analysis, although very accurate, measures only anesthetic dose, not the anesthetic *effect* on the target organ, the brain. Thus, agent-analysis measurements cannot identify alterations in expected levels of hypnosis due to pharmacodynamic variability among patients. Rather, the existence of this variability means that identical drug concentrations commonly produce considerably different hypnotic responses among individuals or within the same person at different times.

Consciousness monitoring continually measures the hypnotic effects of administered anesthetic doses, regardless of pharmacokinetic or pharmacodynamic variability.

Table 3-2. Considerations in anesthetic agent measurement

Measurement of end-tidal inhalation agent concentration is an effective method of confirming agent delivery and assessing anesthetic uptake and distribution. Empiric-dosing regimens to maintain end-tidal agent concentration at certain values (e.g., greater than MAC_{awake}) provide useful guidelines during anesthesia care. However, anesthetic dosing using only this measurement does not necessarily consider the following:

1. Changing requirement due to varying levels of surgical stimulation or adequacy of local anesthetic effect
2. Individual responses and sensitivity to an agent
3. Impact of age, gender, or metabolic rate on anesthetic requirement
4. Synergistic interactions among multiple anesthetic agents
5. Impact of coexisting disease, or preexisting alcohol/drug dependence

For example, use of BIS values and responses as a guide allows the anesthesia provider to administer a particular anesthetic agent at the dose required to achieve the desired hypnotic effect in the *individual* patient.

CONSCIOUSNESS MONITORING DURING TYPICAL GENERAL ANESTHESIA

A "typical" general anesthetic case involves three phases:

1. induction of anesthesia (and frequently airway management)
2. maintenance of anesthesia
3. emergence from anesthesia

Monitoring level of consciousness during all phases of anesthesia can assist in evaluating a patient's current status and will provide a continuous indicator of the hypnotic state.

Most consciousness-monitoring systems display a graphical trend that represents the ongoing calculations of consciousness index during the case. A typical BIS trend obtained during general endotracheal anesthesia is displayed in Figure 3-4. The BIS value itself is displayed as a single value that is calculated from data gathered over the last fifteen to thirty seconds of EEG recording and updated every second. Deriving the BIS Index value from several seconds of EEG data effectively "smooths" the data to prevent excessive fluctuations in BIS values and allows a value to be determined even if the EEG signal is briefly interrupted. When abrupt changes occur in hypnotic state—for example, during induction or rapid emergence—the BIS value may lag behind the observed clinical change by approximately five to ten seconds. A BIS value, although extremely responsive, is not instantaneously altered by changes in clinical status.

Monitoring the BIS trend is particularly useful during surgery. Changing anesthetic dosing to lighten or deepen anesthesia will usually manifest as a slow upward or downward trend, respectively. As seen in Figure 3-4, for example, a small bolus of propofol will be displayed as a short-lived downward dip in the BIS trend. In contrast, a cortical response caused by intense surgical stimulation is often signaled by large, abrupt increases in the BIS trend. This latter trend change is most likely to occur when the anesthetic technique relies heavily on hypnotic agents but includes little or no analgesic component (local analgesia, opioids, or other analgesic agent).

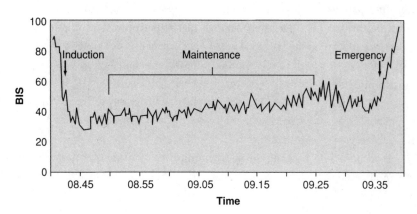

Figure 3-4. BIS trend during a typical general anesthesia procedure.

Clinicians should be cautious about using a particular consciousness-monitor value in isolation as a predictor of patient responsiveness, because *arousal responses to pain are not well correlated with absolute hypnotic effect.* However, BIS monitoring will document the cortical EEG reactivity responses associated with stimulation.

Further, even allowing for the delay associated with signal processing, surgical stimulation can sometimes produce a rapid increase in BIS values prior to the appearance of other clinical signs such as hypertension or movement, facilitating timelier anesthesia management.

Cyclic oscillation in BIS under steady-state conditions may provide an indication of the shifting balance between sensory suppression and sensory stimulation. In volunteer studies, greater BIS variability was observed when sedatives were used alone compared to when an analgesic agent (i.e., alfentanil) was used concurrently.[13]

Consciousness Monitoring During the Induction of Anesthesia

Induction of anesthesia may have individualized goals that are case-specific or patient-specific. **The overall goal of induction is to produce unconsciousness rapidly.**

Another induction goal may be to potentially manage the airway in the unconscious patient and establish adequate anesthesia conditions for surgery. The most common forms of controlling the airway during general anesthesia are either via endotracheal intubation or insertion of a laryngeal mask airway (LMA). In each of these situations, production of certain anesthetic conditions related to the airway need to be ideal. Consciousness monitoring can assist the anesthesia professional to achieve those conditions.

As seen in Figure 3-4, the BIS Index trend clearly displays the effects of anesthesia induction in a patient undergoing hernia repair. Close inspection of the left portion of the trend demonstrates rapid decrease of the BIS Index during induction using **bolus** administration of intravenous hypnotic in preparation for endotracheal intubation.

Consciousness Monitoring During Endotracheal Intubation

During endotracheal intubation, one general goal of the anesthesia provider is to minimize cardiovascular stimu-

lation, thus preventing resultant hypertension and tachycardia. Several strategies are commonly used to blunt the blood pressure and heart rate response, including the following:

1. Sufficient dosing of intravenous induction agent (e.g., propofol, thiopental)
2. Opioid supplementation (e.g., fentanyl)
3. Administration of intravenous or endotracheal lidocaine
4. Administration of antihypertensives (e.g., esmolol)
5. Alternative intubation methods (e.g., fiberoptic intubation)

With the use of these concomitant medications, however, the potential for hypotension during the induction period may also increase (*vide supra*).

BIS responses to stimulation associated with laryngoscopy and intubation can be markedly attenuated in a dose-dependent fashion with opioid administration, for example, fentanyl or remifentanil. It should be noted that a single BIS value during the induction period is unable to predict subsequent BIS responses to significant stimulation. For example, in one study examining hemodynamic, BIS, and awareness responses, BIS values less than 60 prior to intubation did not guarantee a lack of arousal responses following laryngoscopy and intubation. The utility of the BIS monitor is greatly enhanced by trending the EMG as a secondary trace. BIS values lag 30 seconds behind real time. Typically, arousal responses are preceded by a spike in (real time) EMG. This study did note that BIS Index was an accurate indicator of current clinical state: arousal responses were observed only in patients with high BIS values.[14]

In other settings, particularly in elderly patients or patients with significant coexisting illness, a gentle induction technique is sometimes used to minimize perturbation of blood pressure and heart rate.

This can be achieved with smaller and/or divided dose administration of induction agent or with low-dose administration of an inhalation agent. During this method of induction, BIS monitoring can measure achievement of the desired hypnotic effect from the various induction protocols.

Consciousness Monitoring During the Maintenance of Anesthesia

In most surgical cases, the "maintenance" phase of anesthesia care is the longest. During this intraoperative period, anesthesia care focuses on the following:

1. Maintenance of an adequate anesthetic state
2. Maintenance of physiologic homeostasis during surgical events
3. Avoidance of potential adverse events
4. Preparation for smooth, rapid emergence

Consciousness monitoring during anesthesia maintenance can help meet these goals of intraoperative care by providing continuous confirmation of hypnotic effect—for all classes of anesthetics, under most operative conditions, and for nearly all types of patients.

Level-of-consciousness monitoring can improve intraoperative decision making. For example, observation of the BIS trend can facilitate diagnostic evaluation of unexpected changes in cardiovascular system reactivity, permitting rapid restoration of homeostasis. Consciousness monitoring can also guide adjustments in anesthesia care—for example, an increase in administered anesthetic dose, analgesic supplementation, or the addition of an antihypertensive. With the addition of consciousness-monitoring information, the anesthesia provider can monitor not only cardiovascular responses but central nervous system—specifically, cortical—responses as well.

Maintenance strategies using BIS monitoring

Two important clinical trials have demonstrated that the adjustment of anesthetic delivery to maintain the BIS Index within a bracketed target range during maintenance of general anesthesia results in improved perioperative recovery patterns as compared to standard anesthesia care.[15, 16] These studies and several others have highlighted the positive patient outcomes realized when consciousness monitoring is combined with assessment of intraoperative hemodynamic data and clinical observations of movement and autonomic response to generate patient-management strategies. Consciousness-monitoring data can ensure that the key anesthetic goals of hypnosis and analgesia are met throughout the maintenance phase.

The integration of consciousness monitoring with other traditional monitoring creates new insight regarding

patient management. Table 3-1 outlines conceptual management strategies based on integration of clinical profile with BIS data for "balanced" anesthesia techniques utilizing hypnotic and analgesic components. Using the BIS value in combination with hemodynamic data improves the rational selection of sedatives, analgesics, and autonomic blockers in what can otherwise be very confusing clinical situations.

Although a BIS value of 45–60 is a typical target during the maintenance phase, the BIS value target range needs to be tailored to the anesthetic technique. For example, in cases of balanced anesthesia involving sufficient analgesia administration or other agents to assure adequate analgesia, the typical target range of 45–60 is most appropriate for general anesthesia. However, for anesthesia techniques that utilize little or no opioid or analgesic supplementation, increased dosing of the hypnotic agent—typically, an inhalation anesthetic—to produce acceptable suppression of noxious stimulation will result in lower BIS values, frequently in the 25–35 range. BIS values in the range of 60–75 may produce excellent results in cosmetic procedures performed with local anesthetic infiltration and intravenous sedation/analgesia administration.[17]

It is again important to note that **reliance on consciousness-monitoring information alone for intraoperative anesthetic management is not appropriate.** Clinical judgment is crucial when interpreting this data. Patient assessment should include evaluation and correlation of level-of-consciousness data with hemodynamic and other monitoring data as well as observation of clinical signs. Consciousness-monitoring data should be thought of as an additional piece of information that must be interpreted in the context of all other information available for patient assessment.

Consciousness Monitoring During Emergence from Anesthesia

Level-of-consciousness monitors document the decreasing effect of anesthesia when agent delivery is reduced or stopped and the patient enters the emergence phase. Because these monitors provide a real-time measure of level of consciousness, it allows the anesthesia provider to fine-tune titration downward according to individual patient response. Consciousness monitoring permits reduction in anesthesia dosing in tandem with the decrease in surgical stimulation, promoting a rapid emergence that avoids premature recovery of consciousness as well as delayed emergence from anesthesia.

As seen in Figure 3-4, in the patient undergoing hernia repair, emergence was heralded by the rapid increase in the BIS Index. BIS monitoring of brain status documented the decreasing anesthetic effect and the increased level of consciousness that correlated with patient eye opening in response to voice command.

Responding to Consciousness-Monitoring Changes During Anesthesia

When consciousness monitoring is used during anesthesia care, it is necessary to note fluctuations in calculated level-of-consciousness values. However, many such fluctuations, like a single fluctuation in blood pressure, are not necessarily clinically significant. However, in some situations, additional assessment is required in response to changes in these values.

Changes in the hypnotic state due to changes in dose and/or patterns of agent delivery will produce changes in the consciousness-monitoring value. Normally, if the change in anesthetic dosing was incremental—for example, slight adjustment in the vaporizer setting or modest changes in intravenous anesthetic infusion dosing—these changes in BIS values are gradual. In contrast, sudden changes would not be expected and would require confirmation and assessment.

CONSCIOUSNESS MONITORING AND GLOBAL CNS FUNCTION

Since the introduction of more routine cortical EEG monitoring using BIS and other consciousness-monitoring technologies, a variety of clinical reports have noted anecdotal benefits offered by this form of brain monitoring.[18] Although consciousness monitoring is not intended to be used for regional ischemia monitoring—for example, during carotid endarterectomy procedures—the relationship of the EEG and to global CNS function does provide an indication of patient response and tolerance to intraoperative conditions. As such, acute variations may alert the anesthesia and surgical teams to changes in the patient condition that indicate the need for additional evaluation of brain status, including adequacy of perfusion.[19]

CONSCIOUSNESS MONITORING AND GLOBAL CNS FUNCTION

Consciousness-monitoring technologies aim to provide a consistent and reliable measure of level of consciousness across a wide spectrum of patients and anesthetic agents. Nevertheless, in certain circumstances, displayed values on consciousness monitors may not be an accurate reflection of the hypnotic state of the patient. As noted earlier, consciousness monitoring is an *adjunct* to clinical judgment, *not a substitute* for it. This section presents certain unusual circumstances that may produce inaccurate readings and the management of those situations.

Most signal artifact in waveforms such as the ECG, SpO_2, or arterial blood pressure is easier to detect than artifact within the EEG waveform. Indeed, with the variable frequency and amplitude of the EEG waveform, the presence of certain types of artifact may be extremely difficult to recognize visually. Most consciousness-monitoring systems utilize a variety of signal analysis methods to detect and reduce extraneous artifacts that contaminate the EEG. For example, many of the improvements in the BIS system over the past decade have been in the area of artifact processing. Despite these improvements, however, artifact produced by some non-EEG signals can potentially interfere with the ability of these systems to render an accurate value. Given this potential for artifact contamination, the clinician must identify situations where the underlying EEG signals—and hence the calculated value—may not accurately reflect the clinical endpoints of sedation and hypnosis.

Inaccurate calculation of level-of-consciousness values due to artifact contamination of the EEG signal may result from electromyogram (muscle) activity, high-frequency artifacts (e.g., from medical devices), EEG variants and signal analysis, and unique pharmacologic responses (electromyogram [EMG]).

The most frequent source of EEG contamination in sedated and lightly anesthetized patients is the EMG. This contamination results from increased tone of the frontalis muscle of the forehead that lies beneath the BIS sensor. Typically, significant EMG activity is present during awake states and during emergence from anesthesia.

The frequency spectrum of endogenous EMG activity partially overlaps with the frequency spectrum of the awake EEG. In order to maximize the sensitivity of BIS to detect wakefulness, high frequency signals are analyzed by the BIS processing system. As a result, in the presence of significant EMG activity, calculated BIS values may tend to be higher—in a range that normally may indicate the potential for inadequate anesthesia—than would actually reflect the true hypnotic state of the patient.[20] As in all clinical situations, patient-care decisions should not be based solely upon the displayed BIS value but rather upon complete clinical assessment of the patient. During intraoperative anesthesia situations where EMG is biasing BIS to a higher value, administration of either increased anesthetic or a muscle relaxant can produce a significant decrease in EMG.

As noted, appearance of high-frequency facial EMG activity commonly occurs during awakening and, in fact, has been incorporated into other consciousness monitors. During emergence from anesthesia, BIS frequently increases in conjunction with this increased EMG activity, although the presence of EMG is not required for BIS to track the return of consciousness.

Although EMG activity can sometimes be seen in the raw EEG trace, typically it is more difficult to discern. Therefore, in situations with the potential for EMG contamination, it is important to note the amount of activity generated by EMG. BIS systems display an EMG parameter that shows total power of electrical activity seen in the frequency bandwidth of 70–110 Hz. When the EMG power exceeds 50 dB, there is greater potential for EMG contamination of the underlying EEG signal.

To further address the problem of EMG contamination, Aspect Medical Systems developed the BIS-XP platform. This system uses dual-channel EEG processing, making it more resistant to the effects of EMG. The potential for spurious BIS values is reduced when using the XP platform; however, it is not eliminated entirely.

EEG Variants and EEG Signal Analysis

Two challenges to any EEG-based assessment of the level of consciousness are the presence of EEG variant activity and the recognition of anesthesia-induced EEG effects. Specifically, these challenges are presented by:

1. Paradoxical delta phenomenon
2. Small-amplitude EEG
3. Epileptiform activity
4. Missed near-suppression

Paradoxical delta phenomenon

In a small percentage of patients, a paradoxical response develops in the EEG during a lightening of anesthesia effect or in response to surgical stimulation. This phenomenon, known as "paradoxical arousal" or "paradoxical delta," is characterized by a slowing of the EEG, with large delta waves.[21] In response to this unusual EEG slowing, the level-of-consciousness value may decrease suddenly.

Small-amplitude EEG

In one case report, an awake individual had a very low BIS value. This was presumed to be the result of EEG variant activity—specifically, a congenital, extremely small-amplitude EEG.[22]

Epileptiform activity

The occurrence of epileptiform activity, for example, during the administration of high concentrations of sevoflurane anesthesia, can also lead to temporal increases in BIS values. In one report, BIS values were appropriately low during administration of high concentrations of sevoflurane. However, with the development of epileptiform activity, BIS values increased abruptly during the epileptic discharge, corresponding to increases in cerebral blood flow (and presumably glucose metabolism) measured with PET scanning.[23] Also of note is the transient dip in BIS following discontinuation of sevoflurane and cessation of seizure activity. In situations of concern regarding sevoflurane administration or potentially local anesthetic toxicity, unexpected increases in BIS, particularly following an increase in the administered dose, should prompt a rapid inspection of the raw EEG to assess for the presence of epileptiform activity.

High-frequency artifacts

A variety of medical devices generate high-frequency signals that can contaminate the EEG signal. If this extraneous artifact is not detected, the inclusion of the high-frequency signal could lead to errors in the calculation of BIS. Some of the devices that have been reported, in rare settings, to produce artifact and resultant inaccuracy of the BIS are listed in Table 3-3.

Table 3-3. External sources of electrical/ mechanical artifact

1. Warming systems (fluid and forced-air warming systems)
2. Circulatory-assist systems (CPB, VAD, ECMO)
3. High-frequency ventilators
4. Suctioning systems
5. Surgical instruments (shavers, drills, radiofrequency devices)
6. Cardiac-pacing devices (pacemakers, defibrillators)

For an external device with the potential to generate artifact, proximity to the EEG sensor increases the risk of EEG signal contamination and effects on calculated values. Therefore, it is critical to consider the physical location of such devices in relation to level-of-consciousness–monitoring system components. To confirm artifact in situations where an external device may be interfering with the level-of-consciousness monitor, temporary cessation of the device usage (if appropriate) may reveal a characteristic pattern of interference.

A few important external sources of artifact noted in Table 3-1 include the following:

1. Pacemakers
2. Medical/surgical devices
3. Electrocautery device

PACEMAKERS. Typically, signals emitted from pacemakers have a high amplitude and regular pattern. As a result, they are readily identified as artifact by most consciousness-monitoring systems and are not processed as EEG. However, in some situations, the programmed pacing rate and current profile causes the extraneous paced signal to be interpreted as an EEG signal. The presence of this artifact influences the BIS value.

MEDICAL/SURGICAL DEVICES. A variety of medical/surgical devices generate high-frequency electrical or mechanical signals and may produce artifacts within the measured EEG. Such devices include fluid- and forced-air–warming devices,[24] intravenous administration devices, mechanical surgical instruments, and cardiopulmonary bypass machine.

ELECTROCAUTERY DEVICES. In many situations, the electrical signature of an electrocautery device is recognized as nonphysiological and is not processed with the EEG data. However, these devices can generate a variety of electrical artifacts that may affect level-of-consciousness monitors as well as other patient-monitoring systems used in the operating room. In situations of prolonged electrocautery, there may be a reduction in the amount of artifact-free EEG available for analysis and calculation of level-of-consciousness value. Most level-of-consciousness monitors include significant mechanisms designed to filter out electrical artifact produced by electrocautery use.[25]

CONSCIOUSNESS MONITORING AND THE "ABNORMAL" BRAIN

Some anesthesia providers have appropriately expressed concern about the accuracy and reliability of the consciousness monitors in patients who have abnormal brain structure or function as the result of injury or disease. This would include patients with clear evidence of CNS disease such as prior cerebral vascular accident with residual neurologic impairment. It would also include patients with systemic illness who may have neurologic implications, for example, those with encephalopathy complicating hepatic or renal disease. Because of limited clinical experience with such patients, level-of-consciousness values should be interpreted cautiously in patients with known neurological disorders. For example, one case series reported response to command at lower BIS values (50–70) in patients while undergoing tumor resection during awake craniotomy.[26] All of these patients were taking anticonvulsant medication. One approach advocated by two authors is to obtain a baseline BIS value prior to induction of anesthesia to determine whether abnormal CNS status may impact the reliability of the consciousness monitor.[27]

BIS and Pharmacologic Responses
Nitrous oxide (N₂O)
The BIS Index is sensitive to the clinical pattern of administration and the relative dosing of N_2O and other anesthetic agents. For example, as a sole agent administered for sedation, N_2O appears to have little sedative effect at concentrations of up to 50%, and the BIS value similarly is unaffected.[28] In one volunteer study, however, administration

of 70% N_2O did produce unconsciousness but without a change in BIS value. A recent paper demonstrated a lack of correlation with OAAS scores during bupivicaine epidural anesthesia with 33%, 50%, and 67% N_2O sedation.[29]

The intraoperative addition of N_2O to inhalation anesthesia has had variable effect on measured BIS values. One study reported a dose-dependent decrease in BIS when 20–60% N_2O was administered, whereas another found no change in BIS with addition of 50% N_2O.[30] In studies with intravenous balanced techniques (propofol/remifentanil or midazolam/fentanyl), the addition of 70% N_2O did not alter BIS with or without surgical stimulation. In a study focusing on the response to laryngoscopy, N_2O administration prevented the movement response but not a hemodynamic response, without changing BIS.[31] Thus, the effect of N_2O administration prevented the movement response but does not *per se* seem to be *nonlinear* with respect to hypnosis, and the contribution to the anesthetic state may be via its potent analgesic effects.

Ketamine

Ketamine, an intravenous anesthetic of unique chemical and pharmacodynamic characteristics, plays an important role in office-based practices as well as cosmetic anesthesia. One of the observed physiologic effects of ketamine is the dose-dependent activation of the EEG (increase in high-frequency activity). Thus, frequently following bolus administration of a clinically effective dose of ketamine (e.g., 0.4–0.5 mg $\cdot$ kg^{-1}), both BIS and Entropy values tend to increase transiently, and bolus administration of ketamine presumably modifies the relationship between these parameters and the level of consciousness.[32]

The timing of administration of ketamine is also important. When smaller dissociative doses of ketamine are administered in the setting of propofol-induced sedation, it has no acute effect on BIS but minimizes the increase in BIS in response to profound stimulation.[33] Following bolus administration of ketamine, BIS values decreased to baseline values during low-dose *propofol*-infusion administration. (1 mg $\cdot$ kg^{-1} $\cdot$ hr^{-1}).[33]

Several reports have described the successful use and clinical utility of BIS during intravenous techniques involving ketamine administration (i.e., dose administration <1 mg $\cdot$ kg^{-1}) with simultaneous propofol administration.[34,35] The clinical application of this technique, including the use of BIS monitoring in the setting of cosmetic surgery, is more fully described in Chapters 1 and 4.

Etomidate

Etomidate, another intravenous anesthetic agent, also has a unique pharmacodynamic profile. Anesthesia induction with etomidate frequently results in skeletal muscle excitation (i.e., myoclonus, tremor, fasciculations). This clinical effect may result in the presence of high EMG activity and thus increased BIS during the period of musculoskeletal excitement. However, following induction (or with the onset of neuromuscular blocking agent activity), BIS will reflect the hypnotic state of most patients. The ability of the BIS Index to reflect the sedative effect of etomidate during induction and allow effective titration of an etomidate infusion has been reported.[36]

CLINICAL MANAGEMENT

In clinical situations where artifact seems likely to have influenced the consciousness-monitor value, the anesthesia provider should review all of the available data collected by the monitoring system. For example, additional data provided by the EMG trend display can be used to evaluate increasing level-of-consciousness values. Where there is concern regarding the accuracy of the currently displayed consciousness value, a simple strategy facilitates a rapid determination of the potential for artifact, including assessment of the signal quality index (SQI), the EMG activity, and the real-time EEG signal. The BIS system continuously calculates a signal-quality index to reflect the amount of quality EEG data entering the BIS system over the previous minute and provides that data on the display monitor. In situations of extraneous artifact correctly detected by the BIS processing system, the SQI will decline rapidly.

Many, but not all, extraneous artifacts have been reported to be associated with increased "EMG" activity as measured by the BIS system. Because the EMG parameter displayed in BIS systems utilizes a high-frequency spectral window (70–110 Hz), many electromechanical devices may generate an artifact that is apparent within the EMG parameter. In addition to assessment of the SQI and EMG parameters, inspection of the current, real-time EEG directly recorded (and displayed on the monitor) may assist in the assessment of the patient and current anesthetic effect. The EEG tracing may reveal a clearly contaminated appearance, thus facilitating the determination that artifact may be affecting the calculation of the BIS. However, some subtle artifacts may not be apparent in the assessment of the EEG recording from the monitor screen.

In situations where the consciousness-monitor value seems discordant with another clinical parameter, EEG assessment can facilitate clinical assessment of the adequacy of anesthetic effect. Typical EEG waveform patterns will be seen frequently and, with experience, are easily recognized (see Fig. 3-2). It is important to note that no single pattern of EEG waveform will always be observed at each BIS value.

The varieties of special situations discussed are important reminders to anesthesia clinicians about the need to always consider level-of-consciousness monitoring an additional parameter used in their assessment and management of patients under their care. **No single monitoring parameter (whether the consciousness-monitor value or another vital sign) should be used alone or in isolation to determine patient care.**

SUMMARY: CLINICAL BENEFITS OF CONSCIOUSNESS MONITORING

The use of level-of-consciousness monitoring supports three primary components of anesthesia care: vigilance, intraoperative patient assessment, and anesthetic agent management.

Vigilance is a cornerstone of anesthesia care. Level-of-consciousness–monitoring technologies provide continuous documentation of central nervous system status during anesthesia care. As such, these monitors provide early indicators of changes in brain effect due to anesthetic dosing and delivery. Level-of-consciousness monitoring can help answer the question: "Is my patient adequately anesthetized?" In the operating room, dramatic changes in blood pressure and heart rate may occur and require the anesthesia professional to make rapid diagnostic assessments and timely interventions. Level-of-consciousness monitoring provides data that can facilitate decision-making and management approaches in many of these situations. **Consciousness monitors are not a substitute for keen clinical judgment.** However, using consciousness monitoring information as part of their assessment, anes-

thesia providers can make more informed decisions about the dosing and balance of anesthetic agents and other adjuvant therapies such as analgesics, local anesthesia infiltration, and cardioactive agents.

Improved anesthetic agent administration is the greatest benefit that results from level-of-consciousness monitoring. Using these new parameters, the clinician can manage patients within the optimal plane of anesthesia effect and reduce the unwanted occurrence of excessive or inadequate anesthetic effect. Clinical investigations of consciousness monitoring during general anesthesia consistently demonstrate approximately a 20% reduction in intraoperative anesthetic use and a consistent reduction in the time for emergence from general anesthesia.[37] With consciousness-monitoring technology, the question— "Am I overdosing my patient?"—is often quite easy to answer.

Emerging data suggests that subtle differences in anesthetic effect may be associated with patient outcomes days, weeks, and even months after surgery.[38] This type of long-term perspective, assessing the impact of anesthesia management, may broaden the scope of positive patient outcomes associated with consciousness monitoring beyond the immediate perioperative period.

Level-of-consciousness monitors allow the anesthesia clinician to trend and manage changes in the hypnotic state during a case. Throughout the period of anesthesia care— during induction, maintenance, and emergence—it highlights the important transitions in level of consciousness and provides valuable patient-management data. Level-of-consciousness monitoring is an important tool to enable the best intraoperative care and postoperative outcomes important in the patient undergoing cosmetic surgery.

REFERENCES

1. Flaishon R, Windsor A, Sigl J, et al.: Recovery of consciousness after thiopental or propofol. *Anesthesiol* 86:613,1997.
2. Gibbs FA, Gibbs EL, Lennox WG: Effect on the electroencephalogram of certain drugs which influence nervous activity. *Arch Intern Med* 60:154,1937.
3. Rampil IJ: A primer for EEG signal processing in anesthesia. *Anesthesiol* 89:980,1998.
4. Sigl JC, Chamoun NC: An introduction to bispectral index analysis for the electroencephalogram. *J Clin Monit* 10:392,1994.
5. Johansen JW, Sebel PS: Development and clinical application of electroencephalographic bispectrum monitoring. *Anesthesiol* 93:1336,2000.

6. Bruhn J, Bouillon TW, Shafer SL: Bispectral index (BIS) and burst suppression: Revealing a part of the BIS algorithm. *J Clin Monit Comput* 16:593,2000.

7. Myles PS, Leslie K, McNeil J, et al.: Bispectral index monitoring to prevent awareness during anaesthesia: The B-aware randomised controlled trial. *Lancet* 363:1757,2004.

8. Glass PS, Bloom M, Kearse L, et al.: Bispectral analysis measures sedation and memory effects of propofol, midazolam, isoflurane, and alfentanil in healthy volunteers. *Anesthesiol* 86:836,1997.

9. Lubke G, Kerssens C, Phaf H, et al.: Dependence of explicit and implicit memory on hypnotic state in trauma patients. *Anesthesiol* 90:1,1999.

10. Struys M, Jensen EW, Smith W, et al.: Performance of the ARX-derived auditory evoked potential index as an indicator of anesthetic depth: A comparison with bispectral index and hemodynamic measures during propofol administration. *Anesthesiol* 96:803,2002.

11. Katoh T, Bito H, Sato S: Influence of age on hypnotic requirement, bispectral index, and 95% spectral edge frequency associated with sedation induced by sevoflurane. *Anesthesiol* 92:55,2000.

12. Nakayama M, Hayashi M, Ichinose H, et al.: Values of the bispectral index do not parallel the hemodynamic response to the Rapid Increase in isoflurane concentration. *Can J Anesth* 48:958, 2001.

13. Bloom M, Greenwald S, Day R: Analgesics decrease arousal response to stimulation as measured by changes in bispectral index (BIS). *Anesthesiol* 85:A481,1999.

14. Schneider G, Wagner K, Reeker W, et al.: Bispectral index (BIS) may not predict awareness reaction to intubation in surgical patients. *J Neurosurg Anesthesiol* 14:7,2002.

15. Gan TJ, Glass PS, Windsor A, et al.: Bispectral index monitoring allows faster emergence and improved recovery from propofol, alfentanil, and nitrous oxide anesthesia. *Anesthesiol* 87:808,1997.

16. Song D, Joshi G, White PF: Titration of volatile anesthetics using bispectral index facilitates recovery after ambulatory anesthesia. *Anesthesiol* 87:842,1997.

17. Friedberg BL: Propofol ketamine anesthesia for cosmetic surgery in the office suite, chapter in Osborne I (ed.), *Anesthesia for Outside the Operating Room. International Anesthesiology Clinics.* Baltimore, Lippincott, Williams & Wilkins, 41:39,2003.

18. England MR: The changes in bispectral index during a hypovolemic cardiac arrest. *Anesthesiol* 91:1947,1999.

19. Billard V: Brain injury under general anesthesia: Is monitoring of the EEG helpful? *Can J Anesth* 48:1055,2001.

20. Bruhn J, Bouillon TW, Shafer SL: Electromyographic activity falsely elevates the bispectral index. *Anesthesiol* 92:1485, 2000.

21. Schultz B, Schultz A, Plein S, et al.: Slowing down of the EEG during hypoventilation in emergence from anesthesia. *Anaesthetist* 40:672,1991.

22. Schnider TW, Luginbuhl M, Petersen-Felix S, et al.: Unreasonably low bispectral index values in a volunteer with genetically determined low-voltage electroencephalographic signal. *Anesthesiol* 89:1607,1998.

23. Kaisti KK, Jaaskelainen SK, Rinne JO, et al.: Epileptiform discharges during 2 MAC sevoflurane anesthesia in two healthy volunteers. *Anesthesiol* 91:1952,1999.

24. Hemmerling T, Fortier JD: Falsely increased bispectral index values in a series of patients undergoing cardiac surgery using forced-air-warming therapy of the head. *Anesth Analg* 95:322,2002.

25. England MD, Mosca S, Wong G, et al.: BIS XP platform performance during electrocautery in cardiac surgery. *Anesth Analg* 94:SCA79,2002.

26. Pemberton PL, Dinsmore J: Bispectral index monitoring during awake craniotomy surgery. *Anaesthesia* 57:1244, 2002.

27. Renna M, Handy J, Shah A, et al.: Does dementia affect the bispectral index? *Anesthesiol* 95:A286,2001.

28. Park KS, Hur EJ, Han KW, et al.: Bipectral index does not correlate with observer assessment of alertness and sedation scores during 0.5% bupivicaine epidural anesthesia with nitrous oxide sedation. *Anesth Analg* 103:385,2006.

29. Rampil IJ, Kim JS, Lenhardt R, et al.: Bispectral EEG index during nitrous oxide administration. *Anesthesiol* 89:671, 1998.

30. Coste C, Guignard, B, Menigaux C, et al.: Nitrous oxide prevents movement during orotracheal intubation without affecting BIS value. *Anesth Analg* 91:130,2000.

31. Hans P, Dewandre PY, Brichant JF, et al.: Comparative effects of ketamine on bispectral index and spectral entropy of the electroencephalogram under sevoflurane anaesthesia. *Br J Anaesth* 94:336,2005.

32. Vereecke HE, Struys MM, Mortier EP: A comparison of bispectral index and ARX-derived auditory evoked potential index in measuring the clinical interaction between ketamine and propofol anaesthesia. *Anaesthesia* 58:957, 2003.

33. Friedberg BL: The effect of a dissociative dose of ketamine on the bispectral index (BIS) during propofol hypnosis. *J Clin Anesth* 11:4,1999.

34. Friedberg BL, Sigl JC: Clonidine premedication decreases propofol consumption during bispectral index (BIS) monitored propofol-ketamine technique for office-based surgery. *Dermatol Surg* 26:848,2000.

35. Friedberg BL, Sigl JC: Bispectral index (BIS) monitoring decreases propofol usage in propofol-ketamine office-based anesthesia. *Anesth Analg* 88:S54,1999.

36. Doenicke AW, Roizen MF, Hoernecke R, et al.: TIVA with etomidate or propofol in day-case surgery: Is the bispectral index a useful parameter to lower the maintenance dose? *Anesth Analg* 88:S470,1999.

37. Liu SS: Effects of bispectral index monitoring on ambulatory anesthesia: A meta analysis of randomized controlled trials and a cost analysis. *Anesthesiol* 101:311,2004.

38. Monk TG, Saini V, Weldon BC, et al.: Anesthetic management and one-year mortality after noncardiac surgery. *Anesth Analg* 100:4,2005.

4 | The Dissociative Effect and Preemptive Analgesia

Barry L. Friedberg, M.D.

INTRODUCTION
THE DISSOCIATIVE EFFECT
PREEMPTIVE ANALGESIA
CONCLUSION

INTRODUCTION

A Medline search for the number of articles that contain "ketamine" yielded 8,553, with 6,905 in English. A Melvyl (University of California system catalog) search for the number of books containing "ketamine" as a word in the title or keyword yielded thirty two, with twenty in English (many are dissertations). A "Google" search for "ketamine" yielded over 250,000 sites. As reported on the World Wide Web, a 50 mg dose of ketamine (route of administration unclear) taken *by itself* produces an "NDE" or "near death experience," whereas a 100 mg dose of ketamine produces an "out of body" experience. In the world of the street drug user, ketamine is a recreational drug with the reputation of unpredictable, nasty side effects. Uncontrolled "street" experimentation produced a "solution" for the nasty side effects commonly referred to as "kitty flipping." "Kitty flipping" is the ingestion of methylenedioxymethamphetamine (MDMA), or "Ecstasy," to produce a positive state of mind before "flipping" to "kitty," a code name for the "k" word ketamine. *MDMA is not to be confused with NMDA, N-methyl D-aspartate, the receptors blocked by ketamine.*

For all that has been written about the drug ketamine, the reader could assume that much is understood. Despite the prodigious output of articles, books, and web sites, ketamine remains maligned, feared, and misunderstood as an anesthetic agent.

Ketamine was originally introduced to the anesthesia profession as a complete, total intravenous anesthetic

agent. Ketamine was supposed to be the magic "silver bullet," for which no other drugs were required. Negative psychotomimetic experiences (in the form of hallucinations or dysphorias) were visited not only on unsuspecting patients but also on unsuspecting PACU personnel. Unhappy PACU staff had to try to manage these wild and unpleasant emergence issues. Quickly, ketamine gained a reputation as an unpredictable agent. At least two generations of anesthesiologists have given ketamine a wide berth.

However, anesthesiologists involved in pediatric burn units find IM ketamine, mixed with atropine, very useful for painless dressing changes in children under the age of nine or ten.

Older children require the concomitant use of benzodiazepines to mitigate the tendency for negative psychotomimetic side effects of the drug. Shortly after ketamine's introduction, the veterinary anesthesia community adapted it. Animals did not complain of hallucinations. It was also virtually impossible to destroy an animal for lack of the correct body weight in the dosage calculation.

Even in the 21st century, anesthesia trainees continue to express concerns about the psychotomimetic side effects of the drug. Ketamine is a protean drug, changing faces within different **contexts**! Ketamine's most beneficial usage is *not* as a solo anesthetic agent but as an adjuvant. In Vinnik's hands, it has been used as a separate bolus *after* a hypnotic level of diazepam had been titrated.[1] Vinnik, a plastic surgeon, described the dissociative phenomenon as "all or nothing" without reference to NMDA receptors. The patient either is immobile for the injection of the local analgesia or is not. Movement with injection implies that more ketamine would be required. After a test dose of 5 mg diazepam, 15 mg diazepam followed to induce a state of hypnosis. *Vinnik administered diazepam through an external jugular IV to minimize the phlebitis seen when using peripheral veins.*

More diazepam in 5–10 mg increments, up to 40 mg total, is given until the desired hypnotic level was achieved. Vinnik's initial dose of ketamine was 75 mg, based on adult brain weights being essentially equal. Ketamine's dissociative effect is independent of *adult* body weight. Administering the 75 mg ketamine dose, Friedberg observed several patients in his first fifty cases emerging with horizontal nystagmus. This undesirable side effect led Friedberg to try a 50 mg dose of ketamine. Horizontal nystagmus may also induce PONV in patients with a positive history of motion sickness.

Vinnik further asserted that there was no upper limit on the amount of ketamine one could use. More ketamine simply meant a longer emergence. This caveat turns out to be true only if one is using a long half-life drug like diazepam. More ketamine does prolong emergence. However, with propofol, the upper useful, aggregate dose of ketamine is 200 mg.[2] In Vinnik's practice, patients were discharged to the care of a nurse for twenty-four hours. Aldrete scores in Vinnik's patients that Friedberg observed would have precluded discharge by most anesthesiologists. When asked if he was concerned about the state of postoperative grogginess of his patients, Vinnik responded that he wanted them sleepy for two to three days to prevent them from undoing his surgery (Vinnik CA, Personal communication, March 1992). Vinnik felt if the patients were too awake after surgery, they would be less inclined to follow their postoperative instructions.

In case #51 (8/24/92), before Friedberg understood the difference between diazepam and propofol protection from ketamine-induced hallucinations, a total of 650 mg ketamine was administered over five hours. During the case, the surgeon refused to give additional local analgesia after the initial injection (see Chapter 1, Table 9). Friedberg was forced to administer progressively more ketamine to compensate for inadequate local analgesia. The patient emerged *three hours* postoperatively. She had severe persistent nystagmus and ultimately experienced emesis. This

negative experience was the last time Friedberg attempted to use his PK MAC technique for that surgeon. Friedberg was forced to reevaluate Vinnik's claim that there was no upper limit on the amount of ketamine one could use, especially when using a short-acting hypnotic propofol.

A forty-two-year-old, Caucasian female patient with a positive history of previous PONV and motion sickness was anesthetized for a rhinoplasty with the MIA™ technique on March 1, 2005. The initial 50 mg of ketamine failed to produce a complete dissociative effect within two to three minutes. A second 50 mg dose of ketamine was administered and an additional two minutes elapsed before the surgeon attempted to inject the local anesthetic. The patient continued to display movement in response to the needle. A third 50 mg dose of ketamine was administered and an additional minute was allowed to elapse. After a total of 150 mg ketamine, the patient was completely immobile for the injection of her breasts. The BIS during the entire sequence of securing the dissociative effect remained below 75. Unfortunately, the surgery was completed an hour after the last dose of ketamine had been administered. The patient emerged promptly but experienced persistent horizontal nystagmus. She experienced hours of PONV at the office, delaying her discharge to home. The patient experienced PONV for approximately six hours total postoperatively. At that time, the PONV spontaneously resolved.

Consider the case duration when pursuing a complete dissociative effect.

In retrospect, this patient probably would have been better served with a less-than-complete dissociative effect. The patient did not experience hallucinations, hypertension, or tachycardia from the ketamine. She had no complaint of postoperative pain. The persistent horizontal nystagmus that produced the PONV could probably have been avoided by accepting a less-than-total dissociative effect for a relatively brief case. Had the case been a four-hour abdominoplasty or a four- to six-hour rhytidectomy, there would likely have been sufficient time for the patient to redistribute and metabolize the ketamine. Fortunately, this patient suffered no negative effect on her surgical outcome. On the first-postoperative-day interview, her sister admitted that they were both so motion sensitive that they had to sit in the front of the bus and use scopolamine (Transderm®) patches wherever they traveled. The

Table 4-1. Essential dissociative concepts

1. Neither the size of the brain nor the number of NMDA receptors varies appreciably in adults.
2. The number of NMDA receptors does NOT vary with body weight or skeletal muscle mass in adults.
3. Ketamine's dissociative effect is independent of adult body weight.
4. Visualize the dissociative effect of ketamine as a "midbrain spinal" (i.e., no afferent signals reach the cortex).
5. Hypnosis first, then dissociation.

patient accepted the author's explanation of her postoperative experience and his apology.

This patient is only the third patient in the author's fifteen-year experience that required more than 100 mg of ketamine to achieve a *complete* dissociative *effect.* Curiously, both of the other two cases were also rhinoplasties. The author's series includes more than 3,000 PK MAC cases (including 1,500 MIA™ technique). Learning is an ongoing process. Our activities are rightly described as the "practice" of medicine, not the "perfection." Patients can continue to teach us, if we listen. Patients will accept less-than-perfect outcomes if some humility is exhibited (see Table 4-1).

Building on Vinnik's work with ketamine, Friedberg substituted propofol for diazepam. Friedberg described the use of a ketamine **bolus** *after* a stable level of hypnosis from propofol had been achieved with a *gradual* propofol induction.[3] Friedberg's PK technique is a MAC or the MIA™ technique when patients are premedicated with po clonidine, the propofol is titrated with a quantitative infusion pump, and the BIS monitors the effect of the propofol (see Appendix in Chapter 1).

THE DISSOCIATIVE EFFECT

The primary site of CNS action of ketamine appears to be the thalamoneocortical projection system.[4] Ketamine selectively depresses neuronal function in parts of the cortex (especially association areas) and thalamus while simultaneously stimulating parts of the limbic system, including the hippocampus. This process creates what is termed functional disorganization[5] of nonspecific pathways in the midbrain and thalamic areas.[6,7] How does the preceding description translate into clinical terms for the anesthesiologist seeking to utilize ketamine?

Visualize the dissociative effect of ketamine as a "midbrain spinal." The ketamine "midbrain spinal" sets the stage for preemptive analgesia (*vide infra*). The cortex cannot respond to (noxious) signals it does not receive! No "wind-up" phenomenon is likely without afferent stimulation.

After obtaining identical dissociative effects with a 50 mg dose of ketamine in 90-pound women and muscular 250-pound men, Friedberg **concluded that the number of NMDA receptors does NOT vary with body weight or skeletal muscle mass in adults.** Investigators attempting to reliably reproduce preemptive analgesia with ketamine doses based on body weight that fall short of saturating the number of NMDA receptors (i.e., the dissociative effect) are doomed to, at best, variably positive[8-13] and, at worst, negative results.[14-19]

A recent negative outcome paper by Vallejo et al.[19] was received for publication in January 2002. Although Friedberg's 1993 paper was cited as a reference in Vallejo et al.,[19] none of his more recent papers were.[2,20] Vallejo et al.[19] were unable to demonstrate a difference in PONV rates. Their negative outcome was not surprising. Both groups received emetogenic isoflurane 0.5–1.5%. Vital signs and visual analog scale scores were utilized as indices of anesthetic depth, not a level-of-consciousness monitor, like the BIS. Vallejo et al.[19] administered ketamine $1-1.5 \text{ mg} \cdot \text{kg}^{-1}$ or doses between 70–120 mg **without** subsequent local analgesia. Friedberg advocates doses of 50 mg ketamine (independent of body weight) **followed by** local anesthesia. Vallejo et al.[19] had no specific endpoint of hypnosis before giving a greater-than-50-mg dose. To no surprise, they reported an elevated heart rate and increased incidence of dreaming in the ketamine group. Friedberg's endpoint of propofol for ketamine administration is precise and reproducible, that is, BIS 70–75. The outcome of Friedberg's approach is the lack of historically described ketamine side effects. Table 4-2 contrasts the number of medications administered by Vallejo et al.[19] with Friedberg's MIA™ technique. By failing to follow the "hypnosis first, *then* dissociation" rule, followed by adequate local anesthesia, Vallejo et al.[19] violated the *entire* algorithm for the successes published by Friedberg.[2,3,20]

Table 4-2. Drugs in Vallejo et al.[19] compared with MIA™ technique[2]

Vallejo et al.[19]	Friedberg MIA® technique[2]
1. Midazolam (1–2 mg) IV	1. Clonidine (0.2 mg) PO
2. Glycopyrrolate (0.2 mg)	2. Glycoprryolate (0.2 mg)
3. Propofol (2 mg · kg⁻¹) monitored by vital signs & visual analog scores	3. Propofol (150 ug · kg⁻¹ q 20 seconds – minibolus) monitored by BIS titrated to <75
4. Ketamine (0.5 mg · kg⁻¹)	4. Ketamine 50 mg IV push
5. d-Tubocuarare	5. Lidocaine with epinephrine (injected to adequate analgesia)
6. SCH	
7. Ketorolac	
8. Isoflurane	
9. Oxygen	
10. Nitrous oxide	
11. Rocuronium	
12. Neostigmine	

Pavlin et al.[14] used a multimodal approach to diminish postoperative pain. Like Friedberg, they used rofecoxib as a preemptive anti-inflammatory drug. *Rofecoxib was withdrawn from the market by the F. D. A. in 2004.* The dose of ketamine Pavlin et al.[14] administered was $0.2 \text{ mg} \cdot \text{kg}^{-1}$. Ketamine was given prior to the skin incision but *after* the afferent stimulus of the local analgesic! This feature of their study design demonstrates their probable belief that a sevoflurane/fentanyl anesthetic would block incoming stimuli to the cortex from the local injection. *GA does not reliably block the entry of all noxious stimuli to the cortex.* Injection of local anesthesia under GA alone will not reliably produce preemptive analgesia.

At $0.2 \text{ mg} \cdot \text{kg}^{-1}$, the average dose of ketamine in the Pavlin et al.'s[14] 82.5 kg patients was **16.5 mg**. This dose of ketamine is highly unlikely to saturate the NMDA receptors in the adult brain. *At best, only 80% of patients will achieve a dissociative effect at 25 mg; 98% of patients obtain a dissociative effect with a 50 mg dose of ketamine.* Because Pavlin et al.[14] were titrating their anesthetic to BIS 44 (compared with Friedberg's reports of 70–75), they *could* have safely given a **50 mg** dissociative dose of ketamine without producing hallucinations, tachycardia, or hypertension. Assuming they *had* given the ketamine prior to the injection of the local, paralyzing their patients would have made it impossible for Pavlin et al.[14] to determine whether their

patients were *immobile* for the injection. Using dissociation for the injection of the local anesthetic would have obviated the need for **opioids**, sevoflurane, endotracheal intubation, *and* neuromuscular blockade.

A **0.6%** PONV rate has been reported in **Friedberg's high-risk** practice,[2] compared with Pavlin et al.[14] reporting a **33%** PONV rate. "High risk" has been defined as non-smoking, female patients with a previous PONV/motion-sickness history having elective cosmetic surgical procedures greater than two hours in duration. Patients perceive PONV on emergence as caused by the anesthetic. In contrast, they do not blame the anesthesiologist for PONV after taking postoperative pain medication! Opioid **avoidance** defines a nonopioid, preemptive analgesia (NOPA) that is essential to the elimination of PONV with the MIA™ technique. Opioid **avoidance** facilitates room air, spontaneous ventilation (RASV) in the majority of healthy patients. Elimination of routine administration of oxygen, a drug that supports combustion or fire, is an obvious safety advantage for laser resurfacing cases.[20]

PREEMPTIVE ANALGESIA

Adequate local analgesia is **mandatory** to facilitate the NOPA of the MIA™ technique. Without a level-of-conscious monitor, like BIS, it is impossible to differentiate between patient movement from inadequate local analgesia and patient movement from inadequate propofol.

Patients receiving Friedberg's MIA™ technique (i.e., BIS 60–75) experienced the lesser trespass than general anesthesia (i.e., BIS 45–60 with systemic analgesia). Propofol was titrated to BIS 60–75 prior to the dissociative effect from the 50 mg ketamine dose. Over 1,500 MIA™ technique patients have experienced no recall of their surgical experience *without* concomitant benzodiazepine administration (see Table 4-3).

Without the ability to differentiate brain-based (implying inadequate propofol) versus spinal-cord–based movement, the anesthesiologist may be hard-pressed to convince the surgeon to inject more local analgesia. Too often, patient movement engenders comments from the surgeon that the patient is "too light." The anesthesiologist's invariable response is "needs more local." Without the ability to measure either component, there can be no resolution of this familiar argument. The "too light" versus "needs

Table 4-3. Essential preemptive analgesia concepts

1. Reproducible preemptive analgesia occurs administering the dissociative concepts.
2. GA does not reliably block the entry of all noxious stimuli to the cortex.
3. Injection of local anesthesia under GA alone will not reliably produce preemptive analgesia.
4. Adequate local analgesia is mandatory to facilitate the nonopioid, preemptive analgesia (NOPA) of the MIA™ technique.
5. Without a level-of-consciousness monitor, like BIS, it is impossible to differentiate between patient movement from inadequate local analgesia and patient movement from inadequate propofol.
6. Insisting on adequate local analgesia during the case minimizes most of postoperative pain-management issues.
7. When BIS is 60–75 with a "zero" EMG and patient movement, the surgeon must be educated to inject more local!
8. Pain signals can be transmitted to the patient's cortex, even in the presence of a vasoconstricted field.

more local" argument becomes circular and unresolvable. Everyone becomes frustrated and the patient suffers needlessly. Demonstrating a BIS 60–75 (with an iso-electric EMG) to the surgeon who may complain about patient movement should provide ample information to defuse the "too light" complaint. The surgeon is correct that the patient is "too light" but incorrect about the etiology. The correct solution 99% of the time is **more** local analgesia!

*The surgical field can be blanched from the epinephrine effect, yet the patient may **still** experience pain.*

This can be very confusing to the surgeon, who observes the epinephrine effect and believes there must be concomitant lidocaine effect. **Only** after three total injections (the initial and two subsequent ones) of local to an area, continued patient movement is managed with an additional 25–50 mg ketamine.

Assuring on adequate local analgesia during the case minimizes most postoperative pain-management issues.

BIS can serve as a "case management" tool. It is critically important for the anesthesiologist trying to provide a value-based service to the cosmetic surgeon to appreci-ate that EVERY cosmetic procedure, *including* abdomino-plasty, **can** be performed successfully solely under local anesthesia! This is true only if the patient is so motivated and the surgeon is very skilled with local anesthesia. Local analgesia with an awake, alert patient is *not* the preferred technique for most surgeons and patients. Despite his service being requested, the anesthesiologist should maintain some perspective and humility when approaching the cosmetic surgical patient.

Commonly, anesthesia services provided in residency-training situations tend to be GA with neuromuscular blockade or major neuraxial anesthesia. The young surgical trainee may be deprived of the feedback to know how well his local analgesia is, or is not, working in these circumstances. Further, the surgical trainee, as well as his anesthesia counterpart, may also be denied the ability to see how few postoperative pain-management issues remain when adequate intraoperative local analgesia is employed under dissociative anesthesia. (See Chapters 9 and 10 for specifics in providing adequate local analgesia for cosmetic surgery.) More importantly, if every procedure **can** be performed solely under local, the anesthesiologist must be able to justify *every* medication administered to the cosmetic surgical patient.

Patient movement occurring at BIS 60–75 with EMG at "zero" (more accurately, 30 on the EMG scale [right side] but reads zero on the BIS scale [left side]) is most likely being generated from the spinal cord level. *When trending the EMG as a secondary trace, it is visually easier to recognize a vertical spike compared to the horizontal factory default setting.* To trend EMG as a secondary trace, go to the advanced screen setup page. Once there, set the "save setting" button after selecting EMG as a secondary trace.

Patient movement with BIS 60–75 and a "zero" EMG defines an adequate level of propofol hypnosis for the MIA™ technique. When patient movement occurs while the BIS is 60–75 and the EMG remains "zero," more local analgesia is the most effective means to preserve the outcome advantages of the MIA™ technique. Spinal-cord–generated movement is devoid of the implication of awareness and recall. While spinal-cord–generated movement may be annoying to the surgeon, it generally does not disrupt the surgical field. *Passive restraints of the patient's arms and legs are recommended with the MIA™ technique. When restraining the arm, pronate it so the wrist is facing the arm board.*

Spinal-cord–generated movement is merely annoying. The same degree of movement could be extremely deleterious for a patient having cerebral aneurysm clipping. Attempts to suppress patient movement with more propofol may be successful but are not productive. Propofol does not block transmission of noxious stimuli to the cortex. Propofol suppression of patient movement will only add to the problems of postoperative pain management. More propofol is only a Band-Aid® when the patient needs a "suture." Attempts to suppress patient movement with more ketamine will often result in exceeding an aggregate dose of 200 mg. Whether ketamine is mixed with the propofol or administered separately, once the 200 mg aggregate dose is exceeded, patients do not emerge quickly or without side effects like horizontal nystagmus. *N. B. This caveat does not apply to cases less than sixty to ninety minutes* without superior outcomes. The anesthesiologist will not be successful in convincing the surgeon or his nurses that the MIA™ technique is a technique to be preferred over opioid-based IV sedation, regional anesthesia, or GA.

The skin is the largest organ in the body. The skin has the largest number of nerve endings. Failure to block negative afferent signals from the skin is a common feature of the negative studies showing failure to obtain preemptive effect with ketamine. *GA primarily depresses the CNS's ability to respond to afferent traffic.* Opioid-based *mu* receptor blockade also fails to prevent the *entry* of noxious, painful stimuli from reaching the cortex. Opioid-medicated, awake patients still acknowledge that they have pain. They state it just doesn't "bother them." Opioids modify only the *affective* response but not the perception of pain. *General anesthesia does not reliably block all afferent stimuli from reaching the brain.* The brain responds to these noxious stimuli by secreting several different polypeptides that are responsible for the "wind-up" phenomenon.[21] After patients emerge from GA, it is apparent that negative signals have reached the cortex. Postoperative pain management continues to be an issue for many patients.[22] Observing patients emerge essentially pain free is one of the hallmarks of the MIA™ technique.

Failure to dissociate prior to stimulation (injection and/or incision) is why a scholarly review of eighty randomized clinical trials, including eight with systemic NMDA receptor antagonists, by Moiniche et al.[23] concluded a negative potential benefit of preemptive analgesia on postoperative pain. The power of this negative review

Table 4-4. Dissociation and preemptive analgesia

1. Variable preemptive analgesic effect with less than a dissociative effect.
2. Time to dissociative effect typically 2–3 min. s/p ketamine injection.
3. **Prevent hallucinations** from ketamine by having a **stable** level of propofol in the brain (BIS 70–75) BEFORE giving the ketamine.
4. Create stable level of propofol with incremental, **not bolus**, induction.
5. No ketamine in the last twenty minutes of a case.
6. 200 mg,[a] in divided doses, is the upper limit of ketamine when using a short-acting agent like propofol.

[a]Especially in motion sickness sensitive patients, consider accepting a less-than-perfect dissociative effect by restricting ketamine dose to 50 mg for cases *less* than ninety minutes.

in *Anesthesiology* was amplified by an insouciant, accompanying editorial. "It is not clear to me that the failure of preemptive analgesia is a great loss in the pragmatic clinical setting."[24] Other studies in the peer-reviewed anesthesia literature beyond the academic purview of *Anesthesiology* **have** confirmed what many clinicians have known for some time.[25–28]

Table 4-4 summarizes the salient points of dissociation and preemptive analgesia with the MIA™ technique. Table 4-5 is included to help *avoid* known, possible errors performing the MIA™ technique. **The worst possible error is to administer ketamine before the propofol.**

A stable, hypnotic level of propofol must **precede** the ketamine if hallucinations are to be avoided. While teaching a resident, Friedberg noted that the resident had administered the ketamine when the BIS was 87. Friedberg moved to rapidly administer propofol to lower the BIS level. Subhypnotic doses of propofol (i.e., BIS >75) fail to block ketamine hallucinations. Predictably, the patient emerged hallucinating. The hallucinations were promptly eliminated with 2 mg IV midazolam **prior** to PACU transport. A calmed patient was then delivered to the PACU. The PACU nurses were spared the emotional trauma of dealing with a hallucinating patient.

The anesthesiologist wishing to perform the MIA™ technique, especially in an institutionally based environment, must avoid traumatizing his supporting PACU staff.

Table 4-5. Errors to Avoid with the MIA™ Technique

1. Ketamine before the propofol: NO
2. Ketamine before LLR/LVR or BIS >75 (i.e., PK MAC *without* BIS): NO
3. Ketamine at BIS >75: NO
4. Bolus propofol induction: NO
5. Inadequate local analgesia: NO, use the power of BIS/EMG
6. Opioids instead of more local analgesia: NO
7. Ketamine instead of more local analgesia: NO
8. Give >200 mg total ketamine or in last 20 min: NO
9. Tracheostomize patient instead of IV lidocaine: NO
10. SCH instead of IV lidocaine: NO
11. Persist trying to obtain complete dissociative effect by administering more than a single 50-mg dose of ketamine for brief cases (i.e., 60–90 min.), especially in motion sensitive patients: NO

Do not permit hallucinations to occur or promptly treat them if they do. Hallucinating patients will only confirm the well-earned, anti-ketamine bias among the nursing staff. Do NOT administer ketamine until the BIS is <75 in the context of a gradual propofol induction.

*If one is performing PK MAC without a BIS monitor, do not administer ketamine until **both** the loss of lid reflex [LLR] and loss of verbal response [LVR].*

Another error is to hasten the induction with a 1 mg · kg^{-1} bolus of propofol. The brain level of propofol will peak and then rapidly decline about the same time the ketamine level is peaking. Ketamine concentration peaking in the brain while propofol concentration is declining from a hypnotic level is functionally the same error as giving the ketamine before the propofol. Both error types set the stage for (avoidable) emergence hallucinations or dysphorias.

As the patient's advocate in the OR, the anesthesiologist must insist on **adequate local analgesia**, either by providing it himself or helping the surgeon understand the need for adequate local. During patient movement, the anesthesiologist should demonstrate the BIS level of 60–75 to the surgeon, who will likely complain about the patient being "too light."

When BIS is 60–75 with a "zero" EMG and patient movement, the surgeon must be educated to inject more local.

The BIS monitor is indifferent to the surgeon's (and the anesthesiologist's) ego. Without the BIS, it may be very difficult to persuade the surgeon to inject more local after the initial injection. It is not uncommon for the surgeon to comment (on the request for more local) that the field is already blanched. The surgeon's (not entirely unreasonable) assumption is that, if the field is blanched from the epinephrine, the patient must also be numb from the lidocaine.

Pain signals can be transmitted to the patient's cortex even in the presence of a vasoconstricted field.

There is no more efficacious IV agent to remedy inadequate local analgesia than *more* local analgesia injected into the surgical field. Only after two subsequent lidocaine injections after the initial one (three total injections) should one administer an additional 25–50 mg ketamine to suppress patient movement.

One of Friedberg's surgeons was not very gifted administering local analgesia. To compensate, this surgeon would inject 1,000 mg lidocaine with epinephrine in *each* breast (as 50 cc of 2%). The total lidocaine dose was 2,000 mg with epinephrine! Most anesthesiologists would be very uncomfortable, at the least, with a surgeon injecting this amount of lidocaine. Working with the MIA™ technique, this surgeon performed over 100 breast augmentation surgeries without any stigmata of lidocaine toxicity. As long as SpO$_2$ >95% and not more than 2,000 mg total lidocaine (typically as 400 cc 0.5%, 200 cc 1%, or 100 cc 2%) is used in the surgical field(s), none of the stigmata of lidocaine toxicity has been observed in Friedberg's experience, either intra- or postoperatively.

Insisting on adequate intraoperative local analgesia for the patient is a *critical* step in creating preemptive analgesia and dramatically reducing postoperative pain-management issues!

CONCLUSION

Preemptive analgesia *does* exist but only under specific and clearly defined, *reproducible* conditions. The dissociative effect is regularly observed when the NMDA receptors are saturated. The dissociative effect sets the stage for reliable preemptive analgesia. There are a finite number of NMDA receptors in the spinal cord and mid-brain. This number does not appear to vary with body weight in adults. A 50 mg IV ketamine bolus will effectively saturate the fixed number of NMDA receptors in the adult brain of approximately 98% of patients.

Very few exceptions will occur (*vide supra*). Completely blocking incoming noxious signals to the cortex using the dissociative effect (the so-called mid-brain spinal) is most likely responsible for the observed preemptive analgesia. "Hypnosis (propofol to BIS <75) first, then dissociation" (50 mg ketamine) eliminates the historically reported undesirable side effects of ketamine.[29]

REFERENCES

1. Vinnik CA: An intravenous dissociation technique for outpatient plastic surgery: Tranquility in the office facility. *Plast Reconstr Surg* 67:799,1981.
2. Friedberg BL: Propofol ketamine anesthesia for cosmetic surgery in the office suite, chapter in Osborne I (ed.), *Anesthesia for Outside the Operating Room. International Anesthesiology Clinics.* Baltimore, Lippincott, Williams & Wilkins, 41:39,2003.
3. Friedberg BL: Propofol-ketamine technique. *Aesth Plast Surg* 17:297,1993.
4. Miyasaka M, Domino E: Neural mechanisms of ketamine-induced anesthesia. *Int J Neuropharmacol* 7:557,1968.
5. Corssen G, Domino EF: Dissociative anesthesia: Further pharmacologic studies and first clinical experience with the phencyclidine derivative CI-581. *Anesth Analg* 45:29,1968.
6. Massopust LC Jr, Wolin JR, Albin MS: Electrophysiologic and behavioral responses to ketamine hydrochloride in the Rhesus monkey. *Anesth Analg* 51:329,1972.
7. Sparks DL, Corssen G, Aizenman B, et al.: Further studies on the neural mechanisms of ketamine induced anesthesia in the Rhesus monkey. *Anesth Analg* 54:1889,1975.
8. Kwok RFK, Lim J, Chan MTV, et al.: Preoperative ketamine improves postoperative analgesia after gynecologic laparoscopic surgery. *Anesth Analg* 98:1044,2004.
9. Menigauz C, Fletcher D, Dupont X, et al.: The benefits of intraoperative small dose ketamine on postoperative pain after anterior cruciate ligament repair. *Anesth Analg* 90:1129,2000.
10. Royblat L, Korotkurutchko A, Katz J: Post-operative pain: the effect of low dose ketamine on general anesthesia. *Anesth Analg* 77:1161,1993.
11. Fu ES, Miguel R, Scharf JE: Preemptive ketamine decreases post-operative narcotic requirements in patients undergoing abdominal surgery. *Anesth Analg* 84:1086,1997.
12. Suzuki M, Tseuda K, Lansing PS, et al.: Small-dose ketamine enhances morphine-induced analgesia after outpatient surgery. *Anesth Analg* 89:98,1999.
13. Pavlin DJ, Horvath K, Pavlin EG, et al.: Preincisional treatment to prevent pain after ambulatory hernia surgery. *Anesth Analg* 97:1627,2003.
14. Adam F, Libier M, Oszustowicz T, et al.: Preoperative small-dose ketamine has no preemptive effect in patients undergoing total mastectomy. *Anesth Analg* 89:444, 1999.
15. Dahl V, Ernoe PE, Steen T, et al.: Does ketamine have preemptive effects in women undergoing abdominal hysterectomy procedures? *Anesth Analg* 90:1419–22,2000.
16. Mathisen LC, Aasbo V, Raeder J: Lack of preemptive analgesic effect of (R)-ketamine in laparoscopic cholecystectomy. *Acta Anaesthesiol Scand* 43:220,1999.
17. Yaksch W, Lang S, Reichhalter R, et al.: Perioperative small-dose S(+)-ketamine has no incremental beneficial effects on post-operative pain when standard-practice opioid infusions are used. *Anesth Analg* 94:981,2002.
18. Van Elstraete AC, Lebrun T, Sanfedo I, et al.: Ketamine does not decrease post-operative pain after remifentanil-based anesthesia for tonsillectomy in adults. *Acta Anaesthesiol Scand* 48:756,2004.
19. Vallejo MC, Romeo RC, Davis DJ, et al.: Propofol-ketamine versus propofol-fentanyl for outpatient laparoscopy: Comparison of postoperative nausea, emesis, analgesia and recovery. *J Clin Anes* 14:426,2002.
20. Friedberg BL: Facial laser resurfacing with propofol-ketamine technique: Room air, spontaneous ventilation (RASV) anesthesia. *Dermatol Surg* 25:569,1999.
21. Thompson SWN, King AE, Woolf CJ: Activity-dependent changes in rat ventral horn neurons in vitro, summation of prolonged afferent evoked depolarizations produce a D-2-amino-5-phosphonovaleric acid sensitive windup. *Eur J Neurosci* 2:638,1990.
22. Cousins MJ, Power J, Smith G: Pain – A persistent problem (Labat lecture). *Reg Anesth Pain Med* 25:6,2002.
23. Moinche S, Kehlet H, Berg J: A qualitative and quantitative systemic review of preemptive analgesia for postoperative pain relief. *Anesthesiol* 96:725,2002.
24. Hogan Q: No preemptive analgesia. Is that so bad? *Anesthesiol* 96:526,2002.
25. Woolf CJ, Chong MS: Preemptive analgesia: Treating postoperative pain by preventing the establishment of central sensitization. *Anesth Analg* 77:362,1993.
26. Ong KS, Lirk P, Seymour RA: The efficacy of preemptive analgesia for acute postoperative pain management: A meta-analysis. *Anesth Analg* 100:757,2005.
27. McQuay HJ: Pre-emptive analgesia: A systematic review of clinical studies. *Ann Med* 27:249,1995.
28. McQuay HJ: Pre-emptive analgesia. *Br J Anaesth* 69:1,1992.
29. Friedberg BL: Hypnosis first, then dissociation. *Anesth Analg* 96:911,2003.

5 | Special Needs of Cosmetic Dental Patients

James A. Snyder, D.D.S.

INTRODUCTION

Cosmetic dental procedures are increasing.[1] Americans have demonstrated their interest in cosmetic medical procedures through their interest in television features, documentaries, and "reality" programming. This programming often features dental procedures ranging from reconstructive maxillofacial surgery through complex dental restorative procedures to simple cosmetic teeth bleaching. Modern dental practice offers many treatment solutions to almost any patient need or desire. Some of these procedures require highly technical and precise care to produce a desirable outcome. The dentist must obtain near-perfect conditions in an otherwise hostile environment.

The primary operating area, a person's mouth, is a small, dark, wet hole with plenty of very delicate, moving parts (see Fig. 5-1). An ill-timed twitch or swallow, a hiccup or sigh, a startled wince and a big problem has been created. Further, in all cases, the treatment objects—tooth, periodontal tissue, dentoalveolar ridge—are tiny. For example, a coronary artery being grafted during coronary artery bypass surgery (CABG) is usually more than 5 millimeters in diameter whereas the distance from the outside of a front tooth to the pulp (nerve) is less than half that.

Modern dentistry is truly powerful. Many cosmetic and restorative treatment options are available from dentists in all parts of the country. Ceramic or polymer laminates (veneers) and crowns can be attached to teeth or titanium implants placed in the bone allowing a fixed, permanent correction for lost, damaged, or irregularly placed teeth. If one does not have enough bone for placement of implants, arrays of bone-grafting procedures are available to replace the lost bone so that dental implants can be placed. Skeletal deformities can be corrected with maxillofacial surgery. Most of these processes can be tedious, and dental treatment is often anxiety-provoking for many people.

FINDING AN ANESTHESIA PROVIDER

There is no American Dental Association (ADA) accredited specialty for anesthesiology! Whereas medicine, nursing, and even veterinary medicine have approved

47

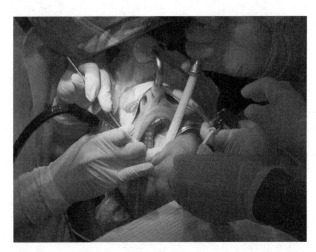

Figure 5-1. The crowded environment of dental work. Note the securing of the endotracheal tube and head wrap.

training and certification programs in anesthesiology, the ADA does not. The ADA is currently the only Department of Education–approved accrediting body for dentists. Although it does not accredit a specialty in anesthesiology, the ADA does have extensive guidelines for the educational requirements expected of providers for all levels of pain and anxiety control in dentistry. The ADA stipulates two years of anesthesia training in Part 2 of the *Guidelines for the Teaching the Comprehensive Control of Anxiety and Pain in Dentistry*. Part 2 is entitled "Teaching the Comprehensive Control of Anxiety and Pain at the Advanced Education Level."[2]

Although the ADA provides guidelines for dental anesthesia training, the ADA has refused to recognize those who have successfully completed that training as specialists in anesthesia. Also, the ADA has not requested that the Commission (CODA) accredit programs that state they meet or surpass those standards. Despite these circumstances, there are trained dentists (and physicians and nurses) who can provide reliable anesthesia care. Further, there are credentials offered that identify dentists with a proper anesthesia background.

The American Society of Anesthesiologists (ASA) requires two or more years (at least twenty-four months) of training solely in anesthesiology for membership. The American Dental Board of Anesthesiology (ADBA) reviews curricula in the dentist anesthesia residency programs. Further, the ADBA examines those completing two years of anesthesia training with a rigorous day-long, vali-

dated oral and written test similar to the one administered by the American Board of Anesthesiology.[3] Success leads to Diplomate status—Board Certification. These persons are Dentist Anesthesiologists (DAs). This is currently the most reliable credential for dentist anesthesia providers.

Board certification as an Oral and Maxillofacial Surgeon (OMS) requires *only* a four-month rotation in anesthesia-related areas. One hundred deep-sedation cases or general anesthetics must be documented.[4]

Some dental graduate programs contain a sedation module or rotation. These vary widely in intensity and duration. Some of the ADA-recognized specialties and many general practice residencies have sedation requirements varying from exposure to competence. A common concern lies in whether a dentist (or nonanesthesiologist physician) trained for a light level of sedation can rescue a patient who inadvertently goes into the next deeper level. These programs vary from a single-day didactic (lecture) to several-days didactic with clinical exposures. The programs are continuing education (CE), not part of a graduate or undergraduate curriculum. The ADA provides detailed guidelines for each level of instruction but has no oversight mechanism.[2] Further, examination of participants is spotty or nonexistent. In-depth exposure to anesthesia and anesthetized patients is very minimal in undergraduate dental education and only slightly greater in most postgraduate dental curricula.[5]

State regulations play an enormous role in the anesthesia strategy for dental patients. Because of the very high risk of patient harm and several high-profile media events following dental-office misadventures, states have sought to regulate anesthesia safety for dental patients. The absence of a professional standard-bearer (i.e., a specialty group such as the American Society of Anesthesiologists [ASA] provides for medicine) and a hodgepodge of legacy anesthesia techniques have made some state laws and regulations highly specific. Providing modern, advanced forms of anesthesia care for dental patients will have to begin with an analysis of one's respective state's laws, regulations, and customs.

Although an increasing number of anesthesiologists and nurse anesthetists have offered their services to dental patients in recent years, the total number of qualified providers to this group of patients is very small. Dentist anesthesiologists have proliferated in states where regulations thoughtfully provide for this higher standard of care but are absent from large blocks of the country. Anesthesiologists and nurse anesthetists may be excluded from conventional practice for dental patients by poorly crafted regulations.[6]

One thing remains constant, regardless of the venue or treatment: general anesthesia or deep sedation (which can quickly change to general anesthesia) *should* be provided by a specialist in anesthesia, that is, an anesthesiologist or dentist anesthesiologist or nurse anesthetist.[7]

DENTISTRY IN THE HEALTHCARE UNIVERSE

What are "Legacy" anesthesia techniques and why do they affect anesthesia practice for dental patients? The Institute of Medicine (IOM) published its study of dental education in 1995 with a 345-page bound volume. Some of its conclusions are instructive in seeking perspective on the differences between dental and medical practices.

On the surface, it would seem there should be little difference in the need and application of anesthesia services. After all, it's only a centimeter from a cosmetic labial procedure to a dental one. This is sometimes a pretty long centimeter. Why would there be such widely different regulations and techniques? One important explanation can be found in some of the IOM conclusions.

"The mission of education is undermined by curricula and faculty that have become out of touch with the needs of students and prospective practitioners, patients, or communities. . . . Further, each mission is weakened by dental schools' isolation from the intellectual and organizational life of the university, from the broader research community, and from the larger health care system. . . .

Dentistry has been relatively slow to support outcomes research, to investigate the rationale for practice variations, and to demand proof of cost-effectiveness for new technologies." [5] "Dental accreditation has been criticized for being inflexible, overly prescriptive, insufficiently independent of dental society leadership, and too focused on process and structure. It is said, thus, to stifle innovation. Further, the current system is criticized as being too little concerned with outcomes."[5] Since the 1995 IOM report, "There is simply no evidence that I know of showing that dental education is following the prescient recommendations of the IOM," former Dean Nash opined in AGD Impact, May 2000.[8] Given this background, it may be easier to visualize why operator-anesthetist strategies, or strategies relying on methohexital, could be still taught through the 1990s. It may also be easier to understand how these practice modes could find their way into a state's legal code.

UNIQUE REQUIREMENTS OF DENTAL PROCEDURES

All dental treatment is in the airway. Aspiration risk is high. Most dental procedures must be accompanied by copious irrigation to cool the rotary instruments (drills) used. The result of all that drilling often causes chips, pieces, and fragments of hard tissue to fly around. Dentists use a lot of very small instruments that can get slippery when wet. Persons with oral guarding, including hyperactive gag reflex, prevent the simplest treatments without a profound level of anesthesia. A small mandibular range of motion or large tongue size may necessitate general anesthetic to gain adequate access to the treatment area. Treatment in close proximity to the airway requires opening the mouth and may require manipulating the head. Either (or both) maneuver(s) may produce a loss of airway patency. These circumstances are not usually issues for other cosmetic procedures, and each has a priority in anesthesia planning.

Sensory perception of the oral and pharyngeal areas is extremely high. Protective reflexes produce very reactive responses to intrusions in the oropharynx. For this reason, it is usually necessary to have a deeper, more complex anesthesia plan than for treatments of seemingly similar acuity on other parts of the body. For instance, a person may permit traction of a skin pedicle after light sedation and local anesthesia infiltrated into the area but react sharply after similar traction of the tongue. Complex muscle and nerve interrelations abound and the autonomic overlay is very present in the head and neck. Many individuals have to compete for a confined space around the patient's head. Current practice puts at least the dentist, a chairside assistant, the anesthesiologist, and everybody's gear, equipment, and instruments in a pretty small space. Some pretreatment choreography is a prerequisite!

Looking at treatment acuity or plan alone can't always determine anesthetic strategy. For instance, a person with hyperactive gag reflex (or Parkinson's tremors) may intend fully to cooperate, require minimal invasive treatment, but require considerable anesthesia management to prevent a tremor or wretch at an inconvenient time (e.g., while the dental drill is spinning at 400,000 RPM near the tongue). Patients manifesting presenile dementia often seem docile but react violently when an oral trespass is attempted. Deeper anesthesia than expected is often needed to obtund this reaction for even the simplest oral examination or treatment.

Dental phobia, "White coat syndrome," fear of needles, fear of pain or the unknown are pretty common in healthcare. Dentistry has its own level of phobia. Dental Phobia is in the DSM,[9] a kind of pantheon of fear. Fear of dental treatment is so universal that it is a common usage metaphor. It is a common plot device for authors and movies (e.g., the 1976 movie "Marathon Man," with Dustin Hoffman and Sir Laurence Olivier). The fear is really, really deep for many people. From where does it come? While the impact of any treatment in the mouth is probably more likely to have negative responses, the answer is most likely that it actually is unpleasant. A majority of the population goes for dental care and discovers that sometimes it sounds bad, tastes worse, and sometimes hurts. When it hurts, it hurts in a sharp, ugly, startling way that leaves an indelible memory, often crossing generations. Regrettably, only a very small percentage of dentists utilize even the most rudimentary pain- and anxiety-control techniques (other than local anesthetic injection). For this reason, patients and their dentists have few options to reduce the likelihood of a bad experience or prevent the repeat of one that has already happened.

Studies show large numbers of the American population do not seek regular dental care.[10–11] These studies usually show that if advanced forms of anesthesia where available, they would seek treatment.[13–15] The offer of competent anesthesia care would likely increase interest in cosmetic dental procedures.

AIRWAY MANAGEMENT

Endotracheal Anesthesia

Anesthesia management for dental procedures requires the usual consideration of operator or surgeon working conditions and patient safety and comfort with the additional concerns highlighted herein, and in addition usually requires managing the airway in a dental office. The concerns outlined would suggest to most anesthesiologists that an endotracheal tube is required—period. Interestingly, most sedation and anesthesia provided for

cosmetic dental procedures do **not** employ an endotracheal tube (*vide infra*). Endotracheal intubation is typically performed with general anesthesia (BIS 45–60 *with* systemic analgesia), not MAC or "deep sedation." An anesthesia machine and all the mandated monitoring are also employed.

Hospitals and stand-alone surgicenters are always equipped with anesthesia machines and ASA-specified monitoring.[7] Increasingly, busy offices have installed them for their anesthesia provider. Further, mobile anesthesia providers have found transportable anesthesia machines and monitors allowing safe, fully compliant anesthetics to be provided almost anywhere. As most who have worked in military field hospitals or third world medical facilities know, what's critical isn't the place but the professionals with the necessary equipment. Modern technique including BIS monitoring, simple end-tidal CO_2 measurement, ultra-short acting agents, and computerized infusion pumps make intubated general anesthesia a practical option.

An obstacle to endotracheal intubation for dental procedures has been the requirement for a nasal approach. Although armored tubes placed orally can be manipulated inside the mouth to allow access for most dental procedures, the constant manipulation increases both intraoperative and postoperative risk. Additionally, tube manipulation increases mouth, throat, and larynx soreness, leading to lower satisfaction levels for patients. Some dental cosmetic procedures may be compromised by the presence of an oral tube. For instance, precise occlusal registration may not be possible and exact lip position cannot be determined. Actually, occlusal registration is the relationship of the teeth in various jaw positions such as protruding or moved laterally. The exact position of tooth cusps and ridges determines function and comfort. *N. B. "Occlusal registration" is the indexing of the relationship of the teeth. It is sometimes called the "bite."* An accurate occlusal registration can have profound influence on the final cosmetic outcome.

DAs and others who have extensive experience providing anesthesia for dental procedures use nearly exclusively a nasal approach. Like most things, experience improves outcomes. A common strategy is to dilate the nasal passage with lidocaine gel or Surgilube™–lubricated straight nasal airways over about five minutes. Three to six increasing sizes are used in the side with the least resistance. Selecting the nasal passage is aided by obtaining a panoramic dental x-ray. The final airway should be one size larger than the planned ET tube. Heating the ET tube in hot water or in the folds of a hot towel is very important in minimizing trauma. Studies of examined optimum time of heating and the minimum temperature have been done.[17] About 45°–50° C is fairly reliable.

ET tube will resist boiling for a short time. However, the patient will be burned if the tube is heated to temperatures in excess of 60° C. This combination of nasal passage selection, dilation, lubrication, and heated tube nearly eliminates the other nasal intubation issue—epistaxis (nosebleeds). Because the entire treatment is around the head and the head is going to be moved during treatment, the properly positioned tube must be secured (see Fig. 5-1). Nasal tubes need to be secure for length (to prevent one-lung ventilation), but they also need to be free from twisting, torquing, rotating, or otherwise spindling or stapling. Tube movement during the procedure can result in nosebleeds after extubation as well.

Patient eye protection is required for dental procedures for all anesthetic levels. Goggles or safety glasses are fine for awake or conscious sedation strategies, but tape, drapes, and/or a specific protective device are needed for deeper levels. There is just too much going on around the head not to protect the patient's eyes. An operator's finger, a flying tooth fragment, a dropped instrument (remember, these things are tiny and slippery), or a drip of some dental material could all easily end up in an unprotected eye. The risk of microbe inoculation of the eye in the dental treatment environment is very high. Ultra high-speed dental handpieces (drills) with copious irrigation to protect the tooth and bone from its heat create a large aerosol cloud filled with everything that could be found in the mouth—virus, bacteria, fungus—a real microbiology workshop. Eye protection has to be considered in securing the nasal tube. After all, there is only so much room and this is also going to be the operating area. Luckily, dental treatment teams usually work at roughly the three and nine o'clock positions around the head, leaving the twelve o'clock position for the anesthesiologist.

Who would have thought the simple endotracheal tube (ETT) could be improved on? Disposable, safer materials, pneumatic cuffs, and size and pressure options for the cuffs all evolved. The RAE™ nasal and then oral curved tubes are a nice convenience, especially for dental and other head and neck procedures. Although there is a massive array of rigid and flexible anesthesia standard connectors allowing almost any conceivable positioning, RAE™ can usually be used without additional connectors to allow improved access to the treatment area. A recent modification in the tip design of the ETT, the Parker,™ reduces trauma during insertion.[18] Tubes shielded from laser are available and are necessary if laser is used in the mouth with an oral intubation.

Muscle-relaxant use is not necessary for intubation. While 50% of DAs routinely intubate, none use muscle relaxants to achieve it.[18] How is this done? Current literature contains numerous successful techniques using high doses of opioids or ketamine. However, the use of topical local anesthesia for the airway has been the favorite technique for DAs.[19] Delivery of lidocaine spray by LTA,™ atomizer, or transcrichoid injection renders the cords nonreactive to the tube passing. A topicalized airway lowers the overall drug requirement for the general anesthesia. Cheaper, faster, better anesthesia and recovery are the desired outcome goals. LTA™ delivery is the most popular route of administration. Delivery of topical lidocaine to the airway requires about five minutes to achieve effect. For those persons with reactive airway, good results have been achieved with 2% lidocaine, 100 mg, .

Even if a muscle relaxant is necessary to the anesthesia plan, recent drug introductions have reduced the concerns. Several rapid-onset, short-acting nondepolarizing muscle relaxants are available. Depending on the procedure duration, it may not be necessary to use a reversal agent if the muscle relaxant was used *only* to facilitate intubation. The presence of nondepolarizers in the anesthesia technique requires the availability of a reversal agent and a peripheral nerve stimulator. Further, an unexpected incomplete reversal could mean a transfer to a nearby intensive care unit.

A common concern of operating dentists is access to the posterior teeth when patients have decreased mandibular range of motion (ROM). Normal adult opening at the incisors is usually about 45–55 mm. However, a massetter muscle spasm or intracapsular temporomandibular joint dysfunctions such as an anteriorly trapped meniscus can dramatically reduce this opening. Muscle relaxants can also improve the ROM. A fully secure airway not only allows a safe and precise anesthetic but also gives the operator the fullest possible treatment technique latitude: exact patient positioning for optimum access, protection from treatment detritus, limitless irrigation, and no treatment interference. A helpful additional benefit of the intubated dental patient is that auxiliary staff need little additional skills to assist for these procedures. Loss of airway due to positioning or contamination is very difficult when compared to other airway techniques.

A common criticism of intubation for dental procedures is that it takes too long. A careful induction of the type described herein takes about fifteen to twenty minutes from entering the operating room to ready for treatment. Although this is probably twice the time needed for a deep sedation, the time is quickly recovered with interest during the treatment time in which interruptions for throat packing, coughing, gagging, or hypoventilation don't occur. Additionally, time is saved due to complete freedom in head position and mouth opening.

Nonintubated Anesthesia

Since most dental anesthesia does not involve endotracheal intubation, how is it done? Although a laryngeal mask airway (LMA)™ —or one of the variations—may be used in a carefully prepared patient while staying short of general anesthesia (Fig. 5-4), the rostral tongue posturing and large oral tube makes most dental treatment more difficult. In limited situations, the LMA™ can be useful. When treatment considerations allow for it, the LMA™ can be used as a "super" throat pack allowing high-volume irrigation or higher protection from bleeding with very small aspiration risk. With the LMA™ properly placed, a small-bore suction can be placed through the nose to the top of the LMA™, then a gauze throat pack placed. This strategy also greatly reduces swallowed blood, thereby decreasing the PONV risk.

Oral pharyngeal airways (and variants like COPA™) are completely in the way during dental treatment. Nasopharyngeal airways lend themselves nicely to MAC or general anesthesia. Dilation with increasing sizes lubricated with lidocaine gel works even if an endotracheal tube is not utilized. Length is also critical when less than general anesthesia is the goal. A too short nasal airway is useless, whereas one that is too long can prevent a working environment if a restless patient coughs or resists.

Topical anesthetics (or local anesthetics) can help with patient tolerance, but they have short action durations. Additionally, the dental treatment requires an open

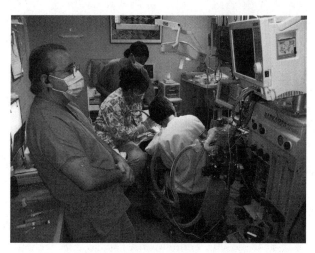

Figure 5-2. Dr. Synder with electronic stethoscope, with both monitors and patient within his eye scan. BIS is 44.

mouth. Occasionally, a perfectly positioned nasopharyngeal airway becomes useless with the mouth open. A big tongue can displace or compress the orifice of the airway. A useful strategy in these cases is to try using a low-pressure endotracheal tube. Position it as if it was a nasopharyngeal airway, inflate the cuff, and cut off the excess. It is possible even to use two nasal airways, connect them with a commercially available adaptor to an anesthesia circuit, and proceed semiclosed. Sometimes there is no exact nasal airway position possible. In those cases, a "go"/"no go" decision is necessary. Cancel, lighten to conscious sedation, or deepen to general anesthesia.

Everything about (dental) anesthesia starts with airway. Because the "prime directive" (protect the airway) and the treatment area are in competition, extra and even extraordinary planning is needed for dental cases (see Fig 5-2). Millions of MAC and general anesthetics are provided for dental patients every year. *Most are done without a fully protected airway!* The public and the profession *believe* these are safely done. Unfortunately, there are no unimpeachable studies verifying this. Further, dentistry has no institutional review of mortality and morbidity, so accurate statistics do not exist. The absence of professional introspection perpetuates empirical practices. Empirical evidence is sometimes dead on. For instance, legend has it that the first defibrillation of a human was done with the energy levels "guessed" based on humans being between mice and horses in size. The "guess," 350 joules, is about what studies verified over time. Good guess! Sometimes, the empirical observation is off the mark. G. V. Black, the

"Father of Modern Dentistry," is reported to have taught that tooth brushing with a hard toothbrush, back and forth, after every instance of eating, leads to good dental health. Black based this observation on those who practiced this ritual. The hard toothbrushers had less dental disease than those who didn't. He failed to notice those who didn't brush at all... ever! No control existed for those that brushed occasionally, brushed up and down, or brushed with implements other than a "brush." The germ theory came later. Food proved much less a problem than the microbes. Hindsight can sometimes be amusing, as the Black anecdote illustrates.

There are some published surveys available on anesthesia-related mortality and morbidity for dental patients.[20] In addition to being *uncontrolled* studies, they contain inconsistencies that the trained observer finds curious. One such survey, the Perrott survey[21] of oral surgeons published in 2003, has been criticized for methodology and integrity. Also worrisome are some of the data reported. Of 24,737 general anesthesia (GA) or deep sedations (DS), 11,138 (or 45%) were done without continuous flow (9,208 with no at all).[21] Also interesting is that 95.5% of the GA/DS were provided by an operator-anesthetist oral surgeon anesthesia "team." The "team" concept is described in the AAOMS guidelines[22] as consisting of three people for GA/DS. However, the Perrott et al. study reports a mean size anesthesia team of 2.7.[21] Another curious finding was that 7.9% of GA/DS were "awake." If 7.9% of these anesthetics clearly failed, why was the dissatisfaction rate only 1.1%? Most interesting was the Perrott et al.[21] conclusion that a 1999 study reporting a 1:1 million mortality rate and a later 2001 study reporting a 1.28:1 million mortality rate proved that mortality provided by oral-maxillofacial surgeons (OMS) has been *decreasing*.[20]

MONITORING

Although there are many monitoring guidelines for anesthesia, the very highest level should always be employed for each level of anesthesia care for all patients—including dental. There is no reason to provide less than the best. (See Chapter 18.) Modern electronics have made it possible to monitor every parameter in practically any situation. Monitoring can be portable, accurate, noninvasive, and inexpensive.

Monitors (and anesthesia equipment) are another area where state regulations play a large role for dental cases. All states currently have laws and/or regulations regarding sedation and anesthesia for dental patients. As discussed herein, these regulations are often very specific. They often have lists of drugs, instruments, and electronic monitors that must be present for various levels of anesthesia. Sometimes the anesthesia levels are defined; however, the definitions may not be clear in the context of current therapeutics (see Appendix 1-1). *Some* states require monitors to be fixed at the treatment site. Portable monitors, regardless of quality, do not qualify! Providing anesthesia for dental patients has to start with individual state regulations. Be prepared to be surprised at what one may find there.

Most parameters are monitored exactly as they would be for any type procedure: pulse oximeter sensor on finger or ear, NIABP cuff on arm, cardioscope electrodes on chest, BIS electrode on forehead, end-tidal CO_2 in the circuit, gas analyzer in circuit, and so forth. What if there isn't a closed system? Many dental cases are done with open or semi-open systems. How can one monitor gases? A monitor with a pump ("side streaming") for its CO_2 and gas bench only needs access to the patient to function. When the circuit is not completely closed, the data is subject to atmospheric corruption, but the "relative" value is still worthwhile. Further, a waveform is created and the alarms can be used.

Creative connections abound, but the use of an 18 ga catheter (*sans* needle) placed in the nose or nasal airway and attached to the luer end of the sample tubing gives a reasonably good result. Once placed, a dental office nitrous-oxide/oxygen hood can be used over it. The result is comprehensive electronic monitoring without an ETT (see Figs. 5-2 and 5-3).

Every monitoring discussion requires a mention of the precordial stethoscope. A heavy metal bell placed on the neck in the sternal notch and attached to tubing and an earpiece or an electronic microphone provides real-time heart and breath sounds. Commercially available radio transmitter and receiver devices provide high-quality audio and freedom of movement.[23] In addition to the information, it provides redundancy because it is separate from a vital-signs or anesthesia monitor. A highly experienced person can detect airway nuance and make a coarse anesthesia depth determination. However, no special training

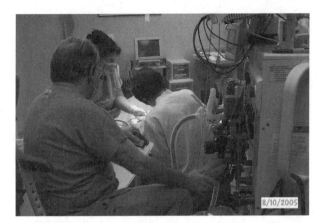

Figure 5-3. Dr. Snyder maintaining a watchful eye on his patient.

is needed to obtain a benefit from the sounds. Coarsely put: sounds are good—silence is bad.

Bispectral (BIS) monitoring[24] is a recent development. (See Chapter 3.) Monitoring the level of hypnosis is highly valuable in anesthesia care. BIS is particularly useful for office-based anesthesia. It makes it possible to achieve amnesia reliably with less than general anesthetic technique. Careful skin preparation and placement of the forehead electrode provides reliable values during any anesthetic for all dental procedures.[25,26] Most patient monitoring results in safer, more precise anesthetics. Once the learning curve is passed, BIS will do this. BIS provides information not available from any other monitoring device. Thoughtful use will result in decreased drug use and faster wakeups and discharges.[27] Best of all, it will allow certainty of amnesia during the procedure. In the end, that is the one thing patients are absolutely, positively expecting.

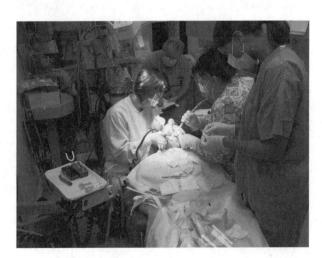

Figure 5-4. Dr. Snyder charting the anesthesia record.

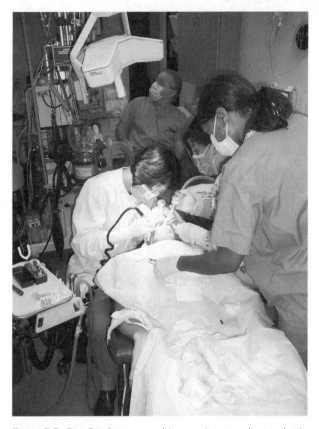

Figure 5-5. Dr. Snyder scans his monitors and anesthesia machine.

ANESTHESIA TECHNIQUE

Any modern technique will do nicely for dental patients. The basic formula (recipe) for anesthesia is as follows:

1. hypnosis + analgesia + muscle relaxation
2. add modern drugs to balance the formula
3. monitor all necessary parameters
4. use local anesthesia liberally
5. supervise 1–4 with anesthesia professional

The majority of anesthesia for dental procedures is deep intravenous sedation without airway protection or ventilatory support. Benzodiazepines in conjunction with opioids have been favored by oral surgeons.[28] Dentist anesthesiologists favor propofol with fentanyl, remifentanil, or ketamine. Benzodiazepines are sometimes used supplementally. Remifentanil is more safely delivered by infusion pump.

In those instances where general anesthesia is planned, after securing the airway, standard inhalation agents are used for maintenance. Desflurane offers very rapid emergence to eye opening, but time to discharge may not be similarly shortened.[29]

ANESTHESIA AND PAIN CONTROL OPTIONS

Years of experience and studies too numerous to count have concluded the same thing: pain is bad. Pain slows recovery.[30] Absence of pain is nearly always the highest criterion (or lowest depending on one's point of view) for patient satisfaction. Every patient believes the fee is too high regardless of what it is. However, a pain-free (or much less pain than anticipated) experience usually yields a satisfied patient. The converse is also true: a near-perfect procedure can be highly underappreciated by a patient having greater than anticipated pain. Patients seeking cosmetic procedures seem particularly demanding of a pain-free experience. Success in this practice requires mastery of pain control.

A thoughtful anesthesia plan can considerably decrease postoperative pain. Dentist researchers pioneered early study of this area. The primary pharmacology tool for studying oral analgesics is the "Cooper—Dionne third molar extraction" model. Dionne[31] demonstrated that the use of pretreatment ibuprofen coupled with long-duration local analgesia nearly eliminated postoperative pain medication needs. Including local anesthetics during and at the end of surgical procedures minimizes neuronal "wind up"[32] and is now accepted practice.

Studies have shown that preoperative acetaminophen, intraoperative low-dose ketamine, and intraoperative low-dose fentanyl have all reduced the need for postoperative analgesia. The use of clonidine as an anesthesia drug is not new among plastic surgeons,[33,34] but it has been getting more use by anesthesiologists recently.[35] Alpha$_2$ adrenergic agonists may open an entirely new pathway for anesthesiologists. For instance, infusion of dexmedotomidine has been used as a sole agent for sedation.[36]

Clonidine has been added to local anesthetics to improve results of regional and epidural blocks for chronic pain or postoperative pain relief.[37,38] Oral clonidine 0.4–0.5 $\mu g \cdot kg^{-1}$ taken ninety minutes prior to induction reduces drug needs for sedation or general anesthesia[35,39] and reduces postoperative pain medication requirements.[39] A recent study demonstrated low pain, low nausea and vomiting, and high satisfaction with general anesthetics using clonidine, low-dose ketamine,

and ketorolac for analgesia.[40] Other studies[35,40] with po clonidine premedication consistently demonstrate a 20% reduction in propofol requirements.

The movement away from opioids, both for intraoperative analgesia and postoperative pain management, has recently hit a snag. The safety of COX-2 inhibitors has been called into question, and some drugs in this class have been withdrawn from the market. Inspection of the mechanism leading to this action suggests that more peripherally acting analgesics such as NSAIDs will also come under scrutiny. Managing postoperative pain with pre- and intraoperative anesthesia strategies may become critical to patient comfort.

The use of opioid analgesics is alive and well in dental practice. However, Moore's recent survey of oral surgery practice showed nearly 93% always or nearly always using opioids as standard postoperative medication.[28]

Pain complaints from lengthy dental procedures originate more often from temporo-mandibular joint and masticatory muscles than from the treatment area. Inflammation after prolonged near-maximum opening of the normally closed mouth is definitely unpleasant. Mouth and face pain is tenacious. There is no way to rest or support a painful TMJ or masseter. Swallowing, speaking, eating, drinking, even lifting, all result in jaw movement. Dexamethasone 8–10 mg IV immediately after induction, is useful in reducing this inflammation and thereby the pain associated with it. Other steroid preparations, adjusted for dose equivalency, may also be useful, but dexamethasone has favorable pharmacokinetics, phamacodynamics, and cost index. Dexamethasone, given early in the anesthesia, also reduces PONV.[41,42] Two patient-satisfaction issues addressed with one drug provides a win-win situation.

POSTOPERATIVE NAUSEA AND VOMITING (PONV)

If pain isn't a patient's highest (or lowest) satisfaction criterion, PONV certainly is. Pain or PONV can make everybody unhappy with the postoperative period. Misery and low satisfaction aren't the only issue with PONV. It can reduce the outcome of many cosmetic procedures, including dental ones. Because the mouth is the primary exit portal in vomiting, dental procedures are especially vulnerable to the damages caused by vomiting. Implants, bone grafts, periodontal plastic surgery, jaw surgery, and extractions will all be adversely affected by vomitus. Outcome is reduced, pain increased, and the misery factor multiplied—a lot of badness.

Another unique requirement of dental procedure anesthesia is that treatment in the mouth increases the likelihood of PONV. Treatment site bleeding or oozing is swallowed, detritus from treatment including organic and inorganic dust is swallowed (or possibly aspirated), treatment often produces edema, prolonged oral opening and manipulation can result in tongue and pharynx edema, and dental treatment involves really bad (or worse) tasting materials. These are all PONV provocateurs.

With all treatment occurring in close proximity to the airway, periods of hypoventilation are likely unless a closed airway system is employed. Periods of elevated $PaCO_2$ can lead to PONV. Most dental anesthetics do not employ ETT or other closed-airway-system devices. For instance, oral surgeons provide the majority of dental anesthetics and rarely use ETT.[20]

Underhydration, intraoperative opioid use, oxygen desaturation, prolonged high nitrous oxide concentration, early ambulation, hypoglycemia, and postoperative opioids have all been implicated in PONV. All of these factors can be common, if unintentional, occurrences in dental cases.[43] In preventing pain and PONV for cosmetic procedures, an ounce of prevention truly is worth a pound (or with inflation these days, a ton) of cure. A thoughtfully crafted anesthesia plan begins prior to induction and extends for twenty-four hours. For instance, techniques using minimal opioids, good hydration, adequate alveolar ventilation, and thoughtful recovery techniques will minimize the first nausea episode. Reducing or eliminating opioids from the anesthesia technique looks like a good idea when considering the PONV concern. Remifentanil is the only exception at this time. However, its rapid elimination and favorable distribution characteristics provide negligible postoperative analgesia.

All antiemetics have vastly superior success rates when administered *before* PONV as opposed to their use as a "rescue" therapy. This includes the newer 5-HT$_3$ inhibitors as well as older drugs. The ReliefBand® electric stimulator device works well when used in advance of an episode. Even the lowly OTC drug, meclizine, is effective if given well in advance of the potential triggering events.

VENUE SELECTION

Treatment outside a hospital has always been popular for cosmetic procedures, and the office is the primary location for dental care. The location where a procedure is done has little to do with successful outcomes. Complex surgeries are successfully done on battlefields, makeshift operating rooms, and in many unusual locations. Good cosmetic and dental results have been achieved for millions outside hospitals. The critical ingredient is the training, experience, and ethics of the professionals involved in the treatment.

Dental procedures require special and unique instruments, materials, and procedures. Few hospitals or stand-alone surgery centers are properly equipped. There are many obstacles. Hospital operating rooms are typically arranged for the surgeons and their assistants to be standing. Dental treatment is almost universally provided while sitting.

Dental treatment requires a lot of little x-rays that cannot be exposed accurately with hospital x-ray units. Even a "dental friendly" operating center can stock only a very limited number of dental supplies and materials.

There are *many, many* materials suitable for almost any dental procedures. The technical nuances of using the materials differ from product to product. Suboptimum outcomes are more likely with dentists using unfamiliar or inexactly selected materials.

There are some devices so unique they are unlikely to be found outside a dental office, for example, a ceramic glazing oven, impression mixing machines, and dental lasers. The latest cosmetic materials and techniques often require unique equipment and materials. Treatment options shouldn't be "square pegged" by a facility's "round hole." Finally, dentists, like most professionals, are most comfortable where they are most familiar. If they do not regularly visit a treatment site outside their own offices, they may not be as efficient.

CONSUMER DUE DILIGENCE

Most cosmetic procedures require a considerable financial commitment from the patient. Patients usually invest considerable time and resources selecting a dentist to give them the very best outcome possible. Comfort is usually a part of the calculation. Finding a compatible anesthesia provider to complement the procedure must be part of the equation.

Questions to ask of the anesthesia provider are the following:

1. Is this true "conscious" sedation? (Which means I will be lightly sedated, still respond to verbal commands, and be able to breathe normally without snoring.)

2. Is this a deep sedation technique? (I will not respond to verbal commands and I may need some airway support, e.g., chin lift, mechanical airways.)

3. Will I be given general anesthesia? (Will I be completely asleep? The intravenous medications may be supplemented with an inhalation anesthetic, and a type of artificial airway will probably be used, e.g., endotracheal tube [breathing tube], LMA.)

4. Who will monitor me during the procedure?

5. Will this person have any other responsibilities beside the anesthetic? (The answer should be "no.")

6. How much training and experience with this type of anesthetic does he/she have?

7. What is the rate of successful completion of planned treatment with this type of anesthetic?

8. What type of monitors will be used? (During conscious sedation, your blood pressure, oxygen saturation, heart rate, and respirations should be continuously monitored. Additional monitors are needed if deep sedation or general anesthesia is planned. State regulations may mandate monitoring for different levels. Call or click one's state health professions agency.)

9. How many drugs will be used during the procedure? (When two or three drugs are used together, it increases the likelihood that your sedation may become deep sedation rather than conscious sedation.)

10. If there were a problem, where would I be transferred? How often do problems happen?

11. Who in the office is CPR and/or ACLS certified?

12. How can I reach the anesthesia provider after hours?[43]

REFERENCES

1. Skidmore S: Toothsome treatments; Smile-conscious consumers are boosting the popularity—and profitability—of cosmetic dentistry procedures. *San Diego Union-Tribune.* May 8, 2005; H-1.

2. American Dental Association: ADA Council on Dental Education. Part Two: Guidelines for teaching the comprehensive control of pain and anxiety at the advanced education level. Chicago: First adopted May 1971; reviewed October 2003.

3. American Dental Board of Anesthesiology: *The ADBA Mission.* Available at www.adba.org/mission.html. Accessed June 14, 2005.

4. American Dental Association: ADA Council on Dental Education. Accreditation standards for advanced specialty education programs in oral and maxillofacial surgery. Chicago: Adopted October 1990; reviewed 1998.

5. Field M, ed.: *Dental education at the crossroads: Challenges and changes.* Washington, DC: National Academy Press; 1995.

6. Florida Statue Title , Chapter 466, Section 0285.

7. American Society of Anesthesiologists: Guidelines for office based anesthesia. Reviewed 2000. Available at www.asahq. org/publicationsAndServices/office.pdf. Accessed June 21, 2005.

8. Diogo S: Reconcilable differences?: Dental, medical education remain at odds. *AGD Impact* 28:14,2000.

9. American Psychiatric Association: *Diagnostic and Statistical Manual of Mental Disorders,* 4th ed., text revision. Section 300.29 Specific Phobia of blood-injection-injury type. (443–450) Washington, DC: American Psychiatric Association, 2000.

10. Milgrom P, Garcia RI, Ismail A, et al.: Improving America's access to care: The national institute of dental and craniofacial research addresses oral health disparities. *JADA* 135:1389,2004.

11. Doyle N, Thompson L, Anderson D, et al.: The use of general anesthesia to facilitate dental treatment. *Gen Dent* 51:464, 2003.

12. Newman JF, Gift HC: Regular pattern of preventative dental services: A measure of access. *Soc Sci Med* 35:997,1992.

13. Dionne RA, Gordon SM, McCullagh LM, et al.: Assessing the need for anesthesia and sedation in the general population. *JADA* 129:167,1998.

14. Yagiela JA: Office-based anesthesia in dentistry. Past, present and future trends. *Dent Clin North Am* 43:201,1999.

15. Gordon SM, Dionne RA, Snyder J: Dental fear and anxiety as a barrier to accessing oral health care among patients with special health care needs. *Spec Care Dentist* 18:88,1998.

16. Monk TG, Saini V, Weldon BC, et al.: Anesthetic management and one-year mortality after non-cardiac surgery. *Anesth Analg* 100:4,2005.

17. Kim YC, Lee SH, Noh GJ, et al.: Thermosoftening treatment of the nasotracheal tube before intubation can reduce epistaxis and nasal damage. *Anesth Analg* 91:698,2000.

18. Kristensen MS: The Parker flex-tip tube versus a standard tube for fiberoptic orotracheal intubation: A randomized double-blind study. *Anesthesiol* 98:354,2003.

19. ASDA membership survey, 2004.

20. Oral and Maxillofacial Surgery National Insurance Company: Anesthesia Morbidity and Mortality: 1988–2001. Rosemont, IL: OMSNIC, 2002.

21. Perrott DH, Yuen JP, Anderson RV, Dodson TB: Office-based ambulatory anesthesia: Outcomes of clinical practice

of oral and maxillofacial surgeons. *J Oral Maxillofac Surg* 61:983,2003.

22. Parameters of care for oral and maxillofacial surgery: A guide for practice, monitoring and evaluation. *J Oral Maxillofac Surg* 53:5S,1995.

23. NovaMed: Lifesound heart and breath sound monitoring system: The gold standard in telemetric auscultation. Available at http://www.novamed-usa.com/LifeSound%20Heart%20&%20Breath%20Monitor.html. Accessed July 7, 2005.

24. Aspect Medical Systems: An important refinement in brain monitoring. Available at www.aspectmedical.com/assets/documents/pdf/or_brochure.pdf. Accessed June 20, 2005.

25. Mak S, Crowley J: The utility of the Bispectral Index vs. standard practice anesthetic care: A meta analysis of randomized trials comparing drug reduction and recovery times. *SAMBA Newsletter* Park Ridge, IL: American Society of Anesthesiologists, 2002.

26. Boodman SG: It knows when you're awake. *Washington Post, Health Section.* November 23, 2004.

27. Song D, Joshi GP, White PF: Titration of volatile anesthetics using bispectral index facilitates emergence after ambulatory anesthesia. *Anesthesiol* 87:842,1997.

28. Moore P: Data presented at ASDA, April 2005.

29. Neumann MA, Weiskopf RB, Gong DH, et al.: Changing from isoflurane to desflurane toward the end of anesthesia does not accelerate recovery in humans. *Anesthesiol* 88:914, 1998.

30. Pavlin DJ, Rapp SE, Polissar NL, et al.: Factors affecting discharge time in adult outpatients. *Anesth Analg* 87:816,1999.

31. Dionne RA, Wirdzek PR, Fox PC, et al.: Anesthesiology suppression of postoperative pain by the combination of a nonsteroidal antidrug, flurbiprofen, and a long-acting local anesthetic, etidocaine. *JADA* 108:598,1985.

32. Jinks SL, Antognini JF, Dutton RC, et al.: Isoflurane depresses windup of C fiber-evoked limb withdrawal with variable effects on nociceptive lumbar spinal neurons in rats. *Anesth Analg* 99:1413,2004.

33. Man D: Premedication with oral clonidine for facial rhytidectomy. *Plast Reconstr Surg* 94:214,1994.

34. Baker TM, Stuzin JM, Baker TJ, et al.: What's new in aesthetic surgery? *Clin Plast Surg* 23:16,1996.

35. Friedberg BL, Sigl JC: Clonidine premedication decreases propofol consumption during bispectral (BIS) index monitored propofol-ketamine technique for office based surgery. *Dermatol Surg* 26:848,2000.

36. Hall JE, Uhrich TD, Barney JA, et al.: Sedative, amnesic and analgesic properties of small-dose dexmedetomidine infusions. *Anesth Analg* 90:699,2000.

37. Gentili M, Bernard JM, Bonnet F: Adding clonidine to lidocaine for intravenous regional anesthesia prevents tourniquet pain. *Anesth Analg* 88:1327,1999.

38. Reuben SS, Steinberg RB, Klatt JL, et al.: Intravenous regional anesthesia using lidocaine and clonidine. *Anesthesiol* 91:654, 1999.

39. Goyagi T, Tanaka M, Nishikawa T: Oral clonidine premedication reduces induction dose and prolongs awakening time from propofol-nitrous oxide anesthesia. *Can J Anaesth* 46:894,1999.

40. Dalsasso M, Tresin P, Innocente F, et al.: Low-dose ketamine with clonidine and midazoalm for adult day care surgery. *Eur J Anesthesiol* 22:67,2005.

41. Wang J, Ho S, Tzeng J, et al.: The effect of timing of dexamethasone administration on its efficacy as prophylactic antiemetic for nausea and vomiting. *Anesth Analg* 91:136, 2000.

42. Henzi, I, Walder B, Tramer MR: Dexamethasone for the prevention of postoperative nausea and vomiting: A quantitative systematic review. *Anesth Analg* 90:186,2000.

43. Snyder JA: Communicating with patients about OBA: SOBA's patient assistance sheet. *Am J Anesthesiol* 591, 2000.

6 | Propofol Ketamine (PK) in the UK, Propofol Ketamine Beyond Cosmetic Surgery

Chris Pollock, M.B.

INTRODUCTION

"Nothing can be said to be certain except death and taxes."[1] Had Benjamin Franklin lived two centuries later, he might have cared to add a third—anesthesia with nausea. It is almost an expectation by both patients with health professionals alike that nausea and vomiting follow general anesthesia: it is the "big little problem," it "goes with the territory." Can anesthesiologists honestly conceive of a day when the emesis basin in the PACU is relegated to the museum? Perhaps not, but how far are anesthesiologists moving toward that halcyon day, and exactly just how serious are anesthesiologists about preventing or even treating postoperative nausea and vomiting (PONV)? Just how close are anesthesiologists to "zero tolerance" using what is currently available? Just how often is the full panoply of the available antiemetics prescribed, and just how often are those that are prescribed administered in a timely fashion and by an appropriate route? Just exactly how seriously are anesthesiologists interested in eliminating PONV?

The risk of PONV is generally conceived as an attribute of the patient with subsidiary risks attached to the **context**, **that is**, the drugs and operation. However, drugs themselves have no executive power. Additionally, it is unusual for a patient scheduled for elective surgery to enter the theater suite with *preoperative* nausea and vomiting. The uncomfortable reality surely must be that the major risk factor for the presence or absence of PONV is the choice of the anesthesiologist. For it is, indeed, he or she who chooses which drugs and which techniques to employ and which to avoid in the perioperative management of that patient. Lastly, it is the anesthesiologist's responsibility to ensure that what has been prescribed for the postoperative management is, in fact, given.

The commonest approach to the PONV problem is to continue giving the standard emetogenic anesthetic and bolt on antiemetic drugs,[2] either as prophylaxis, as rescue medication, or as both. This may lessen the immediate PONV burden but does not abolish it. Reliably continuing this type of strategy into the postoperative period on the ward or at home is problematic.

The other approach is to minimize or eliminate the use of drugs that are known to contribute to PONV, to reduce the baseline, as it were. For this strategy some changes are relatively easy to make, for example, the avoidance of nitrous oxide (N_2O). Thus, in using an inhalational anesthetic technique, adjustments can be made to compensate for the absence of the N_2O without a major alteration in the technique itself. Nowadays, especially with the availability of desflurane and sevoflurane, vapors with relatively low blood gas solubility coefficients, the rate of emergence from anesthesia need not necessarily be prolonged in the absence of N_2O. It is probably this ease of elimination from the anesthetic technique that has focused attention on nitrous oxide as the *bete noir* of PONV, but it is perhaps less of a key player in PONV than has been supposed.[2]

Eliminating anesthetic vapors, by contrast, requires a significant change in both technique and hardware. However, it is the use of opioids that is probably the major contributor to PONV. It is the minimization of their use in the *whole* perioperative period that is the real challenge. The *whole* perioperative period is emphasized as there is little to be achieved by avoiding emetogenic agents *during* the anesthetic and then relying on *postoperative* opioids as the main means of pain control.[3]

John Snow is widely regarded as the father of British anesthesia, but in his own lifetime he was more noted for his epidemiological aptitude. He traced the source of a major outbreak of cholera in London in 1854 to a well. Snow famously interrupted this epidemic by the simple expedient of removing the handle from the water pump in Broad Street, Golden Square, London. Were he alive today how might he have combined his epidemiological and his anesthetic interests in approaching the PONV problem? Would some of the handles be removed from certain drug cupboards in the anesthetic room? Perhaps.

In the United Kingdom, almost all general anesthetics are given within a hospital setting. There is neither an administrative nor a financial incentive to the individual anesthesiologist to eliminate PONV. For a patient operated on in a Day Surgery Unit who has "intractable" PONV, an overnight bed can always be found. *Managing the PONV subsequently becomes somebody else's problem.* It is therefore worthwhile to look to the office-based practitioners for innovative ways around that "big little problem." Early discharge and fully managed PONV is a prerequisite for the office-based practice and commercial survival.

PROPOFOL KETAMINE (PK) ANESTHESIA

Friedberg has reported a twenty-four-hour incidence of PONV of 0.6% in elective cosmetic surgical procedures,[4] a whole order below the 7% result quoted by Eberhart using a total intravenous anesthetic technique along with three prophylactic antiemetics.[5] PK is the immediate heir to the diazepam and ketamine technique devised by Vinnik,[6] which retained the desirable properties of ketamine while abolishing the undesirable dysphoria. Friedberg replaced the diazepam with propofol, which has a far superior pharmacokinetic profile, while still maintaining the taming of ketamine. PK is perhaps more usefully paraphrased as "PK LA," which emphasizes the key part that the *local* anesthesia plays in providing the analgesic component.

Ketamine is a dissociative agent with analgesic activity, but its predominant role in PK is to minimize patient movement in response to the local anesthetic injections rather than to the surgery itself. *Ketamine certainly should not be viewed as an opioid replacement.* Sleep doses of propofol reliably block the unpleasant hallucinogenic hazard of ketamine.[4]

PK was originally conceived for use in office-based elective cosmetic surgery practice, in part to reduce the capital and running costs of providing anesthesia. The potential for PK to substantially improve patient outcomes also makes it highly relevant for hospital-based practitioners.

The PK technique as described is strictly appropriate only for noncavity surgery, with the intraoperative analgesia being provided either by nerve conduction blockade or field block (see Chapters 9 and 10). PK can, however, also be used to considerable advantage in minor gynecological and urological surgery *without* the additional use of local anesthesia. PK anesthesia has been well evaluated for surgery in adults, but the experience in its use in pediatric practice is more limited. PK does appear to compare favorably with more standard anesthetic approaches in this group. Over the last five years, Pollock has had the opportunity to use PK anesthesia for a variety of surgical procedures, both adult and pediatric. The response by patients, surgeons, PACU, and ward nurses has been very positive.

Pollock's English surgeons are more accustomed to operating on patients under general anesthesia rather than under local infiltration anesthesia. So it is prudent for the anesthesiologist to take the responsibility for the infiltration of local anesthetic or nerve block prior to the surgery and to present the surgeon with a patient "as if under GA." Although it may seem obvious, it is imperative that the anesthesiologist discuss with the surgeon beforehand exactly where the initial incision and subsequent dissection is going to be to ensure the correct placement of local anesthetic. If the local anesthetic doesn't cover the whole field of the surgery, no amount of rhetoric about improved postoperative outcomes is going to enamor the surgeon to a technique that does not emulate the conditions of a more standard general anesthetic, namely, a relatively still operating field.

In the United Kingdom and most of Europe, Target Controlled Infusion (TCI) pumps incorporating Diprifuser™ are available to administer propofol from prefilled 50-ml syringes to adults. The Diprifuser™ subsystem and software uses a readable tab on the syringe to identify the propofol concentration as either 1% or 2%. The software includes pharmacokinetic parameters based on a three-compartment model. The variables, which can be keyed in at the beginning of anesthesia, are the patient's age (16–100 yrs.), weight (30–150 kg), and the target blood concentration to be achieved. The pumps offer a choice of rate of induction between 30 seconds and 10 minutes. In these pumps, the typical default settings are 40 years, 70 kg, and $4 \text{ ug} \cdot \text{ml}^{-1}$. Hence, for a more elderly or physiologically brittle patient, a lower blood concentration and a slower speed of induction might be chosen. Although the Diprifusor™ takes care of the time-dependent aspects of the infusion, the anesthesiologist needs to adjust the desired target level of blood propofol in light of the individual patient response to noxious or indeed nonnoxious stimulation. It is analogous to adjusting the dial setting on a plenum vaporizer for an inhalational anesthetic. Biological variability certainly rules out a "one target concentration suits all" approach. The correct concentration for any individual is empirical rather than predictable. Whereas the default setting of $4 \text{ ug} \cdot \text{ml}^{-1}$ propofol manages the majority of adult patients, some will require a $10 \text{ ug} \cdot \text{ml}^{-1}$ setting (or even higher) to prevent intraoperative movement. Without a level-of-consciousness monitor, like the BIS, it is impossible to differentiate spinal-cord–generated patient movement from brain-generated patient movement. Suppressing movement with additional propofol is not as optimal a strategy as empirically injecting more local to the operative field. After completion of the surgery, patients may well then wake up very rapidly after discontinuation of the infusion and be completely pain free. The high concentration requirement may *not* be a result of noxious stimulation within an area uncovered by the local anesthetic block.

REVIEW OF BREAST SURGERY USING PK FROM AUGUST 2000 TO AUGUST 2004 (POLLOCK'S SERIES)

Conduct of the Anesthetic

The majority of the breast procedures were for tumor management both benign and malignant. Without the BIS monitor to guide therapy, one may be hard-pressed to gain the surgeon's cooperation. One suppresses movement at the expense of adding incoming noxious afferent stimulation, which may add to postoperative pain management.

In the anesthetic room, a 22G cannula was placed ideally in the nondominant antecubital fossa. Patients were then given 40 mg bolus of propofol (or titrated up to 40 mg in the elderly or frail) and transferred to the operating theater. There, standard monitoring was attached, oxygen via a Hudson mask at $1 \text{ L} \cdot \text{min}^{-1}$ administered, and the patient turned into the lateral position if intercostal nerve blocks were planned (see Chapter 10). The initial dose of propofol provides significant relief of anxiety and acts as an indicator of the likely sensitivity (or resistance) to the drug. Propofol was then infused using a Diprifusor™ infusion pump set to default values for age, weight, and blood concentration and a 30-seconds induction time. After loss of consciousness, ketamine 50 mg was administered. Local anesthetic was administered either by infiltrating the proposed surgical area or by intercostal blocks performed posteriorly at the angle of the ribs from T6 to T1, with 5 ml injected at each level after negative aspiration for air and blood. Although additional patient positioning is required to perform the intercostal blocks using a posterior approach,[7] it allows access to T1–3. Inasmuch as the depth of the rib is greatest at the posterior angle (about 8 mm), the posterior approach also minimizes the risk of pneumothorax in comparison to the lateral approach.[8] If the surgery was likely to extend to T3 or into the axilla, a supraclavicular block was added. The standard local anesthetic used was a 1:1 mixture of 1% lidocaine with 1:200,000 epinephrine and 0.25% L-bupivacaine.[9] For procedures where large volumes of local anesthetic were necessary (e.g., latissimus dorsi flaps), the lidocaine was omitted and 0.25% L-bupivicaine with 1:200,000 epinephrine was used on its own.

If there was no contraindication, an NSAID was included at some time during the procedure either as rofecoxib 50 mg oral preoperatively or ketorolac 10 mg intraoperatively. With the withdrawal of rofecoxib from the market, parecoxib 40 mg or etoricoxib 90 mg PO are Pollock's current choice of agents.

For patients who would be sat up at some stage during the operation (e.g., breast-reduction patients or patients undergoing latissimus dorsi flap [LDF] breast reconstructions), glycopyrrolate 0.2 mg was used at induction as an antisialogogue to reduce the likelihood of coughing. Its utility in patients who remained supine was less apparent, and thus was not routinely given (see Tables 6-1 and 6-2). Details of the patients' age, weight, propofol usage, and duration of anesthetic are given in Table 6-3. All the patients were ASA 1 or 2, apart from twelve who were ASA 3.

Ketamine 50 mg bolus was adequate for 98% of the patients, the remaining 2% requiring up to 100 mg to minimize movement while injecting the local anesthetic. Intraoperative coughing was a problem in twenty-four patients requiring bolus doses of lidocaine 30–50 mg and increasing the propofol infusion rate to settle. In Pollock's experience, coughing tended to occur early in the anesthetic and did not appear to be more common in smokers compared with nonsmokers. As previously mentioned, the administration of glycopyrrolate did not have an obvious effect in reducing the incidence of coughing. All patients were effec-

Table 6-2. Procedures using PK and intercostals blocks

1. Wide local excisions	332
2. Wide local excisions plus axillary gland sampling	330
3. Mastectomy +/−Prosthesis or tissue expander +/− axillary gland sample	267
4. Mastectomy with latissimus dorsi flap	9
5. Breast reductions (25 bilateral)	32
6. Axillary clearance/sampling	27
7. Breast prosthesis insertion/replacement	149
8. Breast augmentation	10
9. Miscellaneous	24
Total breast surgical procedures	1,439

tively managed by the lidocaine and a transient increase in the propofol infusion rate. None required opioids or paralyzing agents to control it.

At the beginning of the anesthesia, the Diprifuser™ is set for a slow induction over thirty seconds. This typically gives rise to a loss of consciousness after thirty to sixty seconds. Nevertheless, apnea often occurred, but its duration was very brief (less than fifteen seconds), and blood oxygen saturation was well maintained by the prior use of supplemental oxygen through a Hudson mask. No patient required ventilation on account of prolonged apnea. The majority of airways could be maintained by careful positioning of the head. In a few patients (26 of 1,439, or 1.7%), a nasopharyngeal airway had to be inserted, particularly in those procedures where the patient was sat upright.

Although patient movement is not uncommon with PK, its incidence and severity decreased with experience in using the technique. Rarely did patient movement interfere with the conduct of the surgery. Five patients required supplemental opioids (nalbuphine or tramadol along with two antiemetics) during the operation. Only one patient, an LDF procedure, required conversion to a more standard general anesthetic with a laryngeal mask, opiate, paralysis, and ventilation.

Patient Outcomes

Pneumothorax as detected by aspiration of air prior to injecting the local anesthetic occurred in three patients (0.36% of patients, 0.06% per space injected). None of

Table 6-1. Procedures using PK and local anesthetic infiltration

1. Fibroadenomas	109
2. Major duct excision	123
3. Excision male gynecomastia	10
4. Scar revision	17
Total	259

Table 6-3. Surgical procedures

Procedure	Age yrs	Wt kg	Prop mg	T min
1. Excision fibroademona and similar	32 (16–60)	63 (40–109)	373 (174–970)	19 (8–54)
2. Wide local excision c axillary sample	58 (31–86)	69 (41–117)	601 (274–2612)	40 (20–110)
3. Mastectomy +/− axillary sample +/− implant	59 (28–92)	70 (45–130)	775 (240–2653)	76 (22–215)
4. Latissimus dorsi flap +/− mastectomy	48 (36–68)	77 (61–107)	3656 (2400–5132)	335 (180–403)

the patients became symptomatic and were treated expectantly. In other series, the incidence of pneumothorax was as low as 0.073%,[10] but typically they are closer to 2%.[11–13]

One eighty-year-old ASA 3 patient died on the third postoperative day from a stroke. Preoperatively she was in intermittent atrial fibrillation (AF) and heart failure. The procedure was a mastectomy and axillary gland clearance.

There was one instance of awareness during the operation (a mammotome excision of gynecomastia) in a 100 kg male, but without intraoperative discomfort. This probably resulted from the inappropriate reduction in the rate of propofol infusion near the beginning of the anesthetic after 75 mg of ketamine had been administered. There were no reports of unpleasant dreams or feelings on questioning in the PACU. Indeed, most patients experienced decidedly pleasant dreams, although the content was typically mundane. The recall of the dream was rapidly lost soon after awakening. Thus, the timing of questions regarding dreaming will be critical to the response. This may explain the marked discrepancy between this and other reports of an incidence of dreaming in only 1% of patients.[4] Nevertheless, the important observation is that, given the bad reputation of ketamine for emergence dysphoria, there were no such cases in this series. Pollock has related his patients' dreams as being pleasant. It is probably more accurate to state that the patients were in a rather euphoric state[14] and that they were dreaming; the two were not necessarily linked.

Postoperative strong opioids were required in 21% of the patients in the PACU. Using titrated morphine,

the median dose was 6 mg, the maximum 20 mg. All patients receiving morphine were given ondansetron 4 mg and cyclizine (Marazine) 10 mg at the same time. Only two patients required additional morphine during their stay on the ward. Oral codeine or tramadol was available on the ward along with paracetamol (acetaminophen) and an NSAID. Two-thirds of the patients were inpatients and were reviewed the following day (a minimum of fifteen hours postoperatively). The incidence of nausea (requiring treatment with antiemetics) was 2.2% and of vomiting 0.27%. The majority of these episodes appeared to be in association with the use of oral codeine or tramadol postoperatively. This rate is approaching Friedberg's incidence of 0.6%.[4] The comparable incidence of PONV in breast-surgery patients under general anesthesia (GA) and single-level paravertebral block was 33%.[15] With paravertebral block and conscious sedation (CS), the PONV rate was 20%.[16, 17] This rate may relate to the use of opioids as part of the CS technique. The twenty-four-hour PONV incidence after a GA using sevoflurane, fentanyl, and prophylactic ondansetron was 17%.[18]

In the United Kingdom, there is no regulatory advantage in defining a procedure as "deep sedation" as opposed to "general anesthesia" (GA). The two significant distinctions are between conscious sedation, which can be given by a nonanesthesiologist, and general anesthesia, which need be administered by a physician trained in anesthesia. Deep sedation is regarded as a GA. Nonetheless, deep sedation using PK appears to be an optimum mode of management in breast surgery in (a) avoiding the failure rate of 9% using paravertebral block with CS,[17] and (b) the PONV morbidity associated with a more standard GA, or a CS that includes the use of opioids. An additional advantage is the absence of delay between completing the blocks and commencement of surgery. Either the inclusion of lidocaine in the block or the analgesic effect of the ketamine allowed satisfactory operating conditions to be achieved almost straight away after performance of the local anesthetic block, avoiding the twenty-four-minute set up time for CS plus paravertebral block.[19] The time to complete a set unilateral intercostals blocks was typically between 90 and 120 seconds. In using PK and intercostal nerve block, there is a limited increase in setup time compared to general anesthesia, but there is a substantial improvement in the quality and duration of analgesia. The outcome from this approach is a major reduction in the use of perioperative opioids. This minimization of opioid use combined with the avoidance of vapors and nitrous oxide lurches the benchmark for PONV decidedly far to the left.

Intercostal block is neither a widely utilized nor a widely taught procedure in the United Kingdom. The literature enthuses about its use in (a) open cholecystectomy where it reduces opioid requirement (but does not abolish it), (b) in rib fracture management—which rarely comes to the attention of the practicing anesthesiologist, and (c) in thoracic surgery, where its benefit is limited as the posterior branch of the intercostal nerve is better picked up by either an epidural or paravertebral block. In addition, pneumothorax is perceived as a risk better avoided than managed. In reality, the posterior approach to intercostal blockade is surprisingly safe—even in moderately obese patients. Intercostal blockade (a) has a prolonged duration of action, (b) is quick to perform, (c) can be used with a reasonable regard to the infiltration of LA onto the rib, acceptable to an unsedated patient, and (d) has high degree of efficacy. The incidence of pneumothorax is about 1%. The vast majority of patients is asymptomatic and can be managed expectantly.

REVIEW OF PK FOR MINOR GYNECOLOGICAL PROCEDURES

Conduct of the Anesthetic

PK anesthesia as described[4] requires local anesthetic infiltration or nerve block to provide the analgesic platform for the procedure. Nonetheless, for short gynecological procedures with a minimal incisional stimulus, the same technique can be successfully employed without the necessity of presurgical infiltration with local anesthetic. In procedures such as suction termination of pregnancy (STOP), acceptable operating conditions can be achieved, along with a good recovery profile particularly in relation to PONV by using PK. Even for laparoscopic clip sterilization, it is feasible to use PK if the intraperitoneal insufflation of carbon dioxide is not excessive and the surgeon is well skilled.

Patients were given an NSAID if there was no contraindication either as an oral premed (rofecoxib 50 mg) or at induction (ketorolac 10 mg). For the patients who did not receive an NSAID, tramadol 100 mg was given at induction along with 10 mg cyclizine (Marazine) as an antiemetic. Cervical misoprostal was applied two hours preoperatively in patients for STOP. A sedative dose of propofol (40 mg) was given in the anesthetic room, and then the patient was transferred to the operating theater. There standard monitoring was attached, and oxygen $1 \text{ L} \cdot \text{min}^{-1}$ administered through a Hudson mask with gas sampling for the display of expired CO_2. In these relatively short cases, the propofol was titrated manually instead of by Diprifusor.™ Further increments of propofol were administered until loss of consciousness, then ketamine 30–50 mg was given. Further increments of propofol were administered during the procedure to maintain loss of consciousness and in response to excessive movement to the surgical stimulus. It is important not to give large boli of propofol in response to movement but to titrate it in order to avoid apneic episodes. There is often some patient movement (adduction of legs in response to cervical dilatation), but this is rarely of such severity to interfere with the conduct of the procedure.

The anesthetic management for the laparoscopies was similar, but with the addition of 0.5% bupivicaine infiltration of the abdominal wall at the sites of instrumentation. These patients were positioned with a thirty-degree head down tilt (see Table 6-2). **All** the procedures were performed as day cases, and postoperative assessment was limited to six hours after the procedure (see Table 6-4).

Patient Outcomes

Two patients (1.4%) vomited in the postoperative period, one patient in the STOP group, and the other patient after a laparoscopy and tubal clip who had received morphine without antiemetic prophylaxis in the PACU. There were no additional patients with significant nausea requiring medication. No patient experienced dysphoria. This low incidence of PONV in the absence of routine antiemetic prophylaxis is encouraging in a group of procedures that are regarded as being of high risk. As in the breast procedures, the use of ketamine did not precipitate any instances of unpleasant dreams or feelings.

Table 6-4. Details of minor gynecological procedures under PK anesthesia

Procedure	N	Age yrs	Wt kg	Prop mg	K mg	T min
1. STOP,[a] ERPC	117 (14–43)	24 (40–104)	65 (100–375)	187 (35–50)	45 (5–15)	10
2. Lap[b]	22	31 (18–49)	65 (54–95)	302 (227–480)	59 (50–75)	15 (10–24)
3. Hscopy[c]	5	49 (44–52)	78 (72–90)	234 (150–250)	48 (40–50)	12 (10–15)
4. Misc[d]	3	37 (27–48)	86 (73–94)	233 (200–350)	50 (50)	13 (5–20)

[a]STOP—suction termination of pregnancy
[b]Laparoscopy with and without tubal clips
[c]Hscopy—hysteroscopy
[d]Misc.—insertion of coil, balloon endometrial ablation, excision Bartholin's cyst

In principle, any operation that *could* be performed using local anesthesia in a fully cooperative awake child *would* be a candidate for PK plus local anesthetic in the more typical, uncooperative child. The chief issues are (a) does it work in children, (b) how well is the airway maintained, and (c) is it worth the additional effort?

Does it work in children? Yes, but not as smoothly as in adults. In an adult, ketamine 50 mg (less than 1 mg · kg^{-1}) is usually sufficient to prevent significant movement in response to LA infiltration or other moderate noxious stimulus. In children, even with a dose of ketamine of 2 mg · kg^{-1}, there can often be substantial movement. Increasing the dose above 2 mg · kg^{-1} compromises the speed of recovery. Reduce the stimulus of the local anesthetic injection by (a) using of a fine gauge (30 ga) needle, (b) buffering the LA with sodium bicarbonate, and (c) injecting into distensible tissue planes slowly. Airway integrity? Yes, again. As with adults, the key is to titrate the propofol and to eschew large boli in order to minimize the occurrence of central apnea and of glossopharyngeal relaxation. Active laryngeal reflexes as evinced by coughing are present (although not guaranteed). In the few children who developed upper-airway obstruction, a chin lift was all that was required to recover a patent airway. Is it worth the additional effort? There are obviously issues around the debate between an intubated or laryngeal masked airway versus the unintubated airway that only a large comparative study

can address. The avoidance of triggering agents for malignant hyperpyrexia (MH) and the likely greatly reduced PONV are certainly in favor of PK.

REVIEW OF PK IN OTOPLASTY IN CHILDREN

Conduct of the Anesthetic

All the children were admitted to the hospital ward and most were discharged home the same evening. Those that weren't discharged were kept overnight for domestic or transport reasons. Children were unpremedicated but had topical Ametop gel applied over a vein on the dorsum of the hand or in the antecubital fossa. Anesthesia was induced with increments of propofol, and then either a pediatric Hudson mask or nasal prongs were positioned and oxygen 1 L · min^{-1} administered. Ketamine 1 mg · kg^{-1} was given, increasing to 2 mg · kg^{-1} if there was significant movement while the local anesthetic was being infiltrated. The surgeons routinely inject 0.5% lidocaine with epinephrine into the auricle to separate the tissue planes and to improve hemostasis. The injection is usually very stimulating and would require a relatively high dose of ketamine to minimize movement. An additional ketamine bolus would need to be given prior to injecting the second ear twenty minutes or so later. Additional ketamine can be avoided if bilateral auriculotemporal and posterior auricular blocks are performed after induction. These nerve blocks allow

Table 6-5. PK Anesthesia for pediatric procedures 3 unilateral otoplasties

Procedure	N	Age	Wt	Prop	K	T
		yrs	kg	mg	mg	min
1. Oto[a]	85	9.6 (2–15)	37 (13–66)	366 (100–690)	50 (10–10)	52 (22–100)
2. Other[b]	170	8 (1–15)	34 (8–103)	214 (30–802)	37 (10–100)	23 (5–90)

[a]Oto—Otoplasty
[b]See text for details of "Other"

both sides to be injected in quick succession under a single dose of ketamine. Inasmuch as these blocks are less stimulating than the intra-auricular infiltration, the total dose of ketamine can be substantially reduced. The nerve blocks are performed with a 1:1 mixture of 1% lidocaine with epinephrine and 0.25% L-bupivicaine, typically 2–3 ml per side. The subsequent surgical infiltration of the ears with 0.5% lidocaine and epinephrine evokes minimal movement. In addition, bupivicaine provides prolonged postoperative analgesia, minimizing the need for postoperative, emetogenic opioids. The current Diprifusor™ pumps are not suitable for use in children. Hypnosis was maintained by incremental injections throughout the surgery. There were eighty-five children, of whom three had unilateral surgery.

Patient movement during local-anesthetic intra-auricular infiltration was a problem in the earlier patients, but this was largely resolved by the use of the nerve blocks, and thus the ketamine requirements and wake-up time became progressively less. Three children coughed during the early stages of the anesthetic, requiring suction of the oropharynx and cautious deepening with propofol. One child briefly lost his upper airway, which was regained by a chin lift under the surgical drapes. Neither supplemental opioids nor conversion to a GA was required for any of the cases.

Patient Outcomes

Awakening time was highly variable. Some children were chatting while the bandages were being put on, but others took up to fifteen minutes to emerge. The PACU nursing staff tended to allow children to awaken in their own time without exogenous stimulation. A common spontaneous complaint by children on awakening was of double vision and a feeling of dizziness. Horizontal nystagmus was frequently observable, but there were no incidences of vomiting in the PACU. One child said he had had an unpleasant dream. Follow up the following day by phone to the ward or to the home elicited one patient with vomiting (1.2%).

No child required oral opioids postoperatively, and all were managed on oral paracetamol (acetaminophen) and ibuprofen. The type of follow up was not adequate to elicit the presence or absence of dysphoric symptoms.

OTHER PK PEDIATRIC EXPERIENCE

PK anesthesia was used in a further 170 children between one and fifteen years of age for a variety of superficial procedures, including (a) toe straightening surgery, (b) hypospadias repair, (c) excision of skin nevi, (d) scar revision, and (e) the removal of wires or screws after resolution of bone fractures. These were mainly performed as day procedures. There were no management problems during the anesthetic. Again, no patients required oral opioids in the postoperative period, and there were no episodes of vomiting prior to discharge.

CONCLUSION

PK anesthesia is feasible in adult patients and children over the age of one year having superficial surgery, without producing problems relating to airway management or respiratory depression. In all the cases where the upper airway was lost, a simple chin lift was all that was required to restore ventilation. The reliance on long-acting local anesthetics to provide the analgesic platform for the surgery to take place allows the elimination (or minimization) of opioids in the perioperative period and thus avoids significant respiratory depression and unnecessary vomiting. The elimination of triggering agents for MH was certainly reassuring. Some wake-up times in the PACU were perhaps longer than with conventional GA techniques, particularly with the very young, but this did not lead to delayed discharge from the hospital.

PK anesthesia plus local anesthetic infiltration is a serious contender as the technique of choice for optimum patient outcomes with the low risk of PONV—in part from the minimization of opioid use while still maintaining good quality postoperative analgesia. Even latissimus dorsi flap reconstruction of breast defects lasting six hours or more were manageable on single-shot intercostal blockade and PK, with subsequent limited postoperative opioid requirement. There is minimal respiratory depression in comparison to benzodiazepine with opiate sedation.[20] Success with the technique does require close cooperation with the surgeon. *PK anesthesia is best appreciated by surgeons with whom one works regularly,* rather than on an occasional basis. To the unwary, the modest patient movement that may occur may be misinterpreted as an inadequate general anesthesia. With perseverance, the nuances of PK can be mastered, critically altering the "always sick after anesthesia" to the more measured "usually sick after anesthesia, but *not today*! Anesthesia can be different."

REFERENCES

1. Franklin B: Letter to Jean Baptiste Le Roy. In *Writings*. 1789, vol x.
2. Apfel CC, Kortilla K, Abdalla M, et al.: A factorial trial of six interventions for the prevention of postoperative nausea and vomiting. *N Engl J Med* 350:2441,2004.
3. White PF: Prevention of postoperative nausea and vomiting—A multimodal solution to a persistent problem. *N Engl J Med* 350:2511,2004.
4. Friedberg BL: Propofol-ketamine technique: Dissociative anesthesia for office surgery (a 5-year review of 1,264 cases). *Aesth Plast Surg* 23:70,1999.
5. Eberhart LH, Mauch M, Morin AM, et al.: Impact of a multimodal anti-emetic prophylaxis on patient satisfaction in high risk patients for postoperative nausea and vomiting. *Anaesthesia* 57:1022,2002.
6. Vinnik CA: An intravenous dissociative technique for outpatient plastic surgery: Tranquility in the office surgical facility. *Plast Reconstr Surg* 67:799,1981.
7. Kopacz DJ, Thompson GE: Intercostal blocks for thoracic and abdominal surgery. *Techniques in Regional Anesthesia & Pain Management* 2:25,1998.
8. Moore DC, Bush WH, Scurlock JE: Intercostal nerve block: A roentgenographic anatomic study of technique and absorption in humans. *Anesth Analg* 59:815,1980.
9. Badgwell JM, Heavner JE, Kytta J: Cardiovascular and central nervous system effects of co-administered lidocaine and bupivicaine in piglets. *Reg Anesth* 16:89,1991.
10. Moore DC: Intercostal nerve block for postoperative somatic pain following surgery of the thorax and upper abdomen. *Br J Anaesth* 47:284,1975.
11. Moore DC: Intercostal nerve block for postoperative somatic pain following surgery of the thorax and upper abdomen. *Br J Anaesth* 47:284,1975.
12. Bridenbaugh PO, DuPen SL, Moore DC, et al.: Postoperative intercostals nerve block analgesia versus narcotic analgesia. *Anesth Analg* 52:81,1973.
13. Cronin KD, Davies MJ: Intercostal block for postoperative pain relief. *Anaesth Intens Care* 4:25–9,1976.
14. Mortero RF, Clark LD, Tolan MM, et al.: The effects of small-dose ketamine on propofol sedation: Respiration, postoperative mood, perception, cognition, and pain. *Anesth Analg* 92:1465,2001.
15. Kairaluoma PM, Bachmann MS, Korpinen AK, et al.: Single-injection paravertebral block before general anesthesia enhances analgesia after breast cancer surgery with and without associated lymph node biopsy. *Anesth Analg* 99:1837,2004.
16. Coveney E, Weltz CR, Greengrass R, et al.: Use of paravertebral block anesthesia in the surgical management of breast cancer. *Ann Surg* 227:496,1998.
17. Weltz CR, Greengrass RA, Lyerly HK: Ambulatory surgical management of breast carcinoma using paravertebral block. *Ann Surg* 222:19,1995.
18. Jokela MR, Kangas-Saarela TA, Valanne JVI, et al.: Postoperative nausea and vomiting after sevoflurane with or without ondansetron compared with propofol in female patients undergoing breast surgery. *Anesth Analg* 91:1062, 2000.
19. Klein SM, Bergh A, Steele SM: Thoracic paravertebral block for breast surgery. *Anesth Analg* 90:1402,2000.
20. Avaramov MN, Smith I, White PF: Interactions between midazolam and remifentanil during monitored anesthesia care. *Anesthesiol* 85:1283,1996.

7 | Propofol Ketamine Beyond Cosmetic Surgery: Implications for Military Medicine and Mass-Casualty Anesthesia

Joel W. McMasters, M.D., MAJ, MC, U.S.A.

INTRODUCTION

The terrorist attacks of September 11, 2001, forced medical personnel throughout the United States to reevaluate their capabilities for dealing with mass-casualty situations. This included the specialty of anesthesiology, which had to reexamine its readiness for delivering anesthesia in a chaotic environment. Anesthesiologists know that mass-casualty situations challenge health care professionals because of large numbers of patients, time constraints, and limited resources. In settings such as this, there likely would be more patients requiring surgery and anesthesia than there are anesthesia machines and traditional anesthetizing locations. Thus, mass-casualty situations would be better managed if physicians had anesthetic tools that were more versatile and portable. The anesthesia community familiar with total intravenous anesthesia (TIVA) gave Army anesthesiologists ideas for improving mass-casualty anesthesia. Avoiding the need of heavy and bulky anesthesia machines, propofol-ketamine (PK) anesthesia[1–3] and other combinations of intravenous agents seemed ideal for mass-casualty care.

Army anesthesiologists have begun exploring TIVA as a way of delivering anesthesia on the battlefield of the future, where large numbers of casualties could be the norm. In this chapter we examine how PK anesthesia and TIVA are ideally suited for mass-casualty anesthesia.

THE CASE FOR TIVA

Why is TIVA an ideal anesthetic for military anesthesia and mass-casualty situations? TIVA is simple to deliver, as one needs only a working intravenous line and the appropriate drugs. TIVA is more scientific because physicians and researchers have a better understanding regarding the mechanisms of action of these agents. TIVA is safer than inhalation anesthesia because there is no risk of malignant hyperthermia. There is also less myocardial depression with TIVA, again adding to safety. Finally, TIVA is desirable in the military and mass-casualty setting because of its small logistical footprint. Delivering general intravenous anesthesia does not require bulky, heavy, and expensive anesthesia machines that require maintenance and significant oxygen stores. It is easy to see how the four S's of TIVA—Safe, Simple, Scientific, and Small logistical footprint—are suited for mass-casualty anesthesia in the 21st century (see Table 7-1).

The types of injuries seen in terrorist attacks will range from minor to severe. Literally every surgical specialty

Table 7-1. Four "S's" of TIVA

1. Safe
2. Simple
3. Scientific
4 Small logistical footprint

would be involved in treating patients with injuries sustained in a terrorist attack. Regardless of the type of injury, anesthesiologists need methods of anesthetizing many patients in multiple locations, without needing medical gas systems and electricity. Utilizing PK would eliminate the requirement of an operating room and an anesthesia machine, allowing physicians to manage many patients in other areas, quickly and with excellent operating conditions. This approach to delivering trauma anesthesia in difficult settings is safe, simple, and a force multiplier.

HISTORY OF ANESTHESIA IN AUSTERE ENVIRONMENTS

Though anesthesia has a long history of safety, the experience of Bonnano[4] in Africa in the 1990s is probably the best illustration of the simplicity and safety of total intravenous anesthesia. Working with untrained personnel, Dr. Bonnano used ketamine, diazepam, glycopyrrolate, and local anesthesia to safely anesthetize sixty-two patients having sixty-four different surgical procedures. The types of procedures ranged from gastroschisis repair to Cesarean section to amputations. The ages of the patients were from infants to geriatric patients. Time and time again, anesthesia allowed these procedures to be performed on patients without artificial airways. That is, no one was intubated or had laryngeal mask airways (LMA) or anesthesia face masks for these surgeries. All of the patients breathed spontaneously on room air or an air/oxygen mixture. The untrained personnel were taught by Dr. Bonnano to increase the drip rate of the ketamine based on a patient's heart rate or movement with surgical stimulation. With minimal monitoring and untrained personnel, Dr. Bonnano oversaw these sixty-four cases. There were no anesthetic mishaps. This TIVA technique was safe, simple, scientific, and had a small logistical footprint.

THE TRISERVICE ANESTHESIA RESEARCH GROUP INITIATIVE ON TIVA (TARGIT)

The U.S. Army had already begun a massive transformation project prior to September 11, 2001. However, this initiative was largely focused on combat units. The rapid increase in operational tempo of U.S. military medical units following 9/11 required military physicians to begin their own transformation process.

The medical transformation project had to consider the portability or logistical footprint of medical equipment. The long-standing tools and techniques revolving around inhalational anesthesia were recognized as being less than ideal for mass-casualty situations. The weight and cube of anesthesia machines, inhalational agents, and other equipment requires excessive amounts of space on military transport vehicles. Furthermore, electrical and medical gas requirements of anesthesia machines could be problematic in mass-casualty settings. Realizing that TIVA had a smaller logistical footprint, it became a point of emphasis for U.S. Army physicians.

Thus, Army anesthesiologists began a global initiative focusing on TIVA. Following exhaustive reviews of the medical literature and numerous conferences with internationally recognized experts in TIVA, the Army formulated a strategy for implementing TIVA on the battlefield. In March of 2004, the Triservice Anesthesia Research Group Initiative on TIVA, or TARGIT Center (see Fig. 7-1), opened at Brooke Army Medical Center in San Antonio, Texas. The goal of this Army, Air Force, and Navy

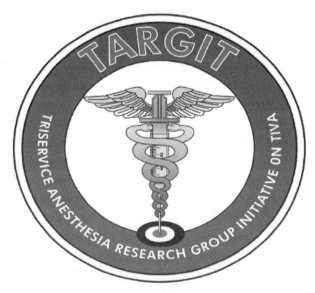

Figure 7-1. TARGIT insignia.

consortium is to improve battlefield anesthesia. In the future, the lessons learned by military physicians at the TARGIT Center will be passed on to our civilian colleagues. Ultimately, patients will benefit from improvements in trauma anesthesia care.

TIVA IN OPERATION IRAQI FREEDOM (OIF)

Though the U.S. military has used TIVA on occasion, inhalational anesthesia has dominated anesthesia practice for years. The TARGIT Center had to demonstrate the simplicity and clinical superiority of TIVA in a combat setting.

Beginning in March of 2003, Army anesthesiologists across Iraq delivered countless numbers of anesthetics to a variety of patients. Although most anesthetics were conducted using isoflurane, TIVA was utilized on occasion. The overall TIVA results were impressive. Patients did well, supplies were conserved, and ketamine was again viewed as being the ideal anesthetic.

In an after-action report describing anesthesia in OIF 2003, Dr. Mark Meeks wrote: "Our unit found the use of ketamine to be extremely beneficial when faced with large numbers of casualties, and a limited amount of medical supplies... patients did not require intubation, or any supplemental oxygen. We saved our meager stocks of medical supplies, such as endotracheal tubes, anesthesia circuits, and cylinders of oxygen."[5] This testimony from the first anesthesiologist to enter Iraq is the best example of the suitability of TIVA for military and mass-casualty anesthesia. Fortunately, the use of TIVA in OIF continued.

Since August of 2004, TIVA has been extensively utilized in Baghdad, Iraq as the anesthetic of choice for craniotomies. This propofol-ketamine-remifentanil (PKR) technique has been used hundreds of times, expertly delivered by an anesthesiologist, and has been named "Cadillac anesthesia."

Describing his experience with TIVA for neuroanesthesia, Grathwohl wrote: "My experience with PKR has been nothing but positive. The setup is simple, meaning it is easy to mix the drugs. Take a 100 cc 1% propofol bottle and add 100 mg ketamine and 2 mg remifentanil. The resulting concentrations are approximately 10 mg propofol $\cdot$ cc^{-1}, 1 mg ketamine $\cdot$ cc^{-1}, & 20 ug remifentanil $\cdot$ cc^{-1}.

"Induce with 50–100 ug fentanyl and 1–2 mg $\cdot$ kg^{-1} propofol. Titrate the 'cocktail' about 70–100 propofol ug $\cdot$ kg^{-1} $\cdot$ min^{-1}. Administer no more than a total of 100–150 mg ketamine for patients under the age of 50. Patients **over** the age of 50 emerge better when limited to a total of 100 mg ketamine. *N.B. This means no more than a total of 100–150 mg of ketamine-containing 'cocktail.' Administer no ketamine in the last twenty minutes of the case.* Do not turn off the 'cocktail' until the initiation of the head dressing. Otherwise, the patients tend to buck on the endotracheal tube when their heads are flexed. They emerge very quickly, in about 5 minutes. Remember to add the remaining of 50–100 ug fentanyl at the end of the surgery. The hemodynamic stability is awesome. I can't remember the last time I had to use neosynephrine. PKR increases the operational tempo of U.S. military medical units."[6]

In the six months before Grathwohl's arrival, over 100 craniotomies were performed with isoflurane fentanyl anesthesia administered by the same nurse anesthetist. On June 2, 2005, Grathwohl[7] summarized his first 100 craniotomies with PKR. The Glasgow Coma Score (GCS) and other neurosurgical trauma severity scores were the same between the two groups of patients. Compared to the previous hundred craniotomies, **half** as many *craniectomies* were required with PKR versus isoflurane fentanyl anesthesia and **half** as many transfusions were required. The isoflurane fentanyl group had twice the postoperative mortality rate compared with the PKR group.

A neurosurgeon deployed to Iraq also has been impressed with TIVA compared with inhalation anesthesia. Poffenbarger[9] wrote: "We have had great brain relaxation with TIVA. I've only had to shoehorn one patient. The wakeups have been crisper than what I am used to and there has been no retching seen with nausea and vomiting. The patients all used to sag hemodynamically with gas anesthesia, but none of that with your technique."

Certainly more will be written about TIVA in Operation Iraqi Freedom, but these early reports are powerful evidence that TIVA can be very effective in trauma anesthesia settings.

The TARGIT Center is now actively involved in clinical research with TIVA. The knowledge being gained will improve the quality of anesthesia being delivered in the combat setting. Since 2003, members of the TARGIT Center at Brooke Army Medical Center have delivered over 1,000 TIVA cases. Regimens using propofol-ketamine (PK), propofol-ketamine-fentanyl (PKF), propofol-ketamine-sufentanil (PKS), and propofol-ketamine-remifentanil (PKR) have been administered and have found niches in everyday clinical practice. PK and PKF are used for many breast surgeries. PKS is often used for abdominal hysterectomies, back cases, and some abdominal general surgery. PKR is most often used for ENT cases with or without spontaneous ventilation. In fact, these techniques have come to be requested on a regular basis by patients and surgeons.

Aside from clinical research, the TARGIT Center is designing a syllabus and educational seminar to teach and train physicians and nurses the science and art of delivering TIVA. In the end, research, education, and implementation of TIVA should make military anesthesia world class.

THE FUTURE OF MASS-CASUALTY ANESTHESIA

The Triservice Anesthesia Research Group Initiative on TIVA is a step in the right direction for improving mass-casualty anesthesia. As physicians, we must be ready to care for large numbers of casualties in any setting. The mass-casualty environment simply might not be able to support inhalation anesthesia. Therefore, TIVA has to be taught and utilized so that our patients will receive the best level of care. As Hutson[10] described, "TIVA is a simple and flexible technique applicable to all surgical case types. It has a small logistical footprint and can be easily administered in any environment independent of electricity and compressed gases. TIVA offers enhanced physiologic stability, fast emergence and reduced post-operative care requirements translating directly into provider efficiency and multitasking." This is exactly the type of impact that anesthesiology can make in preparing the American health care system for possible mass-casualty situations.

SUMMARY

Anesthesiology is a medical specialty that must continually reevaluate it methods. The motto of the American Society of Anesthesiologists is "vigilance." All anesthesiologists should strive to be in a constant state of vigilance. Furthermore, physician consultants in anesthesiology must be forward thinkers. The care provided to patients has to be first class.

Applied anatomy, pharmacology, physiology, and common sense can and will improve patient outcomes. PK anesthesia and other combinations of intravenous agents will be the anesthetics of the future. It is the military's duty to redefine mass-casualty anesthesia care and be ready for any perioperative challenge.

REFERENCES

1. www.doctorfriedberg.com
2. Friedberg BL: Anesthesia for facial cosmetic surgery, chapter in Herlich AN (ed.): *Anesthesia for oral and maxillofacial surgery. International Anesthesiology Clinics.* Baltimore, Lippincott, Williams & Wilkins, 41:13,2003.
3. Guit JBM, Koning HM, Coster ML, et al.: Ketamine as analgesic for intravenous anesthesia with propofol (TIVA). *Anaesthesia* 46:24,1991.
4. Bonnano FG: Ketamine in war/tropical surgery, a final tribute to the racemic mixture. *Internat J Care Injured* 33:323, 2002.
5. Meeks M: 86th Combat Support Hospital After Action Report on Anesthesia in Operation Iraqi Freedom, 2003.
6. Grathwohl K: Personal communication regarding TIVA in Operation Iraqi Freedom, 2004.
7. Grathwohl K: E-mail correspondence from the front. June 2, 2005.
8. Himmelseher S, Durieux ME: Revising dogma: Ketamine for patients with neurological injury. *Anesth Analg* 101:524, 2005.
9. Poffenbarger G: Personal communication regarding TIVA in Operation Iraqi Freedom, 2004.
10. Hutson C: Total intravenous anesthesia in austere environments. *Military Medicine* (in press) 2005.

APPENDIX 7-1
ARMY ENLISTS DOCTOR'S WORK
TO TREAT WOUNDED SOLDIERS
ORANGE COUNTY REGISTER
JUN 25, 2004 6:50 PM EDT

Corona del Mar (AP)

Local anesthesiologist Barry Friedberg is doing his part for our wounded troops in Iraq. And, until a few weeks ago, he didn't even know it. He didn't know it until the Army called him to personally brief doctors at the Brooke Army Medical Center in San Antonio, Texas.

It seems the Army had read about the portability of Dr. Friedberg's anesthesia techniques and were adapting them to their front line hospitals. His procedures eliminate the use of narcotics and don't require the use of oxygen tanks that are difficult to come by in Iraq.

In Texas, a shocked and puzzled Dr. Friedberg said he found himself "amazed" the Army was interested in his procedures. Why? He'd developed them while going from office-to-office anesthetizing patients on whom local cosmetic surgeons were performing tummy tucks and breast implants.

8 | Lidocaine Use and Toxicity in Cosmetic Surgery

Adam Frederic Dorin, M.D., M.B.A.

INTRODUCTION AND OVERVIEW

The use and toxicity of lidocaine in modern cosmetic surgical practice is arguably the most important topic for any anesthesiologist or surgeon working in this field of medicine. Lidocaine toxicity, primarily in the context of suction assisted lipectomy (SAL), lipoplasty, or liposuction, has historically accounted for a significant proportion of patient morbidity and mortality.

This chapter covers lidocaine pharmacology, the history of lidocaine use in the context of cosmetic/plastic surgical practice, and the politics or practical concerns of pushing the envelope toward higher, "megadose" tumescent lidocaine solutions. As there are ample resources to address the basic structure of the lidocaine molecule, and multiple books and articles on the basic science and pharmacokinetics of lidocaine, no space is wasted in displaying this information. Similarly, the related subjects of peribulbar versus topical anesthesia in ophthalmic surgery and transient neurotoxic symptoms in lidocaine spinal anesthesia are not analyzed in this context.

BRIEF PHARMACOLOGY

Lidocaine, an amide molecule synthesized from cocaine, was first applied in the practice of medicine in 1948.[1] As clinical applications and the advancement of medicine expanded the role of lidocaine, this drug found a niche applied topically and subcutaneously for local anesthesia for a variety of surgical procedures. Lidocaine is used intravenously to treat ventricular arrhythmias. Dilute solutions of lidocaine mixed with epinephrine are administered as tumescent solution for liposuction cosmetic surgery. Lidocaine is available as a topical solution (2–4% or 20–40 mg $\cdot$ ml^{-1}), a rectal suppository (10% or 100 mg $\cdot$ ml^{-1}), viscous lidocaine (2% or 20 mg $\cdot$ ml^{-1}), and a jelly (2%); there also exists a topical ointment (5% or 50 mg $\cdot$ ml^{-1}), an aerosol (10%), and a solution for subcutaneous and intravenous administration (0.5–2% or 5–20 mg $\cdot$ ml^{-1}).[2]

Lidocaine displays very good absorption following all routes of administration. Absorption from the oral mucosa avoids first-pass metabolism and is thus very rapid. Absorption from the GI tract undergoes hepatic first-pass metabolism, resulting in only about 35% of ingested lidocaine reaching the systemic circulation.[3] The volume of distribution of lidocaine is 1.6 L $\cdot$ kg^{-1}. In the very young and the very old, this volume of distribution can be significantly higher. The plasma half-life of lidocaine is eight minutes; the terminal half-life of lidocaine is ninety minutes. Plasma lidocaine levels fall rapidly following parenteral administration. Following a bolus intravenous injection, lidocaine has a relatively short duration of action (ten to thirty minutes) due to rapid tissue redistribution. Ninety percent of lidocaine clearance is due to hepatic metabolism, and 10% of lidocaine is excreted unchanged in the urine. The pKa of lidocaine is 7.8. Lidocaine is approximately 50% protein bound.[4]

There are several caveats regarding lidocaine metabolism consistent with basic physiology. Lidocaine blood levels will be elevated in the setting of acidosis (e.g., hypercarbia secondary to inadequate airway management, regional infection, or sepsis) due to decreased protein binding. In addition, there are two major lidocaine metabolites: monoethylglycinexylidide (MEGX) and glycinexylidide (GX). MEGX retains 83% of the activity of lidocaine and has a half-life of two hours; GX is less potent but retains a half-life of ten hours. Both MEGX and GX metabolites add to the therapeutic effects of lidocaine. Both are culpable in the clinical toxic effects of lidocaine.[5]

Lidocaine prevents electrical conduction by stabilizing cell membranes. This is achieved by preventing membrane permeability to calcium-dependent sodium and potassium shifts. These shifts effectively block nerve conduction. In the cardiac muscle, lidocaine blocks both open and inactivated sodium channels, decreasing the slope of phase 4 depolarization and the threshold potential. This decreases myocardial automaticity. In ischemic cardiac tissue, this effect is more pronounced, in effect synchronizing myocardial cells and making reentrant arrhythmias less likely.[6]

LIDOCAINE TOXICOLOGY

In the practice of cosmetic surgery, surgeons and anesthesiologists attempt to calculate the "maximal safe dose" of lidocaine for use in subcutaneous infiltration or tumescent solutions. For simplicity, the historical or time-honored, dose-related toxicity of lidocaine in subcutaneous infiltration will be assessed first. The controversy and facts regarding tumescent solutions will be addressed (vide infra). Prolonged surgical cases involving both SAL or liposuction and other cosmetic procedures (e.g., rhinoplasty and/or breast augmentation) can create complex physiologic scenarios in which determination of the "cutoff" level of safe lidocaine dosing can be a difficult calculation. Subcutaneous lidocaine injection has been limited to 4.5 mg $\cdot$ kg^{-1} without epinephrine and 7.0 mg $\cdot$ kg^{-1} with epinephrine. The addition of epinephrine to a solution of lidocaine will nearly double the duration of lidocaine activity. Lidocaine has inherent vasodilating properties. At the capillary bed level, vasodilation acts to accelerate the "washout" or absorption of lidocaine from injected tissues. The vasoconstriction produced by the addition of epinephrine works to offset vasodilation from the lidocaine. Hence, the analgesic effect of the lidocaine/epinephrine combination is increased. Because of this action, there is a decreased peak blood level of lidocaine. This allows the patient to tolerate the administration of a larger initial dose.[5] The physiologic toxicity of lidocaine will become apparent to the clinical practitioner in the sequence of CNS effects (e.g., mental status changes), and then cardiac deterioration and arrest.

Table 8-1. Blood lidocaine levels and manifestations of toxicity

ug · ml^{-1}	Clinical state in the awake patient
1. 1.5–5.0	Therapeutic
2. 5–10	Dizziness, tinnitus, patient complaint of metallic taste on the tongue, lethargy
3. 10–20	Delirium, disorientation, eventually seizures and coma
4. >20	Probable cardiac arrest

Under both IV sedation and general inhalation anesthesia, the CNS signs tend to be obscured! Only the terminal, cardiovascular signs of toxicity are manifest (i.e., A-V dissociation and hypotension). Under MAC/Sedation, in the context of intermittent benzodiazepine or continuous propofol administration, the seizure threshold of lidocaine will be elevated. An elevated seizure threshold may *potentially* contribute to a false sense of security if the serum and tissue levels of the sedating agents fall more rapidly than the blood level of lidocaine.

The hemodynamic changes associated with lidocaine toxicity are primarily the consequence of direct cardiac effects, resulting in hypotension, A-V block, and asystole.[6] A blood concentration of lidocaine in the range of 1.5–5.0 ug · kg^{-1} is considered therapeutic (see Table 8-1). In an *awake* patient, blood levels in the range of 5–10 ug · kg^{-1} will characteristically result in dizziness, tinnitus, patient complaint of metallic taste on the tongue, and lethargy. These symptoms may be obscured when patients are sedated. At the levels of 10–20 ug · kg^{-1}, the awake patient will experience delirium and disorientation, which will eventually lead to seizures and coma. Finally, blood levels of lidocaine greater than 20 ug · kg^{-1} will significantly predispose a patient for cardiac arrest. The toxicity of lidocaine (not unlike many drugs that undergo hepatic metabolism) will be heightened (and the threshold lowered) in the setting of congestive heart failure (CHF) and liver cirrhosis. (Both heart failure and cirrhosis lead to a decreased clearance of the drug.) The use of some drugs by patients, such as beta-blockers (decreased cardiac output) and cimetidine (cytochrome P450 system), will result in the further enhanced toxicity of lidocaine.[5] *Editor's note: This concern may be more hypothetical than is clinically apparent —BLF.*

Today's patient often takes so many medications, both prescription and herbal, that it can be difficult to fully assess their anesthetic impact in a brief preoperative visit (see Chapter 14 and Appendix A). Some of those medications act as inhibitors of the liver cytochrome P450 (3A4) isoenzyme system. Dorin categorizes these drugs along the same lines as the mechanisms of systemic toxicity that occur with increasing doses of lidocaine. CNS impairment typically occurs first with increasingly toxic levels of serum lidocaine.

Selective serotonin reuptake inhibitors (SSRIs) are a class of antidepressants that inhibit the cytochrome P450 system. This class of drug includes sertraline, paroxetine, norfluoxetine, fluoxetine, fluvoxamine, and citalopram. Newer agents in this class of antidepressants have been appearing on the market on a yearly basis. Other antidepressant medications, such as nefazodone, may also hypothetically affect lidocaine metabolism and potentially predispose to toxic levels of serum lidocaine. The main offending class of agents is the SSRIs.

This is not to suggest that psychiatric medications should be discontinued preoperatively.

It should also not be inferred, with other medications listed herein (e.g., nondiuretic antihypertensives), that patient baseline medications should be suspended prior to SAL or liposuction. Rather, these medications are listed in the context of better understanding the full gamut of physiologic factors influencing potential lidocaine toxicity.

With increasing lidocaine blood levels, cardiac impairment will present itself in lidocaine toxicity after CNS symptoms. Calcium-channel blockers, diltiazem, nifedipine, and verapamil can potentially augment the risk of lidocaine toxicity through inhibition of the liver cytochrome P450 system. Sometimes patients, either preoperatively, intraoperatively, or postoperatively, receive sublingual nifedipine for clinically significant hypertension. How many times does an anesthesiologist or nurse consider the possibility of potentiating lidocaine toxicity when giving nifedipine?

Other types of common patient medications that may justify altering the total dose of lidocaine given intraoperatively fall into the general groups of "bugs and drugs." Along the lines of antibiotics, the "floxin" medications (norfloxacin, ciprofloxacin, and sparfloxacin) and the "mycin" medications (erythromycin and clarithromycin) should be remembered. Antifungals, such as ketoconazole and fluconazole, are also inhibitors of the cytochrome P450 3A4 isoenzyme system. Methadone also inhibits the liver's P450 system as well. Other medications that not uncommonly appear in a patient's preoperative worksheet are tamoxifen, for breast cancer, and methylprednisolone. The immunosuppressant cyclosporine and the antiseizure medication valproic acid should be added to the list of inhibitors of the cytochrome P450 system.

LIDOCAINE TOXICITY: TREATMENT AND EXAMPLES

The appropriate treatment of lidocaine toxicity consists primarily of administering 100% F_iO_2, securing the airway, and providing support of the blood pressure. IV benzodiazepines have been the mainstay of therapy for seizures. Hypotension may be treated with pressors and increasing IV fluids. Atropine may be useful for bradycardia.

Avoid IV lidocaine for the correction of arrhythmias.

Correction of hypoxemia, seizures, acidosis, and hypotension will usually eliminate arrhythmias. Acidosis may be best treated by increasing minute ventilation. Current ACLS guidelines discourage the use of bicarbonate in this setting. Correcting acidosis prevents lidocaine from becoming more available as a free drug in the circulation.

Practitioners should avoid using phenytoin as an anticonvulsant due to its synergistic, untoward cardiac action.[6]

Lidocaine toxicity has been found following every possible route of drug administration or exposure. In children, oral administration has resulted in generalized seizures, with lidocaine levels ranging from 3.8–10.6 ug · kg^{-1}.[7] In the case of a four-week-old infant, seizure, respiratory arrest, and coma resulted from an intravenous dose of 50 mg lidocaine.[8] In this case, the lidocaine peak level reached 5.39 ug · kg^{-1}. In a case of topical lidocaine use by a fifty-five-year-old woman with cutaneous lymphoma lesions, the patient applied 5% topical lidocaine ointment over approximately 60% of her body surface area to treat pruritus. The patient continued this activity for nine days and eventually developed grand mal seizures and a full

cardiorespiratory arrest. The lidocaine level in this patient was measured at 21.2 ug · kg^{-1}.[9]

Before the heated debate about liposuction lidocaine levels surfaced in the mid to late 1990s, a 1991 *American Journal of Cardiology* article foreshadowed the discussions to follow with the report of serious lidocaine toxicity resulting from the subcutaneous infiltration of lidocaine (with epinephrine) in ten patients undergoing cardiac catheterization. Two of these sequential patients became lethargic and had measured lidocaine levels of 6.8 ug · kg^{-1} and 7.2 ug · kg^{-1} following doses of 25 mg · kg^{-1} and 47 mg · kg^{-1}, respectively.[10]

THE POLITICS OF LIDOCAINE TOXICITY AMONG SPECIALTIES

In the early 21st century, there remains a vigorous debate among cosmetic surgical specialties about the terminology of fat removal by aspiration. The parlance of plastic surgeons tends to "suction assisted lipectomy"(SAL) or "lipoplasty," whereas the parlance of cosmetic surgeons tends to "liposuction." Plastic surgeons tend to use the term "wetting solution" in preference to the "tumescent" formula (i.e., 500 mg lidocaine, 1 mg epinephrine, and 12.5 meq $NaHCO_3$ in NSS) promoted by dermatologist Klein in 1987. The finger-pointing and blame-placing regarding "who" has caused "what" complication of lidocaine toxicity continues to the present day.

Patients have experienced death at the hands of **both** dermatologists and plastic surgeons. Williford, commenting on Coldiron et al.,[11] concluded that "ultimately, this debate should not be about the internecine battle: us against them in an Alamo last stand posturing. It should be about honoring the duty of discovering what is most appropriate, cost-effective, efficacious, and safe for our patients"[12] (see Chapter 17). Additionally, tumescent technique with minimal or no sedation is compared against "super wet" technique with major neuraxial or general inhalation anesthesia.

In an article published in 2000, Gorney asserts that "lidocaine toxicity" is probably the second or third most common cause of fatal outcome in lipoplasty.[13] In that same year, a study by Grazer and de Jong of more than 100 liposuction deaths purported to show **no deaths** due to lidocaine toxicity.[14] In a 1999 *New England Journal of*

Medicine article entitled "Deaths Related to Liposuction," Rao[15] reports several deaths associated with tumescent or wetting solutions. Rao makes the observation that the deaths were associated with epinephrine concentrations of 1:2,000,000. *This represents a concentration of 0.5 mg in 1,000 cc in contrast to Klein's recommended 1 mg in 1,000 cc.* The conventional tumescent epinephrine concentration is 1:1,000,000. In one patient who received the 1:2,000,000 epinephrine dilution, the cause of death was exsanguination. Though not conclusively demonstrated, the reduced vasoconstriction provided by the lower epinephrine concentration, when combined with a large-volume liposuction, is suspected as the etiology of the exsanguination. In these cited studies and reports, the lidocaine concentration was 0.1 mg% or lower, in doses less than 60 mg · kg^{-1}. In addition, liposuction was performed within roughly three to four hours of injection, and approximately the same volume of aspirate was removed as was initially infused.

A perusal of the modern literature, as well as articles, web sites, and "blogs," reveals a stark contrast between specialties on the issue of lidocaine-related toxicity in cosmetic surgery (primarily SAL or liposuction combined with additional cosmetic procedures). Cosmetic surgeons tend to blame IV sedation and/or general anesthesia for patient complications.

Following the adoption of pulse oximetry as a standard of care (1990), mortality from anesthesia declined to 1:250,000. Drastic reduction of hypoxic insults and deaths are generally believed to be the cause of the diminished mortality estimate. A proportional decrease in anesthesiologist malpractice premiums followed. Grazer and deJong claimed the anesthesia mortality figure is 1:5,000 or fifty times greater than recognized in the anesthesia community. How can one make sense of the enormous disparity in mortality figures? A possible explanation may be that Grazer and deJong's deaths included those from pulmonary embolism and other non-lidocaine-related outcomes. Pulmonary embolism arises from venous stasis in the leg and deep pelvic veins. Patients are more predisposed to venous stasis when anesthetics that provide profound muscle relaxation (i.e., major neuraxial block or general inhalation anesthesia) are administered. Sequential compression stockings are advocated to minimize leg veins stasis. However, it is presently unknown whether sequential leg vein compression eliminates deep pelvic vein congestion. IV sedation techniques that preserve the normal "muscle pump" of the legs appear to provide a greater margin of safety than relying on the sequential compression stockings.[16] General inhalation anesthesia may still leave the patients in substantial postoperative pain. Patients in pain tend not to ambulate as often or as much as patients who have had preemptive analgesia. Patients medicated with opioids for postoperative pain also tend to ambulate less. Lesser ambulation exacerbates the tendency to venous stasis and potential pulmonary embolic phenomena. Having anesthesiologists present in the surgical suite provides the superb advantage of having a specialized pair of hands to deal with airway complications. The anesthesiologist has an independent focus on monitoring patient vital signs.

Lillis, in the *Journal of Dermatological Oncology* (1988), claimed that 90 mg · kg^{-1} lidocaine was safe.[17] Hildreth, reporting in 1998 at the World Congress of Liposuction on a study that involved thousands of patients, made the claim that lidocaine in doses of 80 mg · kg^{-1} was "safe."[18] The California legislature enacted total liposuction aspirate limit of 5,000 ml. Many plastic surgeons inject approximately the amount they plan to aspirate. In Friedberg's series of patients,[19] female patients weighed an average of 60 kg; 5,000 ml injected with 500 mg lidocaine in each 1,000 ml bag calculates to a lidocaine dose of 42 mg · kg^{-1}. In his clinical experience, the epinephrine-induced delayed absorption of lidocaine contributes to the safety of megadose lidocaine tumescent injection. Further, the seizure threshold of lidocaine is elevated by the concomitant use of continuous propofol at BIS <75. Removing some of the injectate with the aspirate solution also contributes to safety with megadose lidocaine use.

Coldiron et al.[11] reviewed deaths occurring in the office setting using three years of *mandatory* reporting of patient death data from the state of Florida. In contrast, Grazer and deJong's data were derived from a survey based on *voluntary* reporting.[14] The Florida data demonstrate that 42% of those offices reporting deaths and 50% of the offices reporting hospital transfers in the perioperative period were accredited by an independent accreditation agency. In addition, 96% of physicians reporting surgical incidents were board-certified and had hospital privileges. Coldiron et al.[11] concluded that regulatory restrictions on office procedures have little effect on overall patient safety if they fail to identify and address the issue of cosmetic surgeries, in particular, *those that are performed under general anesthesia.*

MEGADOSE LIDOCAINE IN TUMESCENT LIPOSUCTION

Benefits, Pitfalls, and Controversies

The 2000 national statistics for the American Society for Dermatologic Surgeons and the American Society of Plastic Surgeons both put the number of SAL or liposuction procedures performed in the United States at about 450,000.[20] The 2003 census by the American Society for Aesthetic Plastic Surgery (ASAPS) records the number of lipoplasty procedures for that year at 384,626.[21] By all accounts, in recent years, SAL or liposuction ranks as the number one cosmetic surgical procedure performed on an annual basis in the United States.

Tumescent liposuction involves the infusion of a dilute solution of lidocaine and epinephrine into the subcutaneous fat layer. This serves to thicken the fat layer in preparation for aspiration. The physical pressure of the tissue distention in addition to the vasoconstriction from the epinephrine serves to decrease blood loss. Lidocaine provides local analgesia during the procedure and in the immediate postoperative period. Large-volume liposuction procedures (i.e., >4,000 ccs of fat) will likely need to rely on adequate levels of IV sedation, major neuraxial block, or general anesthesia for patient comfort.

Since SAL or liposuction was introduced in the United States in 1983, significant complications, as well as deaths, have been reported in medical journals and the lay press. First, what are the general and somewhat obvious benefits of liposuction with megadose lidocaine? Next, how do some of the pitfalls and controversies impact the use of high-dose lidocaine?

Benefits—practical

The benefits of megadose lidocaine SAL or liposuction build on the inherent appeal of the procedure itself. As an alternative to rigorous dieting and exercise, SAL or liposuction allows patients to quickly shed inches in sculpted areas of the body. Cosmetic surgical patients continue to pay considerable sums of money for SAL or liposuction. Most practitioners would probably agree this patient population is fiercely independent. Cosmetic patients demonstrate the profile of an active, energetic lifestyle. These patients place a high value on time, mobility, and quick postsurgical recoveries. Anything that adds these qualities to the anesthetic side of SAL or liposuction is a value-added component to the patient's perioperative experience. Megadose tumescent anesthesia *is* such a value-added component. The addition of higher total doses of lidocaine to the SAL or liposuction translates, potentially, into greater tissue analgesia. In addition, more areas of work can be performed in one operative setting, and greater volumes of tissues can be infused and aspirated. Pushing the volume/dosage envelope of the lidocaine/epinephrine tumescent solution means a bigger "bang for the buck."

Americans like to accomplish more at whatever they're doing. Likewise, medical practitioners like to get as much of their treatment done in a single patient encounter. With the addition of direct patient remuneration in cosmetic surgeries, the significance of doing (and collecting) more in one visit becomes inherently obvious.

Benefits—clinical

Historically, the injection of fluids has been used to provide a hydrodissection of tissue planes. Hydrodissection predated SAL or liposuction and was never used to facilitate the aspiration of fat. Modern-day liposuction was popularized by Klein, a dermatologist, who reported clinical trials with several liters of a subcutaneous, isotonic injectate containing a very dilute lidocaine (0.05–0.10%) and epinephrine (1:1,000,000) solution.[22] The term "tumescent" gained traction because of the effect the solution had on tissues. Tumescence caused the fatty tissues to become engorged or swell. Vasoconstriction of the subdermal plexus caused the overlying skin to appear blanched. Klein touted his new approach as one that could achieve an independent state of local tissue anesthesia. Klein described his approach as "regional anesthesia." In contradistinction to Klein, anesthesiologists use the term "regional anesthesia" to signify major neuraxial block (e.g., spinal or epidural). Compared to the blood losses not infrequently requiring transfusion with "dry" liposuction, Klein reported nearly bloodless surgery with his tumescent approach.

Klein also reported that postoperative analgesia was reliable and sustained. Tumescent solutions were shown to result in a slower release of lidocaine from injected tissues into the general circulation. As a result, Klein and others demonstrated maximum mean lidocaine serum levels of about 1.3 ug $\cdot$ ml^{-1}, peaking at twelve to fourteen hours after injection and then declining over another six to fourteen hours.[23] The pharmacokinetic profile of tumescent or "wetting" solution is strikingly similar to a one-compartment sustained-release drug model. By relying on the protein/tissue binding characteristics of the lidocaine molecule and the vasoconstrictive qualities of epinephrine, lidocaine is essentially withheld from the general circulation for longer periods of time than conventional local, subcutaneously injected medication.

Benefits—political

One doesn't need statistics or peer-reviewed journals to prove the point that a large percentage of liposuction procedures in the United States is being performed by individuals who are not general/plastic surgery trained. Perusing the advertisement pages of most newspapers and glossy periodicals establishes this point. The list of health care professionals who have incorporated liposuction into their menu of services include dermatologists, otolaryngologists, family practitioners, obstetrician-gynecologists, and others. Klein and other advocates of tumescent technique offered weekend training seminars. Cosmetic as well as some plastic surgeons attended. Prior to 1990, few, if any, plastic surgery residency training programs offered training in "super wet" SAL or tumescent liposuction. Plastic surgeons trained before 1990 were also obliged to learn SAL at weekend courses or even from the sales representatives of companies selling cannulae and suction pumps.

Some have even reported rare sightings of dentists and anesthesiologists performing liposuction. Modern tumescent technique has contributed to the expanded practice settings of SAL or liposuction. Furthermore, the promotion of the tumescent technique has allowed this surgical procedure to safely and successfully adapt to the diverse practice settings of hospitals, freestanding ambulatory surgical centers, and office-based surgical suites.

With improvements in local anesthesia, and the ease with which relatively large volumes of fat could be safely aspirated in one sitting, SAL or liposuction quickly became a cash cow for many physicians. Increasingly onerous paperwork burdens by third-party payers combined with decreasing remuneration for services were additional factors driving many plastic surgeons and other physicians to seek a fee-for-service model in which to practice.

Pitfalls and Complications

In 1999, Grazer and de Jong[14] reported (in a *voluntary* survey of 1,200 cosmetic plastic surgeons) a mortality rate of 19.1 in 100,000 lipoplasty surgeries. This statistic represents 95 reported and verified deaths out of almost 500,000 cases. The total number of SAL or liposuction cases performed in North America over the course of the Grazer and de Jong study period was close to one million cases. The study period was four and a half years.

To put the issue of SAL or liposuction risk and lidocaine toxicity into context, all the potential perioperative surgical complications should be reviewed. Then, the risks related to megadose tumescent liposuction require some assessment.

Hemorrhage

Every surgery can result in hemorrhage. Even a "minor" surgery like a simple mole removal or scar revision in a patient who unknowingly suffers from a blood-clotting deficiency can result in significant blood loss. SAL or liposuction perioperative complications can range from poor wound healing to life-threatening injury. Multiple factors may impact the potential for bleeding in liposuction. Some believe that waiting thirty to forty-five minutes after completing the injection of the tumescent or "wetting" solution provides superior hemostasis. The use of progressively smaller cannula (i.e., 3–6 mm compared with 8–12 mm) probably has contributed to less laceration of larger arterioles. Although underlying and unsuspected coagulopathy may play a role, it is more likely that the undisclosed patient use of herbal, over-the-counter agents (i.e., Ginkgo Biloba, St. John's Wort, garlic, and Vitamin E) are the culprits in excess bleeding (see Chapter 14 and Appendix A). Inappropriate IV fluid therapy may also contribute to a dilutional coagulopathy. Limitation of total volumes in Florida (4,000 ccs fat) and California (5,000 ccs total aspirate) has contributed to the increased safety of SAL or liposuction. *IV fluids need to be administered sparingly, if at all, under these limitations.* Specifically, the potentially lethal formula of replacing 3 ccs of IV fluid for every 1 cc of fat aspirated merits sound condemnation.

All of the preceding factors can have a significant influence on the degree of intraoperative and postoperative bleeding. Compression garments are commonly utilized for SAL or liposuction procedures to help the skin redrape more smoothly. The external pressure tends to obliterate the *potential* third-space effect created by the removal of fat.

One cannot apply the same principles of volume replacement to potential third-space fluid shifts in SAL or liposuction as one would when dealing with extensive skin burns.

No compression garments mitigate the third-space losses in burn victims. Inappropriate, aggressive fluid administration may place the SAL or liposuction patient at risk for fluid overload and dilutional coagulopathy. A drop in oxygen-carrying capacity may occur as the hemoglobin level is diluted by the combined effects of aggressive IV fluids and the reabsorption of nonaspirated tumescent or "wetting" solution.

Dorin was medical director of a high-volume, predominantly cosmetic surgery practice (about seventy-five plastic surgeons) in an upscale metropolitan area. Most of the surgeons were conscientious. Aside from general technique and bedside manners, there were simply some doctors who regularly exercised profoundly poor judgment in their surgical practices. Dorin's facility had a center-based policy based on the 1998 American Society of Plastic and Reconstructive Surgeons (ASPRS) Liposuction guidelines that limited the total volume of injectate and subsequent aspirate to 5,000 ccs. Nevertheless, there were a few cavalier surgeons who continually flouted the guidelines by aspirating as much as 14,000 ml in a given surgical setting! Dorin's ability to insist on compliance with the ASPRS guidelines was compromised in that he was not physically present in those ORs when the guidelines were being violated. Two of these cavalier surgeons eventually had their surgery center privileges terminated by the medical executive committee. One of these surgeons also had several patients admitted to the local hospital emergency room by ambulance. Patients experienced symptoms ranging from severe dizziness *(and an inability to get out of the PACU gurney)* to significant postoperative anemia.

Third-space fluid shifts

Many surgical insults result in the third-space fluid shifts. The degree of the "shift" depends on the degree of tissue damage and the site of the surgery. In SAL or liposuction, the creation of raw, subdermal trauma can be significant. Tissue trauma occurs independent of whether manual or ultrasound cannula are utilized. This injury causes tissues and vessels to lose normal integrity; combined with the risk of extensive and lengthy surgeries that involve large volumes of fat aspiration (i.e., >4,000 ccs), third-space shifts *can* result in serious hemodynamic fluctuations in the postoperative setting. There may be significant electrolyte imbalances. The attentive practitioner will order postoperative labs to quickly identify and correct any disturbances. The practice of applying postoperative compression garments is thought to substantially mitigate the degree of third-space fluid shifts (*vide supra*).

Iatrogenic error

Any surgeon, on any given day, can inadvertently place a liposuction aspiration probe in the wrong place (e.g., intestines, intrapleural, liver, kidney, major blood vessel). Any anesthesiologist or nurse anesthetist, on any given day, can commit the error of inappropriate patient dosing, inappropriate fluid replacement, lack of vigilance in monitoring, poor airway management or planning, and poor patient selection. A patient's choice of medical provider, based on experience and judgment, is invaluable in preventing iatrogenic injury. Despite the marvels of modern medicine, improved surgical techniques, and the computerized advancements in anesthesia monitors, there is **no substitute for good judgment and unwavering vigilance** (see Chapter 18) in the delivery of patient care.

Iatrogenic error can also be more insidious, taking the form of multiple, overlapping therapies and risks. For example, patients undergoing general anesthesia for SAL or liposuction will need, and possibly receive, a lower dose of tumescent lidocaine. Fodor states in his 1999 editorial, "General or epidural anesthesia is used routinely for anything but small extractions, and local anesthetics can be avoided entirely from the infusate."[24] These same patients may be concurrently exposed to increased risks due to the aspiration of greater total volumes. General anesthesia also predisposes patients to venous stasis in the legs and pelvic veins.[16] Stasis may contribute to clot formation and subsequent, sometimes fatal, pulmonary emboli.[16] Utilizing a lower dose of tumescent fluid may translate into greater postoperative patient discomfort. Patients in discomfort tend to limit their activity that exacerbates the tendency for venous stasis and potential clot formation.

Pulmonary edema

Any large volume of tumescent fluid administration, especially in the setting of undiagnosed heart disease/failure, can result in intravascular fluid overload and pulmonary edema. A seasoned anesthesia provider will be attuned not only to the pulse oximeter reading but also to a patient's lung sounds and ease of breathing in the perioperative setting. In an otherwise hemodynamically stable patient, without a history of electrolyte disturbance, a suspicion of intravascular fluid overload may be appropriately mitigated with observation and a small dose of diuretic (e.g., furosemide). Most practitioners would give a dose of 5–40 mg furosemide to start and repeat as necessary over the course of observation. For patients who regularly take furosemide, it would be prudent to use the patient's baseline dose as a starting point for treatment.

Pulmonary embolism

Fat embolism and thomboembolism can be complications of any surgery but should be of special concern in liposuction patients. Lengthy procedures that involve prolonged periods of patient immobilization should be approached with the placement preoperatively of lower extremity compression devices (or, if necessary due to surgical site, rotating compression stockings) to lessen the likelihood of deep venous thromboses. By treating the degree of venous stasis, minimizing caval compression, and applying good surgical fat-aspiration technique, the potential of pulmonary embolism can be minimized. Anesthetic techniques that preserve lower extremity muscle tone (i.e., IV sedation in general and the MIA™ technique in particular; see Chapter 1) may be inherently more advantageous in patients predisposed to the development of deep-vein thromboses (*vide supra*).[16]

Epinephrine toxicity

Anesthesia providers often find it amusing when patients present in the preoperative holding area with a report of "epinephrine allergy." These patients are invariably the victim of some prior dental procedure during which the local anesthetic mixture containing epinephrine resulted in a rather unsettling tachycardia and, possibly, related shortness of breath. Although one may be hard-pressed to find documentation that the body's primary *in-situ* survival drug is inherently "allergenic," experience will yield countless stories of tachycardia and hypertension in the perioperative setting due to the administration of epinephrine-containing local anesthetics. In patients suffering from hypertension and/or pulmonary disease, intravascular epinephrine can be problematic. As Grazer and de Jong have reported,[14] serum epinephrine levels during lipoplasty surgery peaked to 133 ug · ml^{-1} (upwards of five times the normal level) at three hours and returned to normal at a twelve-hour sampling. With each liter of a typical tumescent fluid solution containing 1 mg of epinephrine, the sheer number of annual SAL or liposuction procedures performed is a testament that short-lived supranormal levels of epinephrine are well tolerated by the body.[14]

Lidocaine toxicity

Lidocaine toxicity can result in CNS symptoms and toxicity, followed by cardiovascular toxicity. Because of direct effects on the nervous system, and hepatic enzyme oversaturation, lidocaine toxicity causes depression of the conduction mechanisms of nerve and muscle function. The force of cardiac contraction may also be depressed. Although the absorption of lidocaine following tumescent injection is slow, the potential for drug interaction and overdosage is a real possibility in the perioperative setting.

Controversy—megadosing

A variety of sources (e.g., FDA, PDA, anesthesia textbooks, surgical textbooks) describe a recommended upper limit adult lidocaine dose of 7 mg · kg^{-1} not to exceed 500 mg with epinephrine. Neither the manufacturer of lidocaine nor the U.S. Food and Drug Administration (FDA) have data to support this recommendation. In its 1948 application to the FDA, Astra Pharmaceutical Products, Inc., simply stated that the maximum safe dose of lidocaine is probably the same as for procaine![22] Of further note is that neither the 2005, 2006, nor 2007 PDR (print or electronic version) has any listing for injectabele lidocaine. In stark contrast, studies and common clinical practice have repeatedly demonstrated that doses of highly diluted lidocaine epinephrine or tumescent or wetting infiltration are considered to be safe to levels as high as 55 mg · kg^{-1}.[25]

In preparation for the writing of this chapter, several highly regarded anesthesiologists, with many years and thousands of cases of experience with megadose lidocaine in SAL or liposuction, were consulted. All of them confidently reported having no hesitation (nor personal history of complications) in recommending highly diluted lidocaine doses even in excess of 55 mg · kg^{-1} for SAL or liposuction.

There are several caveats to the recommended use of megadose lidocaine administration. First and foremost is that a dose of 55 mg · kg^{-1} lidocaine is exclusively limited to dilute lidocaine (i.e., 500–1,000 mg lidocaine in 1,000 ccs NSS [Klein] or LR [Hunstad]) that is administered with epinephrine. Second, a dose of 55 mg · kg^{-1} lidocaine is *only acceptable within the* **context** *of tumescent or "wetting" injections for SAL or liposuction.* Third, a dose of 55 mg · kg^{-1} lidocaine applies **only** to surgeries that adhere to prudent guidelines regarding the appropriate total volume of fat aspirate (i.e., 4,000–5,000 ccs), under conditions of adequate anesthesia, monitoring, and *limited* IV fluid management. Sometimes a Foley catheter is used to monitor urine output for large volume SAL or liposuction.

Last to consider are "combined" cosmetic surgical interventions, wherein SAL or liposuction is performed with other procedures in the same setting. In cases involving the administration of normal lidocaine "out-of-the-bottle" concentrations for subcutaneous infiltration (e.g., rhinoplasty, face/neck lift, breast augmentation), all bets are off. REPEAT: ALL BETS ARE OFF! In the scenarios where nondiluted concentrations of lidocaine are injected, the injection of 35 mg · kg^{-1} could easily prove lethal. In addition, be mindful that normal lidocaine pharmacokinetics of absorption and elimination will be at play.

Anesthetic implications
Most of the discussions heretofore address the issue of toxic consequences to lidocaine overdosing. Intraoperatively, prudent anesthetic management should include good intravenous access and standard monitors (EKG, pulse oximetry, blood pressure, temperature monitoring). End tidal CO$_2$ is a standard of care for general anesthetics and strongly recommended for opioid-based IV sedation techniques. Fluid-in/urine-out assessment and aspirate volume tracking are also important. In addition, experienced practitioners will anecdotally report an added value to BIS monitoring under anesthesia. Because CNS toxicity symptoms typically occur prior to end-stage cardiac toxicity in lidocaine overdosing, there may be a potential value to monitoring the brain while under anesthesia for exten-

sive, prolonged SAL or liposuction. Surveyors for JCAHO, AAAHC, and AAAASF often offer the insight that freestanding facilities (especially single-specialty, office-based operating room suites) are notoriously underequipped for emergency contingencies.

From supplies for malignant hyperthermia to difficult airway carts (adult and pediatric) and code crash carts, anesthesiologists, surgeons, and administrators would be well served in seeking and maintaining the standards required for facility accreditation. It takes only one emergency to reveal the deadly vulnerability of a poorly equipped facility. Freestanding operating rooms must be even more prepared and inclusively self-sufficient than hospital-based operating suites. Greater strides in anesthesia-surgeon cooperation, and the more frequent use of local/MAC, regional block, and BIS-monitored PK (propofol-ketamine) MAC anesthetics, have significantly reduced the need to open the crash cart in the first place! Luck always favors the prepared.

Suggestions for Clinical Practice
Lidocaine toxicity in the **context** of megadose lidocaine tumescent solution injection poses far more unique and interesting questions than is observed with simple subcutaneous infiltration of this drug. Tumescent or wetting injection should not be restricted by the overly conservative formerly published PDR guidelines of 7 mg · kg^{-1} or 500 mg total (with epinephrine) maximum dosing.

Preoperative assessment
It is essential that patients undergo a thorough preoperative medical history (see Chapter 14 and Appendix A). All medications used and discontinued within two weeks prior to surgery should be noted in the patient record. Consideration should be taken for these drugs to have a potential effect on the liver cytochrome P450 enzyme system. In addition to the influence these medications may have on lidocaine metabolism and blood levels, a close eye should be trained on all medications given in the immediate preoperative, intraoperative, and postoperative period.

Sound clinical, perioperative management of patients receiving lidocaine, especially in the context of SAL or liposuction, should incorporate careful patient selection criteria. This is an area of anesthesia and surgical care that is often lost in the various discussions and articles on this subject. Once a patient has passed the basic preoperative laboratory and history hurdles, a solid "laying of hands" should establish the suitability of a patient's cardiac, respiratory, and airway status for surgical clearance. Any signs of fever, productive cough, or labored breathing should be cause for concern. Similarly, wheezing, distended neck veins, or significant peripheral edema should raise red flags immediately. Defer and reschedule the case if and when adequate clinical investigation can establish the patient's acceptability for surgery and anesthesia.

SAL or liposuction is not equivalent to cataract extraction or ganglion cyst surgery.

Foresight must be applied to the scheduled surgical procedure. The ambulatory setting does not allow the routine application of invasive monitoring and thus demands a higher degree of scrutiny in choosing appropriate surgical candidates.

A patient's airway should be carefully assessed for adequacy of mouth opening, presence of dentures, veneers or teeth in poor condition, range of motion about the neck, and the ability to tolerate easily LMA or endotracheal intubation. When in doubt of the potential intraoperative patency of a patient's airway, every effort should be made to obtain previous surgical records and/or speak with the anesthesiologist who was involved in the earlier cases.

CONCLUSION

This chapter has touched not only on the basic pharmacology and pharmacokinetics of lidocaine use and toxicity but also on some of the peripheral issues surrounding this important subject. The clinical techniques of tumescent or megadose lidocaine use, SAL- or liposuction-related complications, and some reported cases of lidocaine toxicity have been reviewed. Also discussed were salient perioperative- and facility-related issues that may affect patient outcomes in the setting of SAL or liposuction. These findings suggest that the continued quest for patient safety should not ignore the progressive trends of office-based dermatologists, plastic surgeons, and anesthesiologists who have made significant contributions to patient safety over the past two decades. With patient safety at the foremost, these pioneers have creatively pushed the envelope of the lidocaine dosage and encouraged anesthesiology practices to avoid the use of traditional general inhala-

tion anesthesia. The discussion of lidocaine toxicity and, more specifically, an examination of megadose lidocaine in tumescent liposuction, covers the full gamut of adequate patient evaluation and clinical management skills necessary for the safe and vigilant practice of anesthesia in the outpatient perioperative setting. Although controversy exists around the safety of liposuction and lidocaine dosing, this most popular of cosmetic surgical procedures will continue to grow in numbers, as does experience, understanding, and comfort level with tumescent technique.

REFERENCES

1. Goodman, Gillman: *The Pharmacologic Basis of Therapeutics.* 10th ed. New York, McGraw-Hill, 2001, pp. 374, 961.
2. Ibid.
3. Boyes RN: *The pharmacokinetics of lidocaine in man. Clin Pharmacol Ther* 12:105,1971.
4. Narand PK: *Lidocaine and its active metabolites. Clin Pharmacol Ther* 24:654,1978.
5. Melmon HK: Clinical Pharmacology: *Basic Principles in Therapeutics.* 2nd ed. New York, Macmillan Ltd. 1978, p. 226.
6. Marriot HJ: Lidocaine toxicity. *J Electrocardiology* 7:70, 1974.
7. Smith, M, Wolfram W: Toxicity-seizures in an infant caused by (or related to) oral viscous lidocaine use. *J Emerg Med* 10:587,1992.
8. Jonville AP, Barbier P: Accidental lidocaine overdose in an infant. *J Toxicol Clinical Toxicol* 28:101,1990.
9. Lie RL: Severe lidocaine intoxication by cutaneous absorption. *J Am Acad Derm* 5:1026,1990.
10. Palmisano JM: Lidocaine toxicity after subcutaneous infiltration in children undergoing cardiac catheterization. *Am J Cardiol* 67:647,1991.
11. Coldiron B, Shreve BA, Balkrishnan R, et al.: Patient injuries from surgical procedures performed in medical offices: Three years of Florida data. *Dermatol Surg* 30:1435, 2004.
12. Williford P: Commentary on Coldiron B, Shreve E, Balkrishnan R: Patient injuries from surgical procedures performed in medical offices: Three years of Florida data. *Dermatol Surg* 30:1443,2004.
13. Gorney M: Liability issues in aesthetic surgery. *Aesth Surg J* 2:226,2000.
14. Grazer FM, de Jong RH: Fatal outcomes from liposuction: Census survey of cosmetic surgeons. *Plast Reconstr Surg* 105:436,2000.
15. Rao, RB, Ely, SF: Deaths related to liposuction. *N Engl J Med* 340:1471,1999.
16. Lofsky AS: Deep venous thrombosis and pulmonary embolism in plastic surgery office procedures. *The Doctors'*

Company Newsletter, Napa, CA,2005. www.thedoctors.com/risk/specialty/anesthesiology/J4254.asp

17. Lillis PJ: Liposuction under local anesthesia: Limited blood loss and minimal lidocaine absorption. *J Dermatol Oncol Surg* 14:1145,1988.

18. Hildreth B: Large Volume Liposuction. Presented at the World Congress of Liposuction, Pasadena, CA, October 9–11, 1998.

19. Friedberg BL: Propofol ketamine anesthesia for cosmetic surgery in the office suite, chapter in Osborn I (ed.), *Anesthesia for Outside the Operating Room. International Anesthesiology Clinics.* Baltimore, Lippincott, Williams & Wilkins 41(3):47,2003.

20. www.asds-net.org/liposafety (Am Soc for Dermatological Surgeons); www.plasticsurgery.org/mediactr/natstats (Am Soc of Plastic Surgeons).

21. Cosmetic Surgery National Data Bank 2003 Statistics. New York, NY. *Am Soc for Aesthetic Plastic Surgery*, 2004.

22. Klein JA: The tumescent technique for liposuction surgery. *Am J Cosmet Surg* 4:263,1987.

23. Klein JA: Tumescent technique for regional anesthesia permits lidocaine doses of 35 mg/kg for liposuction. *J Dermatol Surg Oncol* 16:248,1990.

24. Fodor PB: Defining wetting solutions in lipoplasty. *Plast Reconstr Surg* 103:1519,1999.

25. Ostad A, Kageyama N: Tumescent anesthesia with a lidocaine dose of 55 mg/kg is safe for liposuction. *Dermatol Surg* 22:921,1996.

26. Laurito CE: Anesthesia provided at alternative sites, in Barasch PG, Cullen BF, Stoelting RK (eds.), *Clincal Anesthesia*, 4th ed., Philadelphia, Lippincott, Williams & Wilkins, 2001, p. 1343.

9 | Local Anesthetic Blocks in Head and Neck Surgery

Joseph Niamtu, III, D.M.D.

INTRODUCTION

One of the biggest advances in the last thousand years of medical history has been the discovery of local anesthesia. Prior to this, patients had to endure excruciating pain with procedures taken for granted today. Even the toughest patient cannot imagine having a tooth extracted or an extremity amputated with no anesthesia. Prior to the late 1800s, one could get drunk or literally bite the bullet, neither of which had any effect on pain. An interesting article appeared about a .50 caliber bullet found at the site of the Battle of Ox Hill. The 21st Massachusetts Regiment

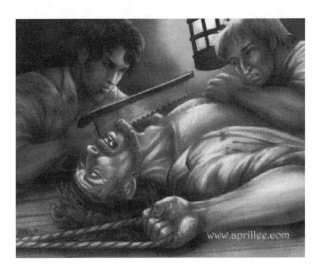

Figure 9-1. Biting the bullet was apparently utilized as a means of pain control prior to the advent of anesthesia.

had fought at a local cornfield with extreme and horrifying injuries. Yet, they had no medical care. The bullet has molar tooth cusp imprints, reportedly from a patient biting during surgery without anesthesia. Figure 9-1 shows an artist's rendition of the horror and panic of such a battlefield amputation, complete with a bullet between the patient's teeth.

Cocaine was the first local anesthetic to be widely used in surgical applications. In the 19th century, it was reported that the Indians of the Peruvian highlands chewed the leaves of the coca leaf (*Erythroxylon coca*) for its stimulating and exhilatory effects.[1-3] It was also observed that these Indians observed numbness in the areas around the lips. In 1859, Albert Niemann, a German chemist, was given credit for being the first to extract the isolate cocaine from the coca shrub in a purified form. When Niemann tasted the substance, his tongue became numb. This property led to one of the most humane discoveries in all of medicine and surgery. Over two decades later, Sigmund Freud began treating patients with cocaine for its physiologic and psychologic effects. While treating a colleague for morphine dependence, the patient developed cocaine dependence.[4]

A resident at the University of Vienna Ophthalmologic Clinic named Koller demonstrated the topical anesthetic activity of cocaine on the cornea in animal models and on himself. In an operation for glaucoma, Koller used cocaine for local anesthesia in 1894.

William Halsted was a prominent American surgeon who investigated the principles of nerve block using cocaine. In November 1884, Dr. Halsted performed infraorbital and inferior alveolar (mandibular) dental block. Halsted also demonstrated various other regional anesthetic techniques. Halsted's self-experimentation with cocaine caused an addiction. After two years of effort to resolve his addiction, he regained his eminent position in surgery and teaching.

Early dentists dissolved cocaine hydrochloride pills in water and drew this mixture up in a syringe to perform nerve infiltrations and blocks. The extreme vasoconstrictive effects of cocaine often caused tissue necrosis but nonetheless provided profound local anesthesia that revolutionized dentistry and medicine forever. Many proprietary preparations of that time period contained cocaine.

By the early 1900s, cocaine's adverse effects became well recognized. These deleterious effects included profound cardiac stimulation and vasoconstriction. Cocaine blocks the neuronal reuptake of norepinephrine in the peripheral nervous system. Myocardial stimulation in combination with coronary artery vasoconstriction has proven lethal in sensitive individuals. Cocaine causes central nervous system stimulation and mood-altering euphoric effect. These effects coupled with the severe physical and psychological dependence proved to be significant drawbacks to cocaine use for local anesthesia.

In 1904, Alfred Einhorn, searching for a safer and less toxic local anesthetic, synthesized procaine (Novocain). Novocain was the gold standard of topical anesthetics for almost forty years when Nils Lofgren synthesized lidocaine (Xylocaine), the first amide group of local anesthetics. Lidocaine provided advantages over the ester group (procaine) in terms of greater potency, less allergic potential, and a more rapid onset of anesthesia.[1,2,5,6]

THE MECHANISM OF ACTION OF LOCAL ANESTHETICS

Local anesthetics block the sensation of pain by *interfering with the propagation of impulses* along peripheral nerve fibers without significantly altering normal resting membrane potentials.[7] Local anesthetics depolarize the nerve membranes and prevent achievement of a threshold potential. A propagated action potential fails to develop and a conduction blockade is achieved. This occurs by the

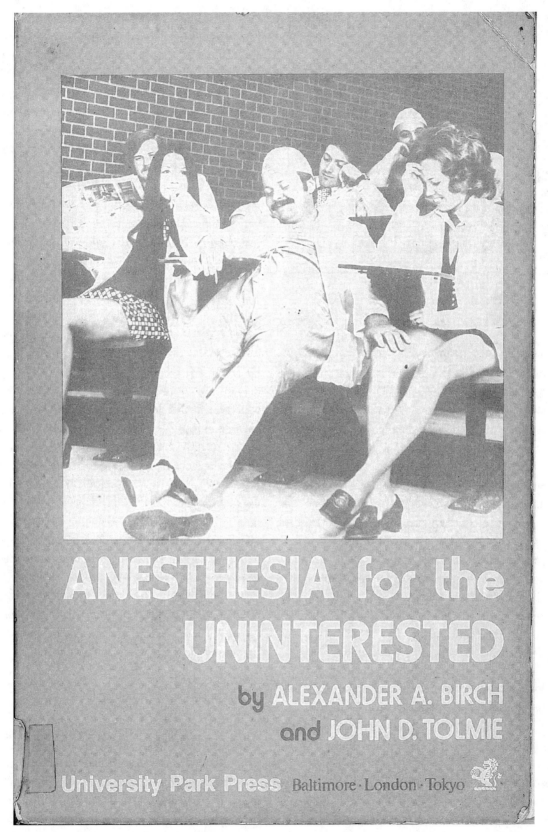

Figure 9-1A. Cover of out-of-print (1976) anesthesia text.

interference of nerve transmission by blocking the influx of sodium through the excitable nerve membrane.[8]

SCIENCE IS SOMETIMES BORING!

When reading the following section, some of the information is clearly boring see Fig. 9-1A. Finite anatomy was boring for most medical and dental students, but it is ultimately *very* important. In order to fully understand how and when to perform a local anesthetic block, one must appreciate the anatomy.

Sensory Anatomy of the Head and Neck

The main sensory innervation of the face is derived from cranial nerve V (trigeminal nerve) and the upper cervical nerves. see Fig. 9-2.

Sensory anatomy of the trigeminal nerve

The trigeminal nerve is the fifth of the twelve cranial nerves. Its branches originate at the semilunar ganglion (*Gasserian ganglion*) located in a cavity (Meckel's cave) near the apex of the petrous part of the temporal bone. Three large nerves, the ophthalmic, maxillary, and mandibular, proceed from the ganglion to supply sensory innervation to the face. Often referred to as "the great sensory nerve of the head and neck," the trigeminal nerve is named for its three major sensory branches. The ophthalmic nerve (V1), maxillary nerve (V2), and mandibular nerve (V3) are literally "three twins" (trigeminal) carrying sensory information of light touch, temperature, pain, and proprioception from the face and scalp to the brainstem. The commonly used terms V1, V2, and V3 are shorthand notation for cranial nerve 5, branches 1, 2, and 3, respectively. In addition to nerves carrying incoming sensory information, certain branches of the trigeminal nerve also contain nerves motor components. *The ophthalmic and maxillary nerves consist exclusively of sensory fibers; the mandibular nerve is joined outside the cranium by the motor root.* These outgoing motor components include branchial motor nerves (i.e., nerves innervating muscles derived embryologically from the branchial arches) as well as "hitchhiking" visceral motor nerves (i.e., nerves innervating viscera, including smooth muscle and glands). The trigeminal nerve exits the trigeminal ganglion and courses "backward" to enter the midlateral aspect of the pons at the brainstem.[9]

The ophthalmic nerve (V1) leaves the semilunar ganglion through the superior orbital fissure. The maxillary nerve (V2) leaves the semilunar ganglion through the foramen rotundum at the skull base, and the mandibular nerve (V3) leaves the semilunar ganglion through the foramen ovale at the skull base (see Fig. 9-3 inset[9]). The remainder of this chapter discusses *only* the sensory components of this nerve system as they relate to local anesthetic blocking techniques for cosmetic facial procedures.

Sensory anatomy of the ophthalmic nerve (V1)

The ophthalmic nerve, or first division of the trigeminal, is a sensory nerve. It supplies branches to the cornea, ciliary body, and iris; to the lacrimal gland and conjunctiva; to the part of the mucous membrane of the nasal cavity; and to the skin of the eyelids, eyebrow, forehead, and upper lateral nose (see Fig. 9-3 V1). The smallest of the three divisions of the trigeminal, it divides into three branches: the frontal, the nasociliary, and the lacrimal.[9] The frontal nerve divides into the supraorbital and supratrochlear nerves providing sensation to the forehead and anterior scalp.

The nasociliary nerve divides into four branches, two of which supply sensory innervation to the face. These two branches are the infratrochlear and the ethmoidal nerves. The infratrochlear nerve supplies sensation to the skin of the medial eyelids and side of the nose. The

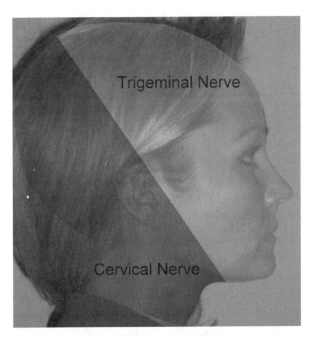

Figure 9-2. Sensory innervation of the head and neck is derived from the trigeminal and upper cervical nerves.

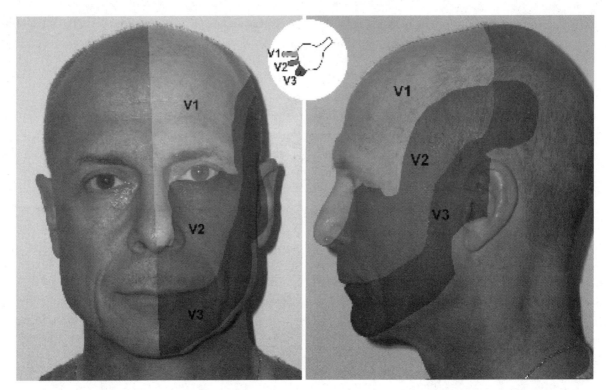

Figure 9-3. Main branches of the trigeminal nerve supplying sensation to the respective facial areas. The inset shows the trigeminal ganglion with the three main nerve branches.

terminal branch of the ethmoidal nerve is called the external (or dorsal) nasal nerve. The ethmoidal nerve innervates the skin of the nasal dorsum and tip. The lacrimal nerve innervates the skin of the upper eyelid.

Local Anesthetic Techniques for the Scalp and Forehead

The frontal nerve exits through a notch (in some cases a foramen) on the superior orbital rim approximately 27 mm lateral to the glabellar midline. This supraorbital notch is readily palpable in most patients. After exiting the notch or foramen, the nerve traverses the corrugator supercilli muscles and branches into a medial and lateral portion. The lateral branches supply the lateral forehead and the medial branches supply the scalp. The supratrochlear nerve exits a foramen approximately 17 mm from the glabellar midline (see Fig. 9-4) and supplies sensation to the middle portion of the forehead. The infratrochlear nerve exits a foramen below the trochlea and provides sensation to the medial upper eyelid, canthus, medial nasal skin, conjunctiva, and lacrimal apparatus.[10]

When injecting this area, it is prudent to always use the free hand to palpate the orbital rim to prevent inadvertent injection into the globe! To anesthetize this area, the supratrochlear nerve is measured 17 mm from the glabellar midline and 1–2 cc of 2% lidocaine 1:100,000 epinephrine are injected (see Fig. 9-5 left). The supraorbital nerve is blocked by palpating the notch (and or measuring 27 mm from the glabellar midline) and injecting 2 cc of local anesthetic solution (see Fig. 9-5 center). The infratrochlear nerve is blocked by injecting 1–2 cc of local anesthetic solution at the junction of the orbit and the nasal bones (see Figure 9-5 right). In reality, one can block all three of these nerves by simple injecting 2–4 cc of local anesthetic solution from the central brow proceeding to the medial brow Figure 9-6 shows the regions anesthetized from these blocks.

Sensory anatomy of the maxillary nerve (V2)

The maxillary nerve or second division of the trigeminal is a sensory nerve that crosses the pterygopalatine fossa before traversing the orbit in the infraorbital groove and canal in the floor of the orbit. It appears on the face at

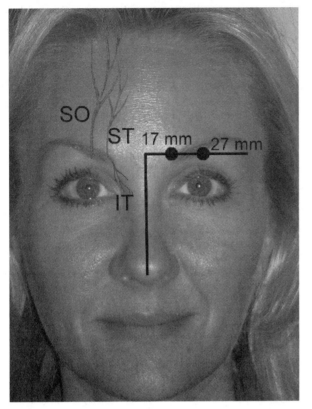

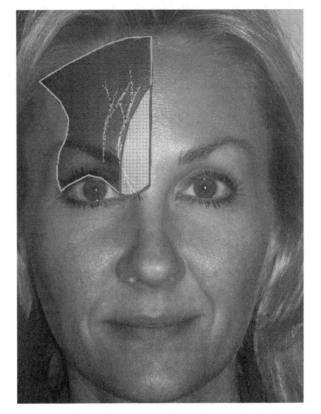

Figure 9-4. The supraorbital nerve (SO) exits about 27 mm from the glabellar midline, and the supratrochlear nerve (ST) is located approximately 17 mm from the glabellar midline. The infratrochlear nerve (IT) exits below the trochlea.

Figure 9-6. The shaded areas indicate the anesthetized areas from supraorbital nerve (SO), supratrochlear nerve (ST), and infratrochlear nerve (IT) blocks.

the infraorbital foramen as the infraorbital nerve.[9] At its termination, the nerve divides into branches that spread out on the side of the nose, the lower eyelid, and the upper lip, joining with filaments of the facial nerve.[9] Terminal branches include the following.

The zygomatic nerve arises in the pterygopalatine fossa, enters the orbit by the inferior orbital fissure, and divides

at the back of that cavity into two terminal branches, the zygomaticotemporal and zygomaticofacial nerves.

The zygomaticotemporal branch runs along the lateral wall of the orbit in a groove in the zygomatic bone before passing through a foramen in the zygomatic bone and entering the temporal fossa. It ascends between the bone and substance of the temporalis muscle and pierces the

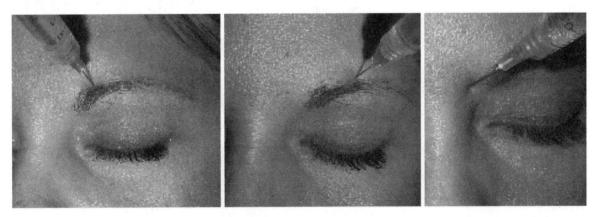

Figure 9-5. The forehead and scalp are blocked by a series of injections from the central to the medial brow.

temporal fascia about 2.5 cm above the zygomatic arch where it is distributed to the skin of the side of the forehead (see Fig. 9-3 V2).

The zygomaticofacial branch passes along the infero-lateral angle of the orbit, emerges on the face through a foramen in the zygomatic bone, and perforates the orbicularis oculi and supplies the skin on the prominence of the cheek (see Fig. 9-3 V2).

As the maxillary nerve traverses the orbital floor and exits the infraorbital foramen, it branches into a plexus of nerves that has the following terminal branches.

The inferior palpebral branches ascend behind the orbicularis oculi muscle and supply the skin and conjunctiva of the lower eyelid (see Fig. 9-3 V2).

The lateral nasal branches (rami nasales externi) supply the skin of the side of the nose (see Fig. 9-3 V2).

The superior labial branches are distributed to the skin of the upper lip, the mucous membrane of the mouth, and labial glands (see Fig. 9-3 V2).

Local Anesthetic Techniques for the Infraorbital Nerve Block

The infraorbital nerve exits the infraorbital foramen 4–7 mm below the orbital rim in an imaginary line dropped from the medial limbus of the iris or the pupillary midline. The anterior superior alveolar nerve branches from the infraorbital nerve before it exits the foramen, and thus some patients will manifest anesthesia of the anterior teeth and gingiva if the branching is close to the foramen. Areas anesthetized include the lateral nose, anterior cheek, lower eyelid, and upper lip on the injected side. This nerve can be blocked either by the intraoral or extraoral route.

To perform an infraorbital nerve block from an intraoral approach, topical anesthesia is placed on the oral mucosa at the vestibular sulcus just under the canine fossa (between the canine and first premolar tooth) and left for several minutes. The lip is then elevated and a 1.5-inch 27 gauge needle is inserted in the sulcus and directed superiorly toward the infraorbital foramen (see Fig. 9-7). The needle does not need to enter the foramen for a successful block. The anesthetic solution needs only to contact the vast branching around the foramen to be effective. It is imperative to use the other hand to palpate the inferior orbital rim to avoid injecting the orbit. Two to four cc of 2% lidocaine with 1:100,000 epinephrine is injected in this area for the infraorbital block.

The infraorbital nerve can also be very easily blocked by a facial approach. This is the preferred route of the author. This may also be the preferred route in dental-phobic patients. A 27 ga 0.5-inch needle is used and is placed through the skin and aimed at the foramen in a perpendicular direction. Two to four cc of local anesthetic solution is injected at or close to the foramen (see

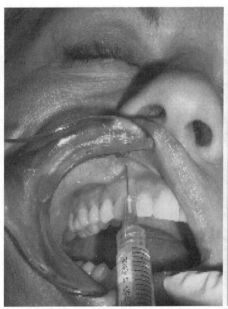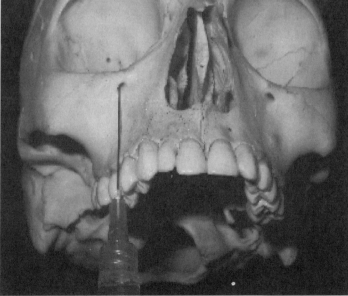

Figure 9-7. The intraoral approach for local anesthetic block of the infraorbital nerve.

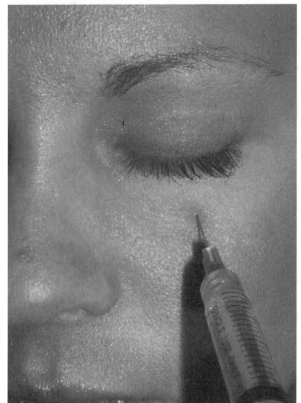

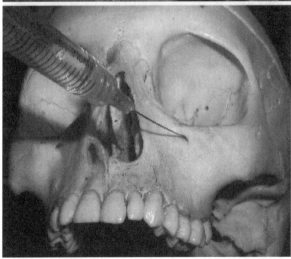

Figure 9-8. The facial approach for local anesthetic block of the infraorbital nerve.

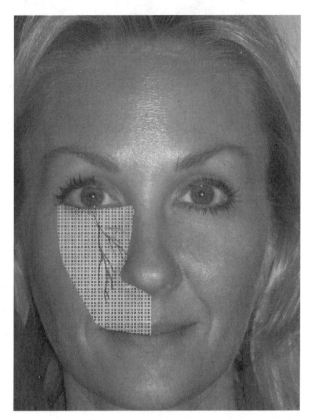

Figure 9-9. Area of anesthesia from unilateral infraorbital nerve block.

Fig. 9-8). Again, the other hand must constantly palpate the inferior orbital rim to prevent inadvertent injection into the orbit.

A successful infraorbital nerve block will anesthetize the infraorbital cheek, the lower palpebral area, the lateral nasal area, and superior labial regions, as shown in Figure 9-9.

The aforementioned techniques provide anesthesia to the lateral nasal skin but does not provide anesthesia to the central portion of the nose. A dorsal (external) nasal nerve block will supplement nasal anesthesia by providing anesthesia over the area of the cartilaginous nasal dorsum and tip. This supplementary nasal block is accomplished by palpating the inferior rim of the nasal bones at the osseous cartilaginous junction. The dorsal nerve (anterior ethmoid branch of the nasocillary nerve) emerges 5–10 mm from the nasal midline at the osseous junction of the inferior portion of the nasal bones (the distal edge of the nasal bones) (see Fig. 9-10). The dotted line in Figure 9-14 shows the course of this nerve under the nasal bones before emerging.

Two often-overlooked nerves in facial local anesthetic blocks are the zygomaticotemporal and zygomaticofacial nerves. These nerves represent terminal branches of the zygomatic nerve. The zygomaticotemporal nerve emerges through a foramen located on the anterior wall of the temporal fossa. This foramen is actually behind the lateral orbital rim posterior to the zygoma at the approximate level of the lateral canthus (see Fig. 9-11).

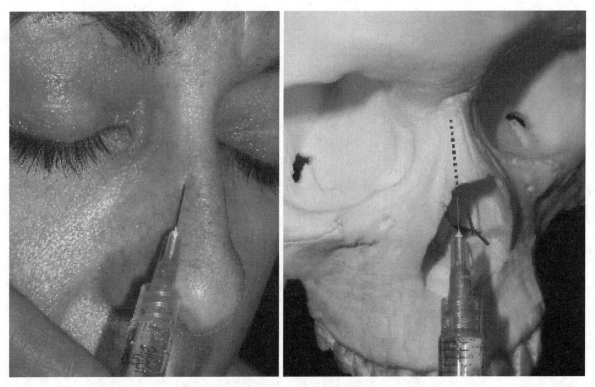

Figure 9-10. The dorsal (external) nasal nerve is blocked subcutaneously at the osseous-cartilaginous junction of the distal nasal bones.

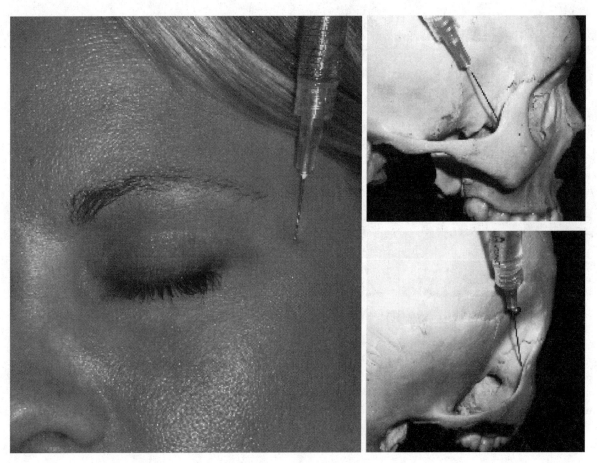

Figure 9-11. The zygomaticotemporal nerve is blocked by placing the needle on the concave surface of the posterior lateral orbital rim.

Injection technique involves sliding a 1.5-inch needle behind the concave portion of the lateral orbital rim. It is suggested that one closely examine this area on a model skull prior to attempting this injection, as it will make the technique simpler.

To orient for this injection, the doctor needs to palpate the lateral orbital rim at the level of the frontozygomatic suture (which is frequently palpable). With the index finger in the depression of the posterior lateral aspect of the lateral orbital rim (inferior and posterior to the frontozygomatic suture), the operator places the needle just behind the palpating finger (which is about 1 centimeter posterior to the frontozygomatic suture) (see Fig. 9-11). The needle is then "walked" down the concave posterior wall of the lateral orbital rim to the approximate level of the lateral canthus. After aspirating, 1–2 cc of 2% lidocaine 1:100,000 epinephrine is injected in this area with a slight pumping action to ensure deposition of the local anesthetic solution at or about the foramen. Again, it is important to hug the back concave wall of the lateral orbital rim with the needle when injecting.

Blocking the zygomaticotemporal nerve causes anesthesia in the area superior to the nerve including the lateral orbital rim and the skin of the temple from above the zygomatic arch to the temporal fusion line (see Fig. 9-12 ZT).

The zygomaticofacial nerve exits through a foramen (or foramina in some patients) in the inferior lateral portion of the orbital rim at the zygoma. If the surgeon palpates the junction of the inferior lateral (the most southwest portion

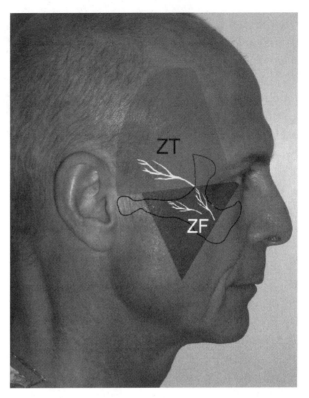

Figure 9-12. The anesthetized areas from the zygomaticotemporal (ZT) and the zygomaticofacial nerve (ZF).

of the right orbit, if you will) portion of the lateral orbital rim, the nerve emerges several millimeters lateral to this point. By palpating this area and injecting just lateral to the finger, this nerve is successfully blocked with 1–2 cc of local anesthesia (see Fig. 9-13). Blocking this nerve will

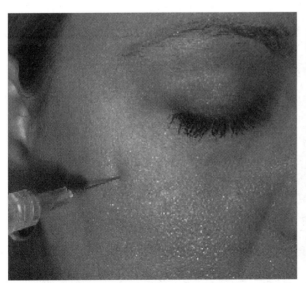

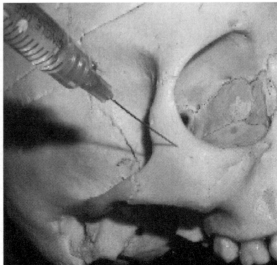

Figure 9-13. The zygomaticofacial nerve(s) is blocked by injecting the inferior lateral portion of the orbital rim.

result in anesthesia of a triangular area from the lateral canthus and the malar region along the zygomatic arch and some skin inferior to this area[10] (see Fig. 9-12).

Total second division nerve block

An efficient and simple technique to obtain hemi midfacial local anesthesia is to block the entire second division or maxillary nerve. This will anesthetize the entire hemimaxilla and the unilateral maxillary sinus by blocking the pterygopalatine, infraorbital, and zygomatic nerves and their terminal branches. This is an easily learned technique involving an intraoral approach at the posterior lateral palate (see Fig. 9-14). The maxillary nerve block via the greater palatine canal was first described in 1917 by Mendel.[11] The greater palatine foramen is located anterior to the junction of the hard and soft palate medial to the second molar tooth (see Fig. 9-14 center). The foramen is usually found about 7 mm anterior to the hard and soft palate junction. This junction is seen as a color change such that the tissue overlying the soft palate is darker pink than the tissue overlying the hard palate. The key to this block is to place a 1.5-inch needle through the greater palatine foramen. It sometimes takes multiple needle sticks to localize the foramen. Due to the need for multiple sticks, the palatal mucosa in this area is first infiltrated with 0.5 cc of lidocaine to facilitate painless location of the greater palatine foramen. A 1.5-inch 25 or 27 ga needle is bent to a 45 degree angle and will usually easily negotiate

the pterygopalatine canal, thereby placing the local anesthetic solution into the pterygopalatine fossa. The course of the maxillary division of the trigeminal nerve (V2) is as follows. The second division of the trigeminal nerve arises from the gasserian ganglion in the medial cranial fossa and exits the skull via the foramen rotundum (see Fig. 9-14 right). The nerve then traverses the superior aspect of the pterygopalatine fossa, where it divides into three major branches: the pterygopalatine nerve, the infraorbital nerve, and the zygomatic nerve.[12] These nerves are targeted in this block.

When the foramen is located, the needle should be gently advanced. If significant resistance is encountered, the needle should be withdrawn and redirected. Approximately 5 percent of the population has been shown to have tortuous canals that impede the needle tip and in some patients this technique is not possible. It is also important to aspirate before injecting to prevent intravascular injection. When the needle is properly positioned (usually at a depth of 25–30 mm), the injection (2–4 ml) should proceed over thirty to forty-five seconds. Transient diplopia of the ipsilateral eye may occur. This results from the local anesthetic diffusing superiorly and medially to anesthetize the orbital nerves. The patient must be assured that if this phenomenon occurs, it is transient. Again, this technique will anesthetize all the terminal branches of the maxillary nerve with a single injection.

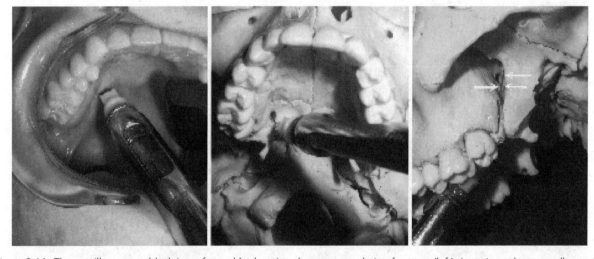

Figure 9-14. The maxillary nerve block is performed by locating the greater palatine foramen (left), inserting a bent needle up the pterygopalatine canal (center) to inject local anesthetic into the pterygopalatine fossa (right). Notice the needle tip in the pterygopalatine fossa on the far right image. As the second division traverses this area, it is blocked at the main trunk.

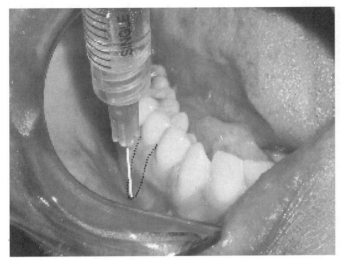 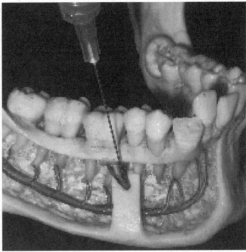

Figure 9-15. The mental foramen is approached intraorally below the root tip of the lower second premolar (left) or from a facial approach (right).

Sensory anatomy of the mandibular nerve (V3)

The mandibular nerve supplies the teeth and gums of the mandible, the skin of the temporal region, part of the auricle, the lower lip, and the lower part of the face (see Fig. 9-3 V3). The mandibular nerve also supplies the muscles of mastication and the mucous membrane of the anterior two thirds of the tongue. It is the largest of the three divisions of the fifth cranial nerve and is made up of a motor and sensory root.[9]

Sensory branches of the mandibular nerve include the auriculotemporal nerve, which supplies sensation to the skin covering the front of the helix and tragus (see Fig. 9-3).

The inferior alveolar nerve is the largest branch of the mandibular nerve. It descends with the inferior alveolar artery and exits the ramus of the mandible to the mandibular foramen. It then passes forward in the mandibular canal, beneath the teeth, as far as the mental foramen, where it divides into two terminal branches, incisive and mental nerves. The mental nerve emerges at the mental foramen and divides into three branches. One branch descends to the skin of the chin, and two branches ascend to the skin and mucous membrane of the lower lip. The buccal nerve supplies sensation to the skin over the buccinator muscle.[9]

Local Anesthetic Techniques for the Mental Nerve Block

The mental nerve exits the mental foramen on the hemi mandible at the base of the root of the second premo-lar (many patients may be missing a premolar due to orthodontic extractions). The mental foramen is on the average 11 mm inferior to the gum line (see Fig. 9-15). There is variability with this foramen, like all foramina. However, by injecting 2 to 4 cc of local anesthetic solution about 10 mm inferior to the gum line or 15 mm inferior to the top of the crown of the second premolar tooth, the block is usually successful. In a patient without teeth, the foramen is oftentimes located much higher on the jaw and can sometimes be palpated. This block is performed more superiorly in the denture-wearing patient. As stated earlier, the foramen does not need to be entered because a sufficient volume of local anesthetic solution in the general area will be effective. By placing traction on the lip and pulling it away from the jaw, the labial branches of the mental nerve can sometimes be seen traversing through the thin mucosa. The mental nerve gives off labial branches to the lip and chin.

When anesthetized, the distribution of numbness will be the unilateral lip down to the mentolabial fold, but many times to the anterior chin and cheek, depending on the individual furcating anatomy of that patient's nerve (see Fig. 9-16). The inferior alveolar nerve also supplies sensory innervation to the chin pad. The mylohyoid nerve may also innervate this area. To augment or extend the area of local anesthesia on the chin, an inferior alveolar nerve (mandibular dental block) block can be performed instead of or with the mental nerve block. Additionally, local skin infiltration in that area may assist.

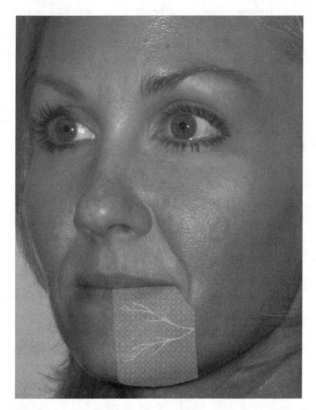

Figure 9-16. This shows the anesthetized areas from a unilateral mental nerve block. Because of various anatomic factors, the area below the mentolabial fold or at the midline may share other innervation.

Local Anesthetic Techniques for the Inferior Alveolar Nerve Block (Intraoral)

Almost every person who has ever been to a dentist has had this block and is aware of its effects, distribution, and duration. This block is technically more difficult to master but is easily learned. The basis of this technique involves the deposition of local anesthetic solution at or about the mandibular foramen on the medial mandibular ramus where the inferior alveolar nerve enters the mandible (see Fig. 9-17).

Detailed description of this technique is beyond the scope of this review article but will be outlined as follows. The patient is seated upright and the surgeon places the index finger on the posterior ramus and the thumb in the coronoid notch on the anterior mandibular ramus (see Fig. 9-17).

A 1.5-inch 27 ga needle is then directed to the medial mandibular ramus at the level of the cusps of the upper second molar and the needle is advanced halfway between the thumb and index finger of the other hand that is grasping the mandible.

Two cc of 2% lidocaine, 1:100,000 epinephrine is then injected in a pumping motion to better the chances of anesthetic solution contacting the nerve and foramen. The needle can be slightly bent as shown in Figure 9-18 to negotiate the sometimes outward curvature of the

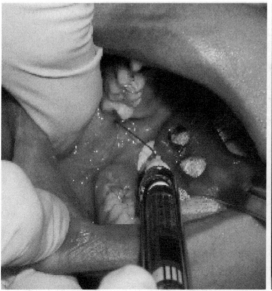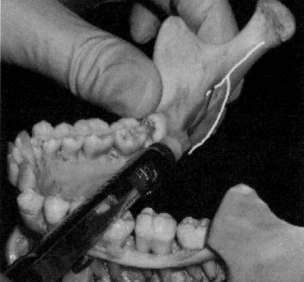

Figure 9-17. The target of the needle in the intraoral inferior alveolar nerve block is at the entrance of the nerve in the mandibular foramen on the medial ramus. The needle can be slightly bent with a medial angle to negotiate the flaring anatomy of the ramus. The mylohyoid nerve (inferior to needle) may or may not be blocked by this technique depending on its level of branching.

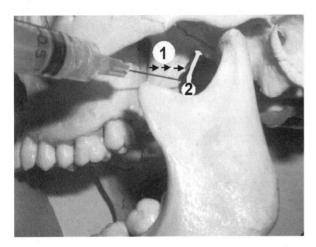

Figure 9-18. The mandibular nerve (V3) block places the local anesthetic just posterior to the lateral pterygoid plate, where the third division of the trigeminal nerve exits the foramen ovale. The needle is walked off the pterygoid plate (1), and the local anesthetic solution is deposited in the region of the third division of the trigeminal nerve (2).

mandibular ramus. The surgeon should first aspirate to avoid intravascular injection. Anesthesia from this block sometimes takes five to ten minutes to take effect. Proficiency in this blocking technique requires practice but is very useful in cosmetic facial procedures. In addition, the ispilateral tongue is usually anesthetized with this block. The area anesthetized includes the lower teeth and gums, the chin, and skin on the lateral chin. The inferior alveolar nerve block frequently includes the mylohyoid nerve. In some patients, the mylohyoid nerve branches above the area of inferior alveolar injection and in this case needs a specific mylohyoid nerve block, as outlined previously.

Local Anesthetic Techniques for the Mandibular Nerve (V3) Block (Facial Approach)

The mandibular nerve can also be blocked from a deep injection as the nerve exits the foramen ovale, posterior to the pterygoid plate[13] (see number 2 in Fig. 9-18). This technique requires more experience and has more potential complications than the intraoral approach.

The technique for performing this block begins with the patient in supine position with the head and neck turned away from the side to be blocked. The patient is asked to open and close the mouth gently so that the operator can identify and palpate the sigmoid notch. This is the area between the mandibular condyle and the coronoid pro-

cess. This notch is located about 25 mm anterior to the tragus. If one places their finger 25 mm anterior to the tragus and opens and closes the jaw, the mandibular condyle can be palpated with the jaw open. When the jaw is closed, the finger will be over the sigmoid notch. A 22 ga, 8-cm needle is inserted in the midpoint of the notch and directed at a slightly cephalic and medial to angle through the notch until the lateral pterygoid plate is contacted (number 1 in Fig. 9-18). This is usually at a depth of approximately 4.5–5.0 cm. Spinal needles frequently have measuring stops that can be adjusted to the position of original contact of the pterygoid plate. The needle is then withdrawn to a subcutaneous position and carefully "walked off" the posterior border of the pterygoid plate (arrows in Fig. 9-18) in a horizontal plane until the needle no longer touches the plate and is posterior to it. The needle depth should be the same as the distance on the needle stop marker when the pterygoid plate was originally contacted. The needle should not be advanced more than 0.5 cm past the depth of the pterygoid plate because the superior constrictor muscle of the pharynx can be pierced easily.[13] When the needle is in appropriate position, 5 cc of local anesthetic solution can be administered. The area anesthetized is shown as V3 in Figure 9-3. Complications include hematoma formation and subarachnoid injection. Again, this block should be learned in a proctored situation and not be attempted by novice injectors.

Sensory anatomy of the scalp

The anterior scalp is anesthetized by injecting the branches of V1 (supraorbital and supratrochlear nerves) and V2 (the zygomaticotemporal nerve). The greater and lesser occipital nerves innervate the posterior scalp. The greater auricular nerve supplies the lateral scalp (see Fig. 9-19).

The greater occipital nerve arises from the dorsal rami of the second cervical nerve and travels deep to the cervical musculature until it becomes subcutaneous slightly inferior to the superior nuchal line.[14] It emerges on this line in association with the occipital artery. The artery is the most useful landmark for locating the greater occipital nerve.

Local Anesthetic Techniques to Block the Scalp

By performing the brow blocks (see Fig. 9-5), the cervical plexus block (see Fig. 9-20), and the zygomaticotemporal

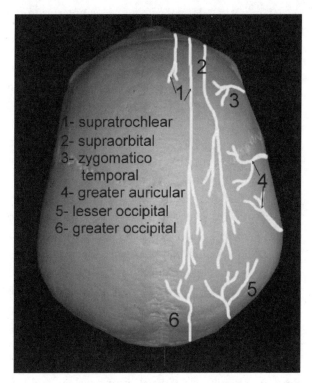

Figure 9-19. Innervation of the scalp where 1 = supratrochlear nerve, 2 = supraorbital nerve(s), 3 = zygomaticotemporal nerve, 4 = greater auricular nerve, 5 = lesser occipital nerve, 6 = greater occipital nerve.

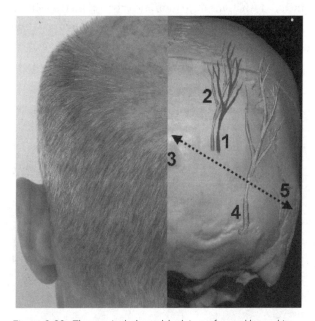

Figure 9-20. The cervical plexus block is performed by making a line from the mastoid process (1) to the level of the transverse process of C6 (2), then finding the point halfway between these two marks (X) just posterior to the sternocleidomastiod (dotted line). Local anesthetic is then injected perpendicularly, superiorly, and inferiorly in this region (the middle picture also shows the greater occipital nerve, which is not part of the cervical plexus.)

block (see Fig. 9-11), most of the scalp is anesthetized, except the posterior area. This is anesthetized by blocking the greater occipital nerve. One can also perform a ring block where wheals of local anesthetic are injected every several centimeters around the entire scalp at about the level of the eyebrows. About 30 cc of local is required to perform a scalp-ring block.

Greater Occipital Nerve Block Technique for Posterior Scalp Anesthesia

The most efficient patient position is sitting upright with the chin flexed to the sternum.[15] The nerve is identified at its point of entry to the scalp, along the superior nuchal line one third to one half the distance between the mastoid process and the occipital protuberance in the midline[14] (see Fig. 9-21). Another measurement for locating the artery is 2.5–3.0 cm lateral to the occipital protrubence.[16] The patient will report pain upon compression of the nerve: the point at which maximal tenderness is elicited can be used as the injection site. A 25 ga 5/8-inch needle is used for the block. The occipital artery is just lateral to the greater occipital nerve and can be used as a pulsatile landmark. Two to four cc of local anesthetic solution can be infiltrated on either side of the artery to ensure proximity to the nerve. Figure 9-22 shows the dermatomes anesthetized by blocking the greater occipital nerve.

Sensory Anatomy of the Neck; Innervation of the Cervical Plexus

The cervical plexus is formed from the ventral rami of the upper four cervical nerves (see Fig. 9-21 center). The dorsal and ventral roots combine to form spinal nerves as they exit through the intervertebral foramen. The anterior rami of C2 through C4 form the cervical plexus. The cervical plexus lies just behind the posterior border of the sternocleido-mastoid muscle, giving off both superficial (superficial cervical plexus) and deep branches (deep cervical plexus). The branches of the superficial cervical plexus supply the skin and superficial structures of the head, neck, and shoulder. The deep branches of the cervical plexus innervate the deeper structures of the neck, including the muscles of the anterior neck and the diaphragm (phrenic nerve) and are not blocked for local anesthetic procedures.

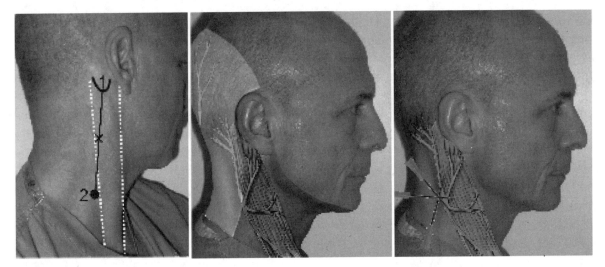

Figure 9-21. The greater occipital nerve is in close approximation to the artery of the same name (1). The nerve can be located by palpating the artery and injecting just medial to it (2). Another landmark is injecting on the nuchal line, one third to one half the distance between the mastoid prominence and occipital protrubence (3 and 5). Number 4 in the diagram shows the lesser occipital nerve.

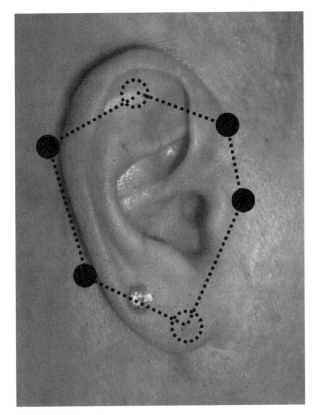

Figure 9-22. Blocking the entire ear (with the exception of the area supplied by the vagus nerve) can be performed by inserting the needle at the black dots and infiltrating along the dotted lines. This will anesthetize the terminal branches of the auriculotemporal nerve, the lesser occipital nerve, and the anterior and posterior branches of the greater auricular nerve. The main trunks of these nerves could be blocked as detailed earlier in this article, but this terminal infiltration technique may be more convenient.

Superficial branches of the cervical plexus include the following.

The lesser occipital nerve arises from the second (and sometimes third) cervical nerve and emerges from the deep fascia on the posterior lateral portion of the head behind the auricle, supplying the skin and communicating with the greater occipital, the great auricular, and the posterior auricular branch of the facial.

The greater auricular nerve arises from the second and third cervical nerves and divides into an anterior and a posterior branch. The anterior branch is distributed to the skin of the face over the parotid gland and communicates in the substance of the gland with the facial nerve.

The posterior branch supplies the skin over the mastoid process and on the back of the auricle, except at its upper part; a filament pierces the auricle to reach its lateral surface, where it is distributed to the lobule and lower part of the concha. The posterior branch communicates with the lesser occipital nerve, the auricular branch of the vagus, and the posterior auricular branch of the facial nerve.

The cutaneous cervical nerve (*cutaneus colli nerve, anterior cervical nerve*) arises from the second and third cervical nerves and provides sensation to the antero-lateral parts of the neck (see Fig. 9-21 center).

Local Anesthetic Techniques for the Cervical Plexus

This technique is used in cosmetic facial surgery to block the superficial branches of the cervical plexus to anesthetize skin of the lateral or anterior neck, the posterior lateral scalp, and portions of the periauricular area (see Fig. 9-2).

The technique involves lying the patient back with the sternocleidomastiod flexed, exposing the mastoid process and the transverse process of C6 (Chassaignac's Tubercle) (approximate level of the cricoid cartilage) (see Fig. 9-21 left). This line is divided in half at the posterior border of the sternocleidomastoid to determine the injection point. Another technique is to simply bisect the distance from the origin and insertion of the sternocleidomastoid without osseous landmarks. The success of this block involves a larger volume of local anesthesia diffusing and spreading out over a larger area rather than absolute accuracy of the nerve position. 3 to 5 cc of local anesthetic solution is injected subcutaneously with the needle perpendicular to the skin. The needle is then redirected superiorly and another 3 to 5 cc are injected. Finally, the needle is then directed inferiorly and another 3 to 5 cc is injected. Figure 9-21 (center) shows the areas anesthetized by a cervical plexus block.

Phrenic nerve involvement is rare with superficial cervical plexus block (more common with deep cervical blocks) but technically possible as C3, 4, and 5 innervate the diaphragm. Healthy patients can tolerate a hemi paralysis of the diaphragm. However, caution must be used in patients with cardiopulmonary problems because assisted ventilation may be required. It must be kept in mind that a bilateral block could potentially de-innervate the entire diaphragm. To prevent unwanted spread of local anesthetic solution, this injection is just subcutaneous in placement and **never done bilaterally**.

Selected Area Blocks
Anesthesia for the ear
Four nerve branches supply sensory innervation to the ear. The anterior half of the ear is supplied by the auriculotemporal nerve, which is a branch of the mandibular portion of the trigeminal nerve. The posterior half of the ear is innervated by two nerve branches derived from the cervical plexus: the great auricular nerve and the lesser occipital nerve (see Fig. 9-22 center). The auditory branch of the vagus nerve innervates the concha and external auditory canal.

Although these nerves can be individually targeted with blocks, a circumferential infiltration (ring block) will anesthetize the entire ear, except the concha and the external auditory canal, which are innervated by the Vagus nerve (CN X). The needle is inserted into the skin at the junction where the earlobe attaches to the head. The anesthetic should be infiltrated while the needle is advanced to the subcutaneous plane. Infiltration is made in a hexagonal pattern around the entire periphery of the ear (see Fig. 9-22). The chonal bowl and external auditory canal will need separate infiltration. One should aspirate (as with all injections) prior to injection to prevent intravascular injection.

Anesthesia for the nose
The nose receives innervation from multiple nerves. The supratrochlear and infratrochlear nerves innervate the root, bridge, and upper portion of the side of the nose. The infraorbital nerve supplies the skin on the side of almost half of the lower nose. The external nasal branch of the anterior ethmoidal nerve (dorsal nasal nerve) exits between the nasal bone and the lateral nasal cartilage to supply the skin over the dorsum of this part of the nose to the tip.

Anesthetic techniques for blocking the nose vary with the type of procedure being performed. To block the external nasal structures (the bridge and tip), bilateral blocks of the following nerves are performed: infraorbital, supratrochlear, infratrochlear, and the dorsal nasal nerves.

For internal nasal surgery such as rhinoplasty or nasal trauma, the aforementioned blocks are performed in conjunction with the following. The second division maxillary block is valuable in providing supplemental anesthesia. This is shown in Figure 9-14. For septal anesthesia, local anesthetic solution is deposited 1 cm in front of the sphenoid rostrum to block the posterior and superior branches of the sphenoplatine nerve (see Fig. 9-23). Bending a 1.5-inch needle will improve visualization while injecting. The infiltrations are performed from posterior to anterior to prevent needle puncture bleeding from obscuring the field. Infiltration can also be made into the inferior turbinates.

Blocking the lips
Minimally invasive cosmetic surgery techniques such as filler injections may require local anesthesia of the lips. Although the doctor could perform bilateral infraorbital and mental nerve blocks, they present disadvantages. Many practitioners are uncomfortable with these blocks,

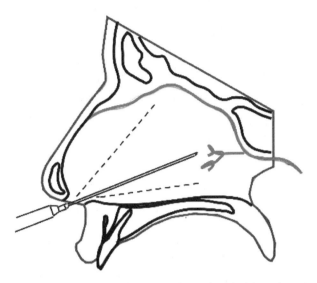

Figure 9-23. Septal anesthesia is performed to block branches of the sphenopalatine nerve and constrict the vascular supply.

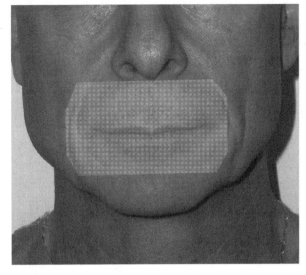

Figure 9-25. This rendition shows the approximate area anesthetized with the vestibular anesthesia technique.

and they can be unpleasant for the patient. In addition, this combination of blocks will render a large area of the face insensate for several hours, which is disconcerting to patients. A simple technique for obtaining anesthesia of the upper and lower lips is to inject 0.5 cc increments of 2% lidocaine with 1:100,000 epinephrine across the vestibule of the anterior maxilla and mandible (see Fig. 9-24). This simple technique is performed as follows. First, topical anesthesia is applied to the anterior and mandibular sulcus for several minutes. Next, a 0.5-inch 30 ga needle is used to deposit 0.5 cc increments of anesthesia in four to five areas between the canine teeth. This technique will provide profound anesthesia in the perioral area, which is usually sufficient for filler injection.

Figure 9-25 shows the area anesthetized by using the infiltration technique in both lips. Obviously, only the upper or lower lip can be anesthetized, respectively. Although profound anesthesia may extend from the nasal tip to the chin, some patients can still feel pain at the lateral portions of the lips but usually tolerate injection.

Tumescent Anesthesia

Dermatologist Jeffery A. Klein, M.D., popularized the concept of tumescent local anesthesia and thereby revolutionized outpatient liposuction as well as enhanced other cosmetic procedures. The word "tumescent" means swollen and firm. By injecting a large volume of very dilute lidocaine (local anesthetic) and epinephrine (capillary

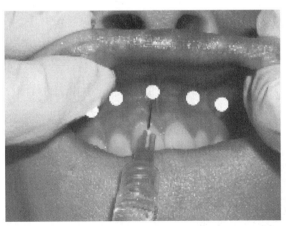
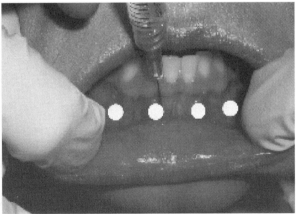

Figure 9-24. A simple vestibular infiltration technique can assist cosmetic techniques such as the injection of fillers.

constrictor) into subcutaneous fat, the targeted tissue becomes swollen and firm, or tumescent. The tumescent technique is a method that provides local anesthesia to large volumes of subcutaneous fat and thus permits liposuction totally by local anesthesia. The tumescent technique may eliminate the need for both general anesthesia and IV narcotics and sedatives.

The tumescent technique for liposuction (1) provides local anesthesia, (2) constricts capillaries and prevents surgical blood loss, and (3) provides fluid to the body by subcutaneous injection so that no IV fluids are needed.[18]

Depending on the clinical requirements, a tumescent anesthetic solution may contain a five- to fortyfold dilution of lidocaine found in commercially available formulations of local anesthesia. Commercial solutions of lidocaine used by dentists and anesthesiologists typically contain 1 gm (1,000 mg) of lidocaine and 1 mg of epinephrine per **50 ml** (2% lidocaine with 1:200,000 epinephrine) of saline. In contrast, tumescent solutions of local anesthesia contain approximately 0.5–1 gm of lidocaine and 1 mg of epinephrine in **1,000 ml** of NSS. This is a twentyfold dilution of the commercial version of lidocaine and epinephrine.[18]

Tumescent liposuction totally by local anesthesia has proven to be extremely safe despite the use of unprecedented large doses of lidocaine and epinephrine. One explanation for this remarkable safety is the extreme dilution of the tumescent local anesthetic solution. Large volumes of dilute epinephrine produce intense constriction of capillaries in the targeted fat, which in turn greatly delays the rate of absorption of lidocaine and epinephrine. Undiluted lidocaine and epinephrine are absorbed into the bloodstream in less than an hour. Tumescent dilution causes widespread capillary constriction that causes the absorption process to be spread over twenty-four to thirty-six hours. This reduces peak concentration of lidocaine in the blood, which in turn reduces the potential toxicity of a given dose of lidocaine (see Chapter 8). Dentists typically use concentrated epinephrine, which may cause a tachycardia, or rapid heart rate, if the epinephrine is rapidly absorbed. When very dilute tumescent epinephrine is used, the widespread vasoconstriction slows the rate of epinephrine absorption, which in turn prevents an increase in heart rate.[18]

Profound vasoconstriction (shrinkage of capillary blood vessels) results from the tumescent infiltration of a large volume of dilute epinephrine into subcutaneous fat. Tumescent vasoconstriction is so complete that liposuction can be done with virtually no blood loss. In contrast, the older forms of liposuction used before the invention of the tumescent technique were associated with so much surgical blood loss that autologous blood transfusions were often routine.

Because the vasoconstriction delays lidocaine absorption, the local anesthetic remains in place in the fat for many hours. This prolonged anesthesia may permit surgery for up to ten hours after infiltration and can provide twenty-four to thirty-six hours of significant postoperative analgesia in some patients.

Maximum recommended lidocaine dosage is 40 mg · kg^{-1} to 50 mg · kg^{-1} for tumescent liposuction when lidocaine is greatly diluted. This is a relatively large dosage compared to the 7 mg · kg^{-1} that is widely accepted as the "safe maximum dose for lidocaine with epinephrine." Anesthesiologists use nondiluted lidocaine for nerve blocks such as epidural blocks.[18]

Because tumescent local anesthesia lasts so long, tumescent liposuction is less painful and more pleasant than liposuction under general anesthesia or IV sedation. With tumescent local anesthesia, patients are able to avoid the postoperative nausea and vomiting associated with general anesthesia or IV opioids. Tumescent anesthesia is so efficient at providing fluid to the body that it is unnecessary to administer IV fluids. There is a risk of dangerous fluid overload if excessive IV fluids are given to a tumescent liposuction patient.[18]

Tumescent Local Anesthesia for Facial Procedures

Although any part of the head or neck can, in theory, be blocked, sometimes it is easier or advantageous to utilize tumescent anesthesia instead of blocks. One big advantage is the simultaneous hemostasis that accompanies the pain control. Head and neck procedures that lend themselves to tumescent local anesthesia include platysmaplasty ("necklift"), rhytidectomy (facelift), brow and forehead lift, and resurfacing procedures. This author utilizes tumescent anesthesia for all of these *except skin resurfacing*. IV sedation with reliance on the potency of ketamine will obtund these patients. Niamtu finds that tumescent local anesthesia distorts the anatomy too much for his preferences. Many practitioners favor this technique with laser resurfacing or chemical peel. Generally, tumescent anesthesia would be combined with selected local anesthetic blocks. This adds extra time, material, and equipment to resurfacing, so Niamtu has not embraced it.

For rhytidectomy, there exist numerous advantages for the use of tumescent local anesthesia. The effects of pain control and hemostasis are obvious. The ability of the engorged tumescent anesthetic solution to hydrodissect the subcutaneous plane is, in Niamtu's opinion, paramount. The efficacy of rhytidectomy hinges on the correct tissue planes being dissected and manipulated. Novice surgeons frequently become confused when specific tissue planes are required. By engorging the subcutaneous plane with 50–100 cc of tumescent anesthesia in each pre- and postauricular areas as well as the 100–200 cc in the submental and cervical regions, the facelift can be performed solely with local anesthesia (see Figs. 9-26 to 9-29).

Blocking the entire face

Although many cosmetic facial procedures are performed with IV sedation or general anesthesia, many can be performed with only local anesthetic techniques if one masters the blocks described in this chapter. Although this author usually uses IV sedation for facelift, chemical peel, and laser resurfacing, he has performed these procedures with *only* local anesthesia. Even when using IV sedation or general anesthesia, a prudent surgeon will utilize local anesthetic techniques. This allows the anesthesia provider to maintain the patient with less IV medication or gas and

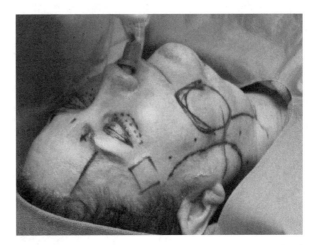

Figure 9-27. The preauricular and jowl tissues are engorged with tumescent in preparation for facelift.

provides superior postoperative pain control. Figure 9-30 shows the various dermatomes providing sensation to the head and neck. By realizing the nerves that supply these areas, a customized "anesthetic map" may be made by the surgeon applicable to the operated areas.

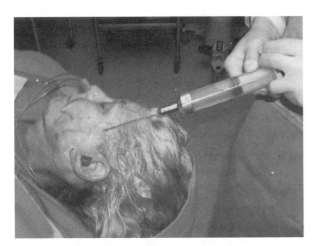

Figure 9-26. Tumescent local anesthesia is infiltrated in the pre- and postauricular areas prior to facelift.

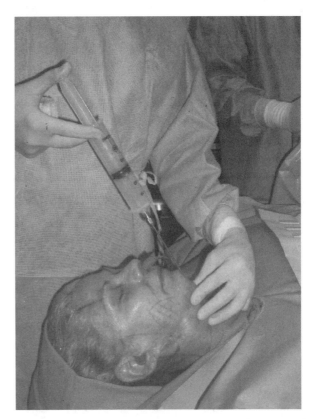

Figure 9-28. The submental area is engorged with 100 cc of tumescent anesthesia in preparation for platysmaplasty.

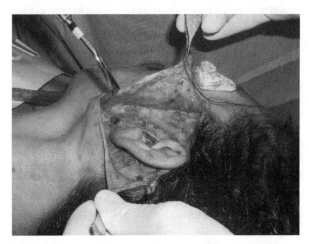

Figure 9-29. The facelift flap is dissected fifteen minutes after tumescent injection to the pre- and postauricular regions. Notice the bloodless field, which speaks for the effectiveness of the tumescent technique.

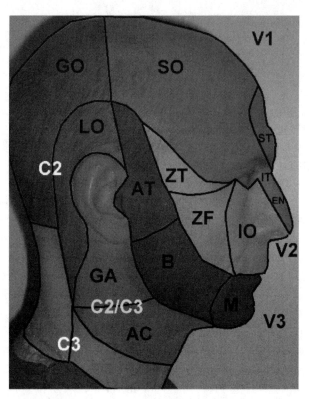

Figure 9-30. The major sensory dermatomes of the head and neck. AC = anterior cervical cutaneous colli; AT = auriculotemporal, B = buccal, EN = external (dorsal) nasal, GA = greater auricular, GO = greater occipital, IO = infraorbital, IT = infratrochlear, LO = lesser occipital, M = mental, SO = supraorbital, ST = supratrochlear, ZF = zygomaticofacial, ZT = zygomaticotemporal.

Using the picture in Figure 9-30, the surgeon can create a formula for which blocks are required for what procedure. An example would be to select a procedure, say endoscopic brow and forehead lift. Look at Figure 9-30 and see what blocks correspond with which dermatomes. For the endoscopic brow, one would need to block bilaterally ST, SO, GO, LO, AT, and ZT. Because of anatomic variables, crossover may be needed with adjacent dermatomes, but Figure 9-30 should be a good map and starting point.

SUMMARY

A firm knowledge of the sensory neuroanatomy of the head and neck can benefit the practice of cosmetic facial surgery for both the surgeon and the patient. Although the pathways of sensation for the head and neck are complex, they can be easily and safely blocked by reviewing the basic innervation patterns shown in Figure 9-30.

The entire sensory apparatus of the face is supplied by the trigeminal nerve and several cervical branches. There exist many patterns of nerve distribution anomaly, cross innervation, and individual patient variation; however, by following the basic techniques outlined in this chapter, the cosmetic surgeon should be able to achieve pain control of the major dermatomes of the head and neck.[19-22]

REFERENCES

1. Hersh EV, Condouis GA: Local anesthetics: A review of their pharmacology and clinical use. *Compend Contin Educ Dent* 8:374,1987.
2. Jastak JT, Yagiela JA, Donaldson D: *Local anesthesia of the oral cavity*. Philadelphia, WB Saunders, 1995.
3. Covino BG, Vassalo HG: Chemical aspects of local anesthetic agents. In Kitz RJ, Laver MB (eds.), *Local Anesthetics: Mechanism of Action and Clinical Use*. New York, Grune & Stratton, 1976; p1.
4. Hersh EV: Local Anesthetics. In Fonseca RJ (ed.), *Oral and Maxillofacial Surgery*. Philadelphia, WB Saunders, 2000; p. 58.
5. Yagiela JA. Local Anesthetics. In Dionne RA, Phero JC (eds.), *Management of Pain and Anxiety in Dental Practice*. New York, Elservier, 1991; p. 109.
6. Malamed SF: *Handbook of Local Anesthesia*, 4th ed. St. Louis, Mosby,1997.
7. Aceves J, Machne X: The action of calcium and of local anesthetics on nerve cells and their interaction during excitation. *J Pharmacol Exp Ther* 140:138,1963.

8. Stricharatz D: Molecular mechanisms of nerve block by local anesthetics. *Anesthesiol* 45:421,1976.

9. Gray H: *Anatomy of the Human Body*, 13th ed. Lea & Febiger, Philadelphia. 1918; p. 1158.

10. Zide BM, Swift R: How to block and tackle the face. *Plast Reconst Surg* 101:840,1998.

11. Mendel N, Puterbaugh, PG: *Conduction, Infiltration and General Anesthesia in Dentistry*, 4th ed. Dental Items of Interest Publishing Co. 1938; p. 140.

12. Mercuri LG: Intraoral second division nerve block. *Oral Surg* 47:9,1979.

13. Brown DL: *Atlas of Regional Anesthesia*. Philadelphia, WB Saunders, 1999; p. 170.

14. Bonica TT, Buckley FO: *Regional anesthesia with local anesthetics*. In *The Management of Pain*. 1990, p. 1883.

15. Wheeler AH: Therapeutic Injections for Pain Management. 2001 www.emedicine.com/neuro/topic514.htm#target10.

16. Gmyrek R: Local Anesthesia and Regional Nerve Block Anesthesia. 2002 www.emedicine.com/derm/topic824.htm.

17. Larrabee W, Msakielski KH: *Surgical anatomy of the face.* New York, Raven Press, Ltd., 1993; p. 83.

18. http//www.liposuction.com. Accessed 2-8-05.

19. Niamtu J: Local anesthetic blocks of the head and neck for cosmetic facial surgery, Part I: A review of basic sensory neuroanatomy. *Cosmet Dermatol* 17:515,2004.

20. Niamtu J: Local Anesthetic blocks of the head and neck for cosmetic facial surgery, Part II: Techniques for the upper and midface. *Cosmet Dermatol* 17:583,2004.

21. Niamtu J: Local anesthetic blocks of the head and neck for cosmetic facial surgery, Part III: Techniques for the maxillary nerve. *Cosmet Dermatol* 17:645,2004.

22. Niamtu J: Local anesthetic blocks of the head and neck for cosmetic facial surgery, Part IV: Techniques for the lower face.*Cosmet Dermatol* 17:714,2004.

Local Anesthetics and Surgical Considerations for Body Contouring

Rodger Wade Pielet, M.D.

INTRODUCTION

A significant number of techniques for proper infiltration of local anesthetic for body contouring procedures can be summarized on three levels. First, establish preemptive analgesia and adequate vasoconstriction at all incision sites. Second, provide both anesthesia and vasoconstriction in all planes of dissection and manipulation. Third, facilitate vasoconstriction to all vascular beds supplying the surgical planes of dissection. The third objective is best accomplished by having an understanding of the musculocutaneous and fasciocutaneous vascular anatomy. In many cases, these vascular pedicles are in close proximity to the sensory nerves; but often, they need to be addressed as distinct anatomic areas. A significant amount of local infiltration occurs prior to the surgical scrub and preparation. This allows for an appropriate amount of time to elapse for adequate analgesia and vasoconstriction.

Breast augmentation, for example, is the second most requested surgical procedure in many aesthetic surgery practices. Although there is no dominant vascular supply to the breast (Maliniak, 1943), the main contributors are perforators from the internal mammary artery, the lateral thoracic artery, and intercostal vessels (Fig. 10-1). There are also perforators from the thoracoacromial and thoracodorsal vessels to the pectoralis major muscle. This understanding is important when performing either sub-glandular or submuscular augmentation mammoplasty with or without mastopexy.

The glandular tissue receives its sensory innervation from the lateral mammary rami of the third through sixth intercostal nerves and medial mammary rami of the second through sixth intercostal nerves (Fig. 10-2). A very separate anterior branch of the fourth intercostal nerve supplies sensation to the nipple. The nipple and areolar complex are always supplied by sensory nerves were seen through the depths the glandular tissue and not by superficial nerves (Fig. 10-3).

LOCAL ANESTHESIA

For proper analgesia as well as vasoconstriction at the incision sites, Pielet prefers the use of 1% lidocaine with epinephrine (1:100,000). This is preferable to the use of bupivicaine with epinephrine because the potent and prolonged vasodilitation of bupivicaine seems to outlast the effects of the epinephrine and there is a slightly higher increase of delayed postoperative bleeding *Editor's note: Bupivicaine does not have vasodilating properties.* Bupivicaine for postoperative pain management is discussed later in this chapter. Either 0.5% or 1% lidocaine with epinephrine is injected to infiltrate the areas of vascular perforators or planes of dissection when necessary.

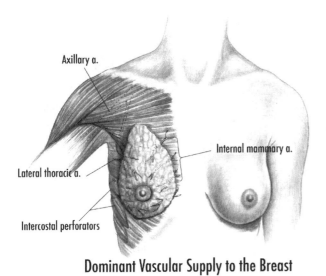

Dominant Vascular Supply to the Breast

Figure 10-1. Dominant vascular supply to the breast.

Numerous authors have written about the use of tumescent fluids to infiltrate the superficial and deep layers of fat when performing liposuction. Tumescent infiltration is also useful in other procedures, such as breast reduction and abdominoplasty. The typical tumescent solution consists of 50 cc of 1% lidocaine plus 1 mg of epinephrine per liter of normal saline or Lactated Ringers solution. Other surgeons may choose to add up to 12.5 cc of 8.4% sodium bicarbonate as well as various concentrations of hyaluronic acid. Pielet has not found either bicarbonate or hyaluronic acid to be necessary.

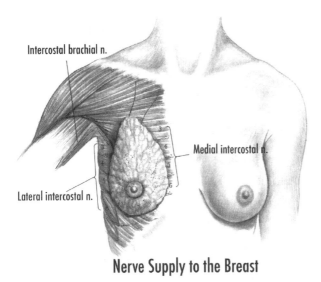

Nerve Supply to the Breast

Figure 10-2. Nerve supply to the breast.

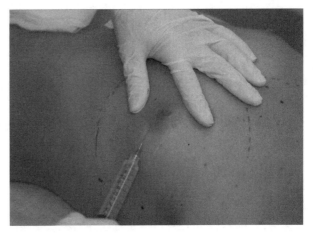

Figure 10-3. Local anesthetic injection to the incisional area for periareolar breast augmentation.

When considering liposuction, for example, it is important to have continuous communication with one's anesthesiologist. Factors that must be monitored during these procedures include the starting hematocrit of the patient, the volume of tumescent fluid infiltrated, volume of fat aspirated, volume of crystalloid administered through the IV, and the amount of lidocaine used.

A useful rule of thumb predicts that if a lidocaine-epinephrine solution is injected in the amount of 15–30 cc per 100 cm^2 of the area to be treated, the hematocrit will fall approximately 1% for every 150 cc of fat aspirated. For example, if 1,500 cc fat were removed by liposuction, the hematocrit would be expected to fall by approximately 10% (Hetter, 1989). A one-to-one volume of fluid is injected equal to the amount of lipo-aspirate from any given area. Depending on the size of liposuction, this often involves amounts of lidocaine that far exceed the limits thought to be toxic (see Chapter 8). Because there is delay in the peak levels for several hours after injection, lidocaine doses as high as 35 mg $\cdot$ kg^{-1} have been found to be completely safe in an outpatient setting (Klein, 1990) (see Chapter 8).

BREAST AUGMENTATION AND PECTORAL AUGMENTATION

The three most common incision sites for breast augmentation include the inframammary fold, the peri-areola, and the axilla. Pielet prefers to perform pectoral augmentation entirely through an axillary incision. Pielet does not perform the transumbilical approach (TUBA),

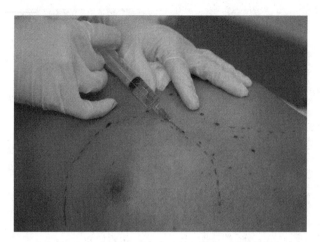

Figure 10-4. Parasternal injection of local anesthesia for breast augmentation.

as this offers no real advantage over other incision sites. Following infiltration of the incision areas, the medial parenchymal breast tissue is infiltrated to block the neurovascular perforators arising from the internal mammary artery above the ribs (Fig. 10-5). This seems to be equally effective as distinct, individual intercostal blocks and does not carry the added minimal risk of pneumothorax, which is slightly more common in very thin individuals. All injections can be accomplished with approximately 10–15 cc of 1% lidoocaine with epinephrine per side. *Editor's note: At least 50–70 cc of 0.5% lidocaine with epinephrine is more effective. Dr. Pielet is a plastic surgeon and client of Dr. Barinholtz (Chapter 11). Inadequate local analgesia is a reasonable explanation for Barinholtz inability to avoid opioids with the MIA™ technique.* Some surgeons may wish to use a dilute tumescent solution in the subglandular or subpectoral spaces.

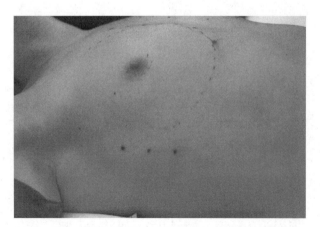

Figure 10-5. Marking for lateral intercostals injections in the anterior axillary line for breast augmentation.

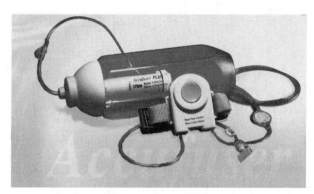

Figure 10-6. Accufusor® pain pump.

Following dissection of the pocket and assurance of meticulous hemostasis, a small catheter is placed in the pocket. The catheter is later connected to a postoperative pain pump delivering a constant infusion of 0.25% bupivicaine to each side. Some devices include an additional patient-controlled bolus (Fig. 10-6). It is also effective to place approximately 5–10 cc of 0.25% bupivicaine in the pocket if the patient does not wish to have catheters emerging from the skin for a few days after she goes home. *Editor's note: Up to 50 cc of 0.25% bupivicaine (125 mg) is considered a safe dose more effective analgesia will result from using 20–25 cc per breast pocket.* Bupivicaine used in these applications has not demonstrated an increased risk of postepinephrine, rebound vasodilatation, or hematoma.

REDUCTION MAMMAPLASTY AND MASTOPEXY

These two operations are performed in a very similar manner. If one considers the breast simplistically, it is comprised of an "outer skin envelope" and "inner stuffing." The stuffing is basically made up of parenchyma, fat, and sometimes an alloplastic implant above or below the pectoralis major muscle. There are several different procedures, techniques, and potential scar configurations based on the patient's needs and surgeon preference. In general, a breast reduction involves the removal of both components, skin and stuffing, whereas a breast lift is usually the removal of skin only.

Most procedures require some degree of skin-flap elevation above the parenchyma. The nipple/areolar complex remains attached to the underlying parenchyma in order to preserve neurovascular continuity. The exceptions to this principle are extremely severe cases of symptomatic macromastia. In this instance, the resultant pedicle would be insufficient to maintain the blood supply to the nipple/areola. The second exception would be for patients whose medical or social (i.e., smoking) history precludes adequate vascularity and/or safety. In these situations, an en-bloc amputation of the skin, breast tissue, and fat with replacement of the nipple/areolar complex is performed as a free graft.

Regardless of the procedure, all incision sites are infiltrated with 0.5% or 1% lidocaine with epinephrine. If any area is to be de-epithelialized, intradermal placement of dilute local with epinephrine is administered. This facilitates the process of epidermal removal and aids in hemostasis of this very vascular plane. The area of the capsule of the breast that is the plane in which shin flaps are elevated is infiltrated. These flaps are elevated only as necessary to accomplish proper redraping of the skin around the parenchymal pedicle. It is important to elevate skin flaps to only within approximately 1 cm of the pectoralis fascia. This dramatically decreases postoperative pain. Any rent in the fascia, either sharply with scissors or with electrocautery, or stimulation of the fascia and underlying muscle produces significant increases in postoperative pain and should be avoided.

SUCTION-ASSISTED LIPECTOMY

Liposuction remains one of the most commonly performed surgical procedures in this country. For most patients, the postoperative recovery and pain is directly proportional to the magnitude of the procedure. In addition to the principles discussed above, it is important to adequately infiltrate the treated areas and allow sufficient time for vasoconstriction. It is possible to perform fat aspirations in the range of 4–6 liters or more on an outpatient basis using these techniques. *Editor's note: Complications increase as volumes aspirated exceed 5,000 cc.* The incision port sites are infiltrated with either 0.5% or 1% lidocaine with epinephrine prior to the surgical prep. There are several published methods for preparation of the tumescent solution. Very low concentrations of epinephrine (1:400,000–800,000) will provide adequate vasoconstriction. There are also many different recommendations for the amount of fluid instilled into each area. In general, a 1:1 ratio of infiltrated fluid to the volume of anticipated fat removal is utilized. Other surgeons choose to use a 'super-wet' technique.

In mid-2004, Pielet started using Vaser[3] Assisted Liposelection (VAL) in addition to the standard tumescent infiltration. The VAL has revolutionized the practice of liposuction. VAL has significantly reduced the use of intraoperative opioids as compared to other methods of tumescent liposuction, including other applications of ultrasonic technology. Decreased opioid requirement is likely related to lesser tissue trauma and increased precision. More harsh techniques require more vigorous action in both tunneling with the cannula as well as application of ultrasonic energy. This decreased precision often results in placement of the tip of the cannula *beyond* the area infiltrated with the local anesthetic-containing tumescent solution. This, obviously, negates the concept of preemptive analgesia and also increases opioid requirements, intraoperative discomfort, and postoperative pain. Because there is more precision, less tissue trauma, and minimal opioid requirements, patients actually complain of *less* postoperative pain.

ABDOMINOPLASTY AND CIRCUMFERENTIAL BODY LIFT AND THIGH LIFT

There is enough similarity between these two procedures to discuss proper infiltration of local anesthetic solutions. Either of these procedures is combined with various elements of liposuction, and the principles outlined previously also apply in this situation. The areas of the incisions are infiltrated in the skin as previously described. For abdominoplasty, a skin flap is elevated up to the level of the costal margin. To facilitate abdominoplasty, tumescent solution is infiltrated for vasoconstriction and preemptive analgesia, just above the fascia in addition to any areas subjected to suction lipectomy (Fig. 10-7).

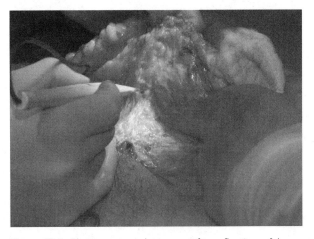

Figure 10-7. Electrocautery device use for reflection of lower abdominal skin flap for abdominoplasty.

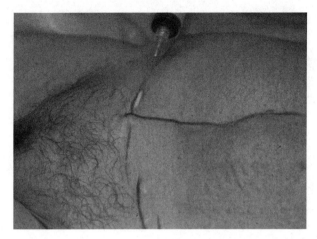

Figure 10-8. Skin infiltration prior to incision for abdominoplasty.

Modest amounts of fat may be aspirated along with subdermal tunneling to facilitate the dissection (Fig. 10-8). Electrocautery may be used to develop a skin flap which is elevated up to the level of the costal margin (Fig. 10-9). *Editor's note: Sometimes the level of analgesia from the tumescent fluid is insufficient for the patient to tolerate the electrical stimulus. Supplementing the tumescent with subfascial injection of the rectus sheath may block the perforating fibers from the midline branch of the intercostals nerves. Additionally, it may be helpful to proceed with blunt finger or scissor dissection to develop the flap. Lastly, one can resort to an additional bolus of 50 mg ketamine to avoid abandoning an intravenous anesthetic; i.e. MIA™ technique (see Chapter 1) or intravenous general anesthesia (see Chapter 11).—BLF*

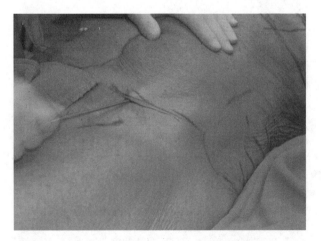

Figure 10-9. Subdermal tunneling (with possible modest liposuction) prior to reflection of skin flap for abdominoplasty.

Once again, great care is taken to dissect the flap slightly above the fascia, attempting to avoid cutting or stimulating the fascia or underlying muscles. This is important for three reasons. First, it allows visualization of vascular perforators. They are cauterized or ligated before they can retract into the fascia. Cut, retracted vessels complicate the task of achieving hemostasis. Second, reduced stimulation and trauma to the fascia and muscle decreases pain. And third leaving a very thin but well-vascularized layer of loose areolar tissue appears to decrease the incidence of postoperative seroma formation. This is particularly helpful since the advent of more aggressive liposuction of the abdominoplasty flap and adjacent areas. The placement of closed-suction drains is a matter of preference and the decision is usually made intraoperatively.

The majority of postoperative pain is initially related to the fascial plication of the abdominal wall. There is a divergence of opinion as to whether or not the imbrication of the rectus fascia, the "internal corset" of the abdominoplasty, requires "muscle" relaxation. Those who believe muscle relaxants are required (see Chapters 11 and 13) also tend to believe the rectus muscle itself is being brought to the midline. Lengthy experience with PK MAC/MIA™ technique for abdominoplasty (see Chapters 1 and 4) has reproducibly obtained adequate muscle relaxation for fascial imbrication *with* adequate local analgesia. After a few days, most patients complain less about this area and more about the areas treated with liposuction.

Formerly, multiport Accufuser catheters were placed along the fascia for postoperative pain management, but an increase in the incidence of seromas was consistently observed despite the use of drains. It is unlikely that this is related to the small amount of fluid infused over time but rather is due to the extreme effectiveness of these pain-control devices. Essentially, the patient is extremely comfortable in the immediate postoperative period to such an extent that they are excessively mobile and shearing forces develop between the abdominal wall in the elevated skin flap. This appears to be the etiology of the higher incidence of seromas. A slight amount of discomfort does lead to splinting and better effective immobilization of the abdominal wall in the first few days after surgery. The aggressiveness of the liposuction of the lateral flank/hip area through the abdominoplasty incision may also facilitate seroma formation. The two most important factors to decrease perioperative pain are elevation of the skin flap just above the fascia and placement of a 25–50 cc bolus of 0.25% bupivicaine in the fascia and the incision prior to closure.

The thigh lift, both medial and lateral, essentially involves extensive tumescent liposuction, blunt dissection, and mild elevation of skin flaps. All of these techniques were outlined earlier in this chapter.

MISCELLANEOUS ALLOPLASTIC BODY AUGMENTATION

In addition to the breast augmentation and pectoral augmentation discussed previously, there has been a considerable increase in the number of requests for both calf augmentation as well as buttock augmentation. In essence, the dissection for calf augmentation is entirely above the gastrocnemius muscle through an incision in the popliteal fossa. Again, the incision line is injected *prior* to surgical preparation and a small amount of dilute local and aesthetic is injected into the subcutaneous space where the implants are to be placed. This is often performed as a purely cosmetic procedure with the placement of one or two implants on each side. It is also performed as a unilateral procedure in individuals with either developmental or traumatic asymmetry.

There are many different approaches for buttock augmentation. Some surgeons prefer a supragluteal or

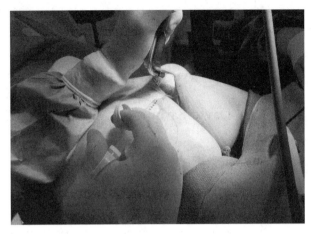

Figure 10-10. The entire pocket is elevated and corresponds precisely to the preoperative markings. This technique aids in hydrodissection, elevation of the plane, hemostasis, and perioperative pain management.

infragluteal incision as well as a single midline incision. Pielet prefers bilateral paramedian incisions, as they seem to yield the most acceptable cosmetic and functional result. Dissection is carried down to the muscle and a subepimesial plane is dissected. Rather than injecting a bolus of local anesthetic into the respective pocket, sequential aliquots of dilute lidocaine with epinephrine are injected into the undulating epimesium between the muscle fibers (see Fig. 10-10).

11 | Intravenous Anesthesia for Cosmetic Surgery

David Barinholtz, M.D.

INTRODUCTION

In the 1840s came the first case reports of successfully anesthetizing patients for surgical procedures. The agents used were *inhalational* agents, specifically diethyl ether and nitrous oxide. Crawford Long, Horace Wells, and William T. G. Morton will forever be credited with bringing the benefits of anesthesia to patients undergoing surgery.[1,3] No longer would surgical patients needlessly suffer. In this era, the only ways to deliver an anesthetic systemically was by inhalation or ingestion (hollow needles had not yet been invented). Inhalation agents provided a rapid, reliable, predictable way to anesthetize patients compared with ingesting alcohol and/or opiates. Hollow needles were introduced in the late 1800s.

Although various injectable adjuncts such as opiates, sedative/hypnotics, dissociative agents, and muscle relaxants were developed in the early and mid 20th century, inhalation agents (i.e., nitrous oxide and the halogenated ether derivatives such as halothane, ethrane, isoflurane) were the mainstays of anesthesia until the 1980s. However, they were far from ideal. Inhalation agents (volatile) are fraught with a myriad of side effects, such as myocardial depression, hypotension, arrhythmias, and postoperative nausea and vomiting (PONV). Anesthesia was very risky until the 1980s. The combination of cardiovascular effects of inhalation agents, the routine use of muscle relaxants, and lack of sophisticated monitoring devices other than ECG, NIABP, and spirometry (in addition to the finger on the pulse, stethoscope, and direct observation) was the underlying reason. Anesthetic-related death rates were generally quoted in the 1-in-10,000 range. With millions of anesthetics being performed annually, the main focus of the anesthesia community was to improve patient safety as opposed to minimizing undesirable side effects such as prolonged anesthetic effects and PONV.

Many things happened in the 1980s to revolutionize anesthesia care. The first commercially marketed pulse oximeter, the Nellcor N-100, was introduced in 1984. Pulse oximetry dramatically reduced the incidence of adverse hypoxic events. Not until 1990 did the ASA deem pulse oximetry a "standard of care." It was intuitively obvious to early technology adapters that knowing the patient's state of oxygenation instantaneously was infinitely preferable to relying on clinical signs and/or blood gases. Nonetheless, it was most disappointing that it took the ASA six years to deem SpO_2 a standard of care. Capnography became a standard of care, dramatically reducing the incidence of unrecognized esophageal intubations. The adoption of these two innovations, along with a large influx of very highly trained anesthesia providers into the profession, is widely believed to be responsible for the dramatic reduction in anesthetic-related mortality.[4] By the mid-1990s, anesthetic-related mortality rates had decreased to approximately 1 in 250,000.[5]

Another seminal event in the late 1980s that revolutionized anesthesia, especially ambulatory anesthesia, was the introduction of propofol.[6] Propofol was the first (and still the only) rapid, ultra–short-acting sedative/hypnotic with a lack of cumulative effects.[7] Propofol could be administered continuously for prolonged anesthetics and still allow patients to awaken rapidly without prolonged somnolence (or "hangover").[8,9] It is this quality, as well as an inherent antiemetic effect, that has made propofol such a popular agent for outpatient anesthesia.

By the mid-1990s, anesthesia care was extremely safe and reliable, especially for healthy people having outpatient surgery. The most popular anesthetic technique was the "balanced" anesthetic. This technique takes advantage of the utility of volatile agents combined with intravenous agents for analgesia and muscle relaxation. Most of these patients were intubated, paralyzed, and mechanically ventilated. Although this technique is safe and reliable, it has its limitations. Prolonged effects of volatile agents (even desflurane and sevoflurane), muscle relaxants, and opioids caused prolonged recovery times and a high incidence of undesirable side effects such as PONV. Also, analgesia was totally dependent on systemic opioids. Surgeons and anesthesiologists were at odds about the use and safe doses of local anesthetics (see Chapter 8). Systemic NSAIDs were reported by some to increase hematoma formation. Loss of NSAID analgesia meant increased reliance on opioids and opioid-related PONV. There had to be a better way.

In 1997, Barinholtz left the hospital-based anesthesia world. After five years in academic anesthesia, the rapidly expanding area of office-based anesthesia captured his interest. Armed with the same knowledge as his colleagues, Barinholtz set out to develop an anesthesia practice outside of the hospital setting that took advantage of all the technologic and pharmacologic advances to provide the safest state-of-the-art office-based anesthesia practice. For the first time in his career, Barinholtz began to question *everything* he did and *why* he did it. Does every patient need to be intubated? Does every intubated patient need to be paralyzed? Are intravenous agents (e.g., propofol) better than volatile agents? Is a 20% PONV rate acceptable? Are some of the techniques Barinholtz administered more for *his* convenience than for the best interest of the *patients*?

Some of Barinholtz's first clients were plastic surgeons. When he first started working with them in their office-based surgical suites, he soon discovered that providing a *safe* anesthetic wasn't good enough. The "standard" propofol induction, LMA placement, maintenance with sevoflurane while judiciously titrating fentanyl, and a dose of droperidol, was safe and reliable. Most patients were discharged in less than two hours. Frequently, rescue antiemetics and opioids were being administered in recovery. The biggest complaints were related to PONV and pain management. *Better outcomes were demanded!*

The cosmetic surgery patient is not like a typical "elective" surgical patient. The cosmetic surgery patient isn't having surgery for a medical condition. These patients desire to look better and expect to feel better. A patient having surgery for a medical condition is most concerned about getting better. In contradistinction, a cosmetic surgery patient will tend to be highly critical of *every* aspect of care preoperatively, intraoperatively, and postoperatively, *in addition* to the achievement of the desired cosmetic result. Once through this process, the cosmetic surgical patient will ultimately answer the question, "Was it worth it?" A rocky perioperative course due to anesthesia can reflect poorly on the surgeon. Conversely, a wonderful anesthetic experience will reflect very positively on the surgeon and the anesthesia provider. Optimizing every aspect of anesthetic care, from the preoperative evaluation through the postoperative follow-up, became the new goal.

What follows is the distillation of eight years of experience in office-based elective cosmetic surgery. What evolved was a propofol-based, intravenous anesthetic, guided by neurophysiologic monitoring, with minimal airway intervention and judicious use of local anesthetics. Based on vastly improved PONV rates and minimal postoperative pain management, Barinholtz's approach provides an anesthetic for the cosmetic surgery patient superior to the former "standard" (*vide supra*).

THE IDEAL ANESTHETIC

For more than 150 years, the professionals who have dedicated their careers to caring for people during one of the scariest, most stressful and anxiety-provoking experiences of their lives have strived to do so with caring, compassion, and above all safety.

What would the ideal anesthetic look like? In a perfect world, the ideal anesthetic would have the following characteristics:

1. SAFE—0% morbidity/mortality rate.
2. QUICK—minimum of time to achieve the desired effect and wear off just as rapidly.
3. EASY/RELIABLE—simple to administer and have very predictable effects.
4. EMERGENCE—wear off quickly without undesirable side effects.
5. ANALGESIC—pain-free experience.
6. AMNESTIC/SEDATIVE/HYPNOTIC (same category because patients make no distinction among the three)—from a patient's perspective, as long as they have no memory of anything they don't desire to remember perioperatively, it makes no difference to them if they were actually *completely asleep*.
7. NO MOVEMENT—although this may not be the largest preoccupation from an anesthesiologist's point of view, it is the single largest issue for a surgeon. Patients talking during their surgery is an additional issue. Whereas a patient may not be aware or care if they are babbling incessantly during surgery, it is very distracting and will upset even the most tolerant surgeon.

No one agent or technology will achieve all seven of these objectives. However, application of the current pharmacologic agents and anesthetic monitoring technologies comes very close.

COMBINING AGENTS—COMPONENT THERAPY

The best argument for an intravenous anesthetic regimen is that one has independent control over every anesthetic variable. Balanced anesthesia or TIVA relies on hypnosis augmented by the addition of analgesics and muscle relaxants. In contrast, an inhalational anesthetic provides hypnosis, analgesia, and a degree of muscle relaxation as an all-in-one package. A sedative/hypnotic such as propofol will provide only unconsciousness and/or amnesia. Dissociative agents (e.g., ketamine) and/or opioids will provide systemic analgesia. If a small amount of skeletal muscle relaxation is necessary for a rectus muscle repair, for example, a small, subparalyzing dose of a short-acting nondepolarizing agent (e.g., rocuronium) provides the desired effect without paralyzing the diaphragm, avoiding the need for intubation and positive pressure ventilation. Adjuncts such as intravenous anticholinergics, antiemetics, and vasoactive agents such as labetolol, esmolol, and ephedrine provides unparalleled control over every aspect of anesthetic effect and side effect. More recently utilized agents, such as the centrally acting alpha$_2$ agonists clonidine and dexmetetomodine, promise to improve the anesthetic even more. In order to optimize the anesthetic, neurophysiologic monitoring for depth of anesthesia and liberal use of local analgesia are essential.

ANESTHETIC AGENTS FOR TOTAL INTRAVENOUS ANESTHESIA (TIVA)

Benzodiazepines

For many years, preoperative administration of diazepam for anxiolysis and perioperative amnesia was a mainstay of most anesthetic regimens. In more recent years, the more potent, shorter-acting, and more amnestic midazolam replaced diazepam. For many, midazolam is still part of virtually every anesthetic. Although a reliable amnestic, it does have its drawbacks. In an elegant Level 1 study, Oxorn[10] demonstrated a lack of propofol sparing effect with 2 mg midazolam premedication in a nonopioid anesthetic. Oxorn reported that midazolam has an antianalgesic effect.[10,11] When administered PO for pediatric patients, even for propofol/sevoflurane-based anesthetics it can be the rate-limiting factor in recovery.[12] For GI procedures, the use of even modest doses of midazolam, with or without opioids, can result in prolonged sedation and/or amnesia. Patients often cannot recall results discussed with the gastroenterologist after the procedure. In contrast, patients receiving propofol, *without* benzodiazepines, for these procedures not only remember results discussed postoperatively but also recover much more quickly. With the more widespread adminstration of centrally acting alpha$_2$ agonists such as clonidine[13]

and dexmetetomidine, which provide excellent anxiolysis, the role of benzodiazepines is being called into question.

Alpha$_2$ Agonists

Clonidine

Although developed as an antihypertensive agent, clonidine has attracted the interest of the anesthesia community for many years. Over the past fifteen years, clonidine has been administered by intravenous, epidural, spinal, and intra-articular routes.[14–18] Clonidine accentuates and spares concomitantly administered anesthetic agents.[19,20] Clonidine is particularly well suited for use in cosmetic surgery patients.[21,22] Its sedative and anxiolytic effects make it an ideal preoperative agent, obviating the need for midazolam. Its sedative and analgesic effects help minimize propofol usage,[23–25] as well as opioids, thus minimizing PONV. Its prolonged antiadrenergic effect helps control blood pressure perioperatively, thus theoretically minimizing chances of hematomas postoperatively. Clonidine has some limitations and concerns, however. Administered orally (usually in the 0.1–0.3 mg range),[26,27] it must be given thirty to sixty minutes prior to surgery. Once given, the dose cannot be titrated. Although generally predictable, the desired de facto tranquilizing effect is not always achieved. Clonidine 0.2 mg will achieve a 2.5–5.0 ug · kg^{-1} blood level in patients weighing between 95–175 pounds. De facto tranquilization is nearly always achieved with a therapeutic dose. Alternatively, sometimes the effect is more dramatic than desired, requiring increased perioperative fluids and occasional use of adrenergic agents to support blood pressure (Table 11-1).

Dexmetetomidine

This centrally acting alpha$_2$ agonist, FDA-approved for sedating ICU patients, is eight times more potent than clonidine.[28] Recently, Mayer[29] at the University of Illinois and Shapiro[30] at Harvard have been involved in clinical trials in the perioperative use of dexmetetomidine. This rapidly acting (approximately ten minutes), short-acting, intravenous agent shows great promise in outpatient anesthesia.[28] Currently, however, its use is cost-prohibitive in the price-sensitive world of cosmetic surgery.

Table 11-1. Anesthetic agents for total intravenous anesthesia (TIVA)

Class	Drug	Site-of-action	Principal effect	Role in component therapy
Benzodiazepines	Midazolam	Bdz/gaba receptors	Amnesia/anxiolysis/sedation	Preoperative anxiolytic/amnestic
Alpha$_2$ agonists	Clonidine (exists in PO/IV form usually administered PO)	Alpha$_2$ receptors in CNS	Anxiolysis/sedation/analgesia decreases adrenergic output	Preoperative anxiolytic intraoperative sedation/ analgesia
	Dexmetetomodine (8X more potent than clonidine IV infusion)	Alpha$_2$ receptors in CNS	Anxiolysis/sedation/analgesia decreases adrenergic output	Preoperative anxiolytic intraoperative sedation/analgesia
Sedative/hypnotic	Propofol	Cerebral cortex	Sedation/unconsciousness	Main sedative/hypnotic/volatile equivalent
Dissociative agent	Ketamine	NMDA receptors	Dissociation/analgesia	Dissociative/analgesic
Opioids	Fentanyl Sufentanil Alfentanil Rein Sentanil	Narcotic Receptors	Systemic analgesia	Systemic analgesia
NSAIDs	Ketorolac COX-2s Celecoxib, Rofecoxib, Valdecoxib (all oral except valdecoxib-IV)	Cyclooxygenase inhibitors	Anti-inflammatory analgesia	Limited because of antiplatelet effect recent concerns with COX-2s
Para-aminophenol derivatives	Acetaminophen	Inhibits central prostaglandin synthesis	Analgesia	Limited 2° to limited effectiveness and hepatotoxic concerns

116

Propofol

In 2007, no discussion of anesthesia for cosmetic surgery can be complete without including propofol. A derivative of isopropylphenol, propofol has single-handedly revolutionized outpatient anesthesia. With propofol as the principal anesthetic agent, aided by judicious use of small amounts of opioids and ketamine and guided by neurophysiologic monitoring, a reliable TIVA is possible. In Barinholtz's practice, every cosmetic procedure, from facelifts to abdominoplasties to breast reductions to prone liposuction, is performed with a propofol-based anesthetic with no more airway intervention than an oropharyngeal airway. The success of this technique depends on the clinical vigilance of the anesthesiologist as well as neurophysiologic monitoring and local anesthetics.

Ketamine

Developed in the 1960s and popularized as a pediatric and veterinary anesthetic agent, ketamine was largely overlooked for use in cosmetic surgery until recently (see Chapters 1 and 4).

Historically, large doses of ketamine administered to pediatric and trauma patients (2–4 mg · kg^{-1}),[31] frequently without amnestics such as midazolam, resulted in profound dysphorias and/or hallucinations. Because of unpredictable outcomes, ketamine fell out of favor with anesthesiologists (*vide supra*).

In the 1990s, some began mixing smaller amounts of ketamine with propofol with impressive results.[32,33] Total doses of ketamine of less than 1 mg · kg^{-1} administered by bolus **or** continuous infusion in the presence of adequate propofol thynosis attenuates the response to local anesthetic injections and minimizes opioid requirements.

In fact, PK MAC in the presence of clonidine premedication, BIS-monitored propofol to 60–75, and adequate local anesthesia obviates the need for opioids altogether.[34]

Opioids

Unfortunately, in Barinholtz' practice, despite the use of clonidine and ketamine in conjunction with propofol, the complete elimination of opioids has not been possible. The surgeons, although adept at administering local anesthetic agents for the most part, aren't perfect. Plastic surgeons take exception to interrupting surgery to administer more local. Rather, they insist on increasing the depth of the anesthetic. Perhaps, with more surgeon education, the

benefits of more local over increasing anesthetic depth will be worth the very modest amount of time required to do so.

Barinholtz' surgeons don't view PONV as a large problem. If PONV were a large problem for plastic surgeons, they would acquiesce to attempts to minimize if not eliminate opioids. However, Macario's studies have shown PONV is a large issue for patients.

With aggressive antiemetic strategies (vide infra), patients experience approximately 1% incidence of PONV in the immediate postoperative period. Nonetheless, elimination of PONV is only one reason to eliminate opioids. The addition of systemic analgesia transforms deep sedation into intravenous general anesthesia. Opioids depress the laryngeal or "life-preserving" reflexes thereby increasing the probability of aspiration. Opioids depress respiration mandating the routine administration of supplemental oxygen and monitoring of EtCO2. Supplemental oxygen is a fire hazard in the presence of lasers and electrocautery devices particularly around the face. Lastly, opioids fail to block noxious input to the brain from the surgical field.

Interestingly, virtually all of the PONV that occurs in these patients happens after taking postoperative opioids at home (i.e. postdischarge or PDPONV). The surgeons could certainly minimize patient calls related to PONV as well as to pain if they adopted more local-analgesia-based strategies, both intra- and postoperatively (vida infra). Opioids will continue to be part of Barinholtz' anesthetic practice for the foreseeable future. However, the following technique has evolved to specifically minimize opioid requirements for all types of cosmetic surgery.

Nonopioid Analgesics

There are primarily two types of nonnarcotic analgesics used for the purposes of preventing and treating perioperative pain.

Acetaminophen

A derivative of para-aminophenol, acetaminophen is effective as an antipyretic and analgesic for mild to moderate pain. Commonly used to treat headaches and mild arthritic pain, its role in cosmetic surgery is limited. The maximum recommended dosages are not very effective in preventing or treating pain associated with cosmetic procedures.[35] Exceeding the maximum doses can be hepatotoxic and is not recommended.

Nonsteroidal anti-inflammatory drugs (NSAIDs)

The prototypical NSAID, ibuprofen, has been used for many years as an effective analgesic for even moderate to severe pain. In addition to its analgesic effect, ibuprofen is a potent anti-inflammatory. Anti-inflammatory action is an especially desirable feature that keeps swelling to a minimum after dental/oral surgery as well as facial cosmetic procedures. In the late 1980s, an injectable NSAID, ketoralac, was introduced. The use of this drug soared. It appeared that eliminating opioids was finally possible. However, case reports began to appear in the surgical literature of postoperative bleeding complications linked to the use of ketorolac (as well as other NSAIDs).[36, 39] Whether a justified indictment or not, most cosmetic surgeons will not allow their patients to take NSAIDs within two weeks of surgery (before or after), let alone administer them perioperatively.

In the mid-1990s, a subclass of NSAIDs was developed.[40] The cyclooxygenase subtype 2 inhibitors (COX-2) take advantage of the fact that there are different types of prostaglandins mediating inflammation and coagulation. Two subtypes of cyclooxygenase act on arachadonic acid to form prostaglandins. By inhibiting cyclooxygenase-2 (and not cyclooxygenase-1), the prostaglandins that are responsible for pain and inflammation are not formed. However, the prostaglandins responsible for proper platelet function, formed through the action of cyclooxygenase-1, are uninhibited. The result is an NSAID that treats pain and inflammation without inhibiting platelet function. Celecoxib was the first FDA-approved COX-2 inhibitor, though it was originally developed to treat arthritis pain without analgesia. Next, rofecoxib (Vioxx®) proved even more effective for postoperative pain.[41, 45] Many practitioners, even cosmetic surgeons, began adopting the use of rofecoxib perioperatively because it eliminated the fear of bleeding complications. Results were promising. Then, an even more potent COX-2 inhibitor, valdecoxib, was introduced specifically for postoperative pain. The results of clinical trials were impressive comparing valdecoxib.[46] An injectable form of valdecoxib, parecoxib, was in phase 3 clinical trials and showed promise as a convenient perioperative analgesic.[47]

Unfortunately, in 2004, amid reports of cardiac deaths associated with the **chronic** use of Vioxx®, Merck removed it from the market.[48] As more data surfaced, valdecoxib was also voluntarily withdrawn. Currently, celecoxib (Celebrex®) is the only commercially available COX-2 inhibitor. It is not as effective as either rofecoxib or valdecoxib for postoperative pain, and there are now concerns regarding this whole class of drugs.[49] It is probably most prudent at this time to avoid their routine use perioperatively until more research is done.

Adjunct Agents

Table 11-2 summarizes adjunct agents utilized in component intravenous anesthesia. These agents are used mainly to offset effects of the previously-mentioned agents. Glycopyrrolate is administered to minimize secretions, especially when using ketamine. The adrenergic agents (ephedrine or epinephrine) can be used to offset the cardiovascular effects of propofol, opioids, and, occasionally, clonidine. The beta-blockers (and alpha/beta-blockers) can be used to offset effects of epinephrine (from local anesthetic injections) and cocaine. Titrated judiciously, one can avoid significant tachycardia, bradycardia, hypertension, or hypotension (Table 11-2).

Rocuronium

Virtually every cosmetic surgical procedure performed in an office-based setting is conducted with a spontaneously breathing, nonintubated patient. Muscle relaxants are not routinely utilized, except in one specific instance. Specifically, rocuronium is administered for the rectus muscle repair portion of an abdominoplasty.

Nondepolarizing muscle relaxants inhibit the nicotinic cholinergic receptors at the neuromuscular junction in direct competition with acetylcholine relative to the concentration at the site. Different muscle groups have varying concentrations of cholinergic receptors. Therefore, it is possible to *partially* paralyze some muscles without affecting others in a clinically significant way (e.g., relaxing some muscles without completely paralyzing the patient). Because the muscle with the highest concentration of cholinergic receptors is the diaphragm, it requires the highest concentration of nondepolarizing agent to paralyze it. A dose of rocuronium exists that will effectively relax the rectus muscle for surgical repair without affecting diaphragmatic function. The ideal dose is approximately 25% of an intubating dose (or 10 mg of rocuronium for a 70-kg adult). Administered a few minutes prior to muscle repair, it gives the surgeon ideal circumstances (virtually

Table 11-2. Adjunct agents

Class	Drug	Site-of-action	Principal effect	Role in compotent therapy
Anticholinergic	Glycopyrrolate	Muscarinic receptors	Antisialogogue	Drying agent
Steroid	Dexamethasone	Cells medating inflammation CNS	Anti-inflammatory antiemetic	Anti-inflammatory antiemetic
Butyrophenones (dopaminergic antagonists)	Droperidol	Dopamine receptors	Antiemetic	Antiemetic
5HT$_3$ antagonists	Ondansetron	5HT$_3$ receptors	Antiemetic	Antiemetic
Beta-blockers	Esmolol	B-adrenergic receptors	Decrease heart rate	Decrease heart rate response to epinephrine in local and /or cocaine
Alpha and beta blockers	Labetolol	Alpha and beta adrenergic receptors	Decrease heart rate decrease blood pressure	Offset effects of epinephrine and/or cocaine
Adrenergic agent	Ephedrine	Direct beta agonist indirect alpha and beta agonists CNS	Increase heart rate increase blood pressure antiemetic	Offset hypotensive effects of anesthesia antiemetic
Adrenergic agent	Epinephrine	Direct alpha and beta agonist	Increase heart rate increase blood pressure	Offset hypotensive effects of anesthesia
Nondepolarizing muscle relaxants	Rocuronium	Nicotinic-cholinergic receptors	Muscle relaxation	Relax rectus muscle for repair

identical to conditions encountered in the intubated, paralyzed, positive-pressure ventilated patient) to complete the repair. Since rocuronium is so short acting and there is usually at least one hour between the muscle repair and the conclusion of surgery, it has not been necessary to administer reversal agents. Also, this technique avoids a completely paralyzed patient and the associated risks (airway, DVTs, awareness). Muscle *relaxation*, not paralysis, is administered. In hundreds of cases done with this technique in the past eight years, no patient has required intubation or become paralyzed at these doses. Succinylcholine (SCH) is available in Barinholtz's practice, but its use is relegated to that of an emergency drug only.

The remaining adjunct agents are addressed in the section on antiemetics.

THE AIRWAY CONTINUUM AND IDEAL AIRWAY MANAGEMENT

The area of anesthesia that causes some of the most controversy and is a significant factor in anesthetic-related morbidity and mortality is airway management. Prior to the invention of the cuffed endotracheal tube (ET) by Guedel,[50] patients were not routinely intubated for surgery. Along with the ET and the discovery of muscle relaxants,[51] routine intubation with paralysis even for minor surgeries became commonplace.[52] Mask ventilation, especially for short procedures such as myringotomy and cystoscopy, was still common. However, by the early 1990s, the overwhelming majority of patients receiving general anesthesia were intubated with an endotracheal tube.

In the early 1990s, a revolutionary airway device was introduced in the United States. Developed by Brain in Great Britain, it was called the laryngeal mask airway (LMA).[53,54] This device gave practitioners an intermediate choice between mask ventilation and endotracheal intubation. Over the past fifteen years, the LMA has gained widespread acceptance worldwide, especially in the ambulatory anesthesia arena. The LMA gives practitioners the ability to maintain a patient's airway, reliably deliver oxygen (and other gases), and monitor end-tidal CO_2, all without the need for paralysis. Its success has spurred a host of similar devices claiming similar advantages, for example, the cuffed oropharyngeal airway (COPA®) and laryngeal Combitube. Both the COPA® and the Combitube® claim

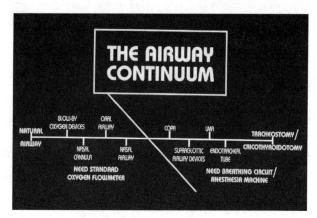

Figure 11-1. The airway continuum.

to offer most of the advantages of endotracheal intubation without the invasiveness. However, all are deeply situated in the pharynx (stimulating all the pharyngeal reflexes). A 15 mm breathing connection facilitates coupling to an anesthesia breathing circuit and, ultimately, an anesthesia machine. Does the patient *always* need a supraglottic device situated deep in the pharynx in order to maintain an airway during deep sedation? Do all airway devices require a 15 mm connector? The answer to these questions is no.

One method to explain and illustrate the concept is to introduce the airway continuum (see Fig. 11-1). The continuum is simply a line that from left to right represents increasing airway invasiveness. On the left is the untampered natural airway and on the right is the most invasive airway intervention, tracheostomy. In between are nasal cannulae, oral and nasal airways, the supraglottic devices, and endotracheal tubes. The continuum is divided into left and right halves. The right half is the side on which all the devices have a 15 mm connection for a breathing circuit. These devices have the advantage of attaching to a fresh gas source, the ability to monitor end-tidal CO_2, and providing the ability for positive-pressure ventilation. However, the presence of a 15 mm connector and the absence of opioids means that patients can breathe, with or without supplemental oxygen, spontaneously through a supraglottic device *without* being connected to an anesthesia circuit. Less is more.

The left half essentially comprises nasal cannulae, oral airways, and nasal airways. Whereas nasal cannulae attach to an oxygen source, traditionally oral airways and nasal trumpets don't. Also, none of these devices conveniently provides the ability to monitor end-tidal CO_2.

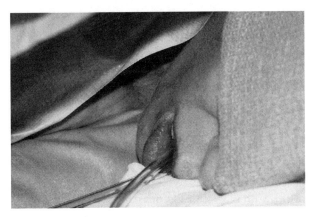

Figure 11-2. Patient with modified oral airway in place for prone liposuction.

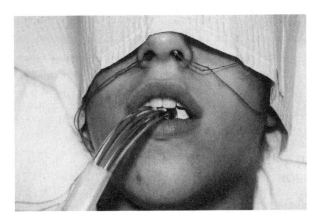

Figure 11-3. Patient with modified oral airway in place for rhyrtidectomy.

Recently, nasal cannulae that simultaneously deliver oxygen and provide for end-tidal CO_2 monitoring have become commercially available. Several years ago, Mallinkrodt patented a device fashioned as a nasal trumpet with the ability to administer oxygen and sample CO_2. One can fashion an oral airway device that can simultaneously deliver oxygen and sample end-tidal CO_2. Figure 11-2 shows a standard Guedel oral airway, flanges trimmed to allow placement behind the teeth, with two lengths of oxygen tubing placed into the opening in the airway: a short length situated distally in the airway that can easily attach directly to a male adapter for end-tidal CO_2 monitoring, and a longer length with the standard 5 in 1 connector, or "Chistmas-tree" adapter, compatibility to attach to an oxygen flowmeter. In the past six years, this device has been employed in thousands of cosmetic procedures. These

procedures include blepharoplasty, endoscopic browlift, rhytidectomy, rhinoplasty, breast augmentation, breast reduction, mastopexy, abdominoplasty, body lift, and liposuction (including prone and lateral cases) (see Fig. 11-2, 11-3, and 11-4). This device facilitates the maintenance of a patent airway, the reliable delivery of oxygen, and the reliable monitoring of end-tidal CO_2 (see Fig. 11-5).

There are two potential criticisms. First, this device does not protect the airway. Second, one cannot immediately ventilate the patient if necessary. These criticisms are valid and underscore the importance of choosing appropriate candidates without anticipated airway difficulty and who are not at risk for aspiration (i.e., GERD). Also, one must have the personnel, drugs, supplies, and equipment (including Ambu® bag, intubation equipment, LMAs, cricothyroidotomy kit, and jet ventilator) to deal with

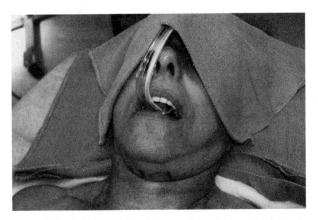

Figure 11-4. Patient with modified oral airway in place for breast augmentation, breast reduction, mastopexy or abdominoplasty.

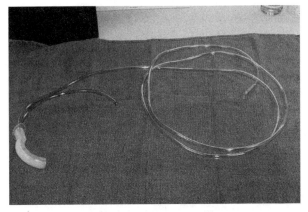

Figure 11-5. Modified oral airway with tubing to sample CO_2 and deliver oxygen.

every airway eventuality as described in the ASA difficult-airway algorithm.[55] Properly prepared, there is no reason every skilled anesthesia provider cannot reproduce Barinholtz's success in applying this technique. No patient has suffered a serious complication with resulting harm from its application in Barinholtz's practice.

THE ROLE OF NEUROPHYSIOLOGIC MONITORING IN TIVA

Since its first practical applications more than 150 years ago, anesthesia care has had three main goals, namely, (1) make patients unconscious/unaware of the gruesome experience of having surgery, (2) immobilize the patient so the surgeon can operate, and (3) don't kill the patient.[56] Historically, issues such as pain control and PONV prevention were distant to these fundamental concerns.

While great strides have been made Because the 1840s in all three of these areas, a review of the improvements of the past fifty years is appropriate. Approximately fifty years ago, curare, and subsequently, its derivatives, came into clinical use. For procedures that require immobility, there is a specific drug, receptor, and monitoring model. As far as anesthetic mortality, the necessary technologies have been developed to directly monitor and address the concerns germane to this issue, specifically, ECG, NIABP, SpO_2, and $EtCO_2$ (Fig. 11-6).

However, between 1842 and 1996, there was no way to directly monitor the patient's level of unconsciousness. There has been an overwhelming amount of attention in the anesthesia community, as well as the lay press, regard-

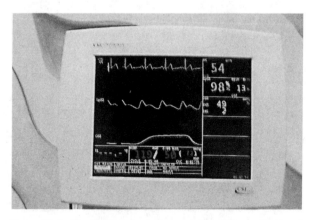

Figure 11-6. Monitor screen during sedation with modified oral airway. *N.B.* True end-tidal CO_2 tracing.

ing the issue of "awareness under [general] anesthesia." The more germane issue for office-based as well as other anesthesiologists is the much more common occurrence of overanesthetizing patients. However, patients have also heard the stories of awareness under anesthesia. Dozens of accounts from patients of their own experiences (or those of a close friend or relative) have been related to Barinholtz. He is frequently asked how he can "make sure" this won't happen to them. The fact that patients are not paralyzed or intubated is of great reassurance to them. Routinely monitoring with BIS is an additional source of reassurance.

The techniques described in this chapter rely on intravenous anesthesia in spontaneously breathing, nonparalyzed, nonintubated patients. Awareness is not a significant concern as these patients can move (or even talk) if they want or need to do so. Despite the fear of undermedicating, the much more likely (and common practice) issue is that of overanesthetizing.

Overmedicating produces more undesirable anesthetic side effects (e.g., hypotension) intraoperatively, more PONV, prolonged recoveries, and wasted drugs. In Barinholtz's anesthesia practice, all drugs, supplies, and equipment are the anesthesiologist's responsibility. Furthermore, the anesthesia provider must be physically present until all patients are recovered and discharged. It makes not only good clinical sense but good business sense to employ neurophysiologic monitoring. In the seven years since employing BIS monitoring, propofol usage has decreased by 20%. Patients rarely spend more than one hour recovering, even after a prolonged (six-hour) anesthetic. The foundation of the anesthetic care provided to Barinholtz's cosmetic surgery patients is the utilization of the TIVA technique in conjunction with BIS monitoring.

Finally, *directly* monitoring the effects the anesthetics have on the target organ—the brain—is more accurate than indirect indices of anesthetic depth. The historically used, *indirect* (and frequently inaccurate) cues to assess depth of anesthesia such as heart rate, blood pressure, tearing, and patient movement are no longer as relevant to decision making as is the measure of the cerebral cortical level of hypnosis (see Chapter 3).

Development of the BIS (and similar competing technologies, such as PSA 4000 and Entropy) and refining the technology (i.e., the BIS-XP platform) are great advancements for anesthetic care. Anesthesiologists should embrace BIS monitoring. Although BIS is not a perfect technology, neither is ECG, NIABP, or pulse oximetry. BIS provides valuable, reliable, reproducible data to help guide anesthetic care. Certainly, monitoring the EEG effects of anesthesia makes more sense than recent attempts to develop technologies to monitor and maintain fixed blood concentrations of anesthetic agents.[57,58] A given concentration of agent in the blood may still have a wide range of clinical effects on different patients. It is important to monitor the effect on the brain *directly* (see Chapter 3).

THE ROLE OF LOCAL ANESTHETICS

Administering propofol and ketamine, supplemented by alpha$_2$ agonists and opioids, *can* provide a TIVA without relying on local analgesia. However, this is not an advisable approach to the care of the cosmetic surgery patient. Intraoperatively, one would have to anesthetize the patient much more deeply. Although ketamine can be used to provide some analgesia, opioids could not be avoided. Postoperatively, pain relief would be completely dependent on opioids. Prolonged recoveries, high PONV rates, and inadequate (certainly suboptimal) pain relief would be the outcome. In order for the patient to have an optimal experience, adequate local analgesia must be utilized.

Years ago, it was a struggle to get surgeons to employ local analgesia as part of the surgical procedure. How many anesthesiologists have heard their surgeon say, "Why do I need local? That's what you're here for." Luckily, today's enlightened cosmetic surgeon knows that employing local analgesia is a valuable and necessary adjunct for the ultimate success of the surgery. The concept of preemptive analgesia is well established in both the anesthesia and surgical literature.[59–62]

Postoperative local analgesia is achieved by using a long-acting local anesthetic, such as bupivicaine, in the operative field before closing. Alternatively, placing a continuous infusion of local anesthetic postoperatively in the form of one of many commercially available pain-pumps will minimize, if not eliminate, the requirement for opioids.

Treating postoperative pain with local anesthetics, instead of opioids, results in more effective pain relief.

The patient is made more mobile (minimizing risks of thromboembolic phenomena), less prone to PONV and postoperative hematomata, and less likely to experience postoperative hypertension secondary to pain (again, minimizing the risk of a hematomata). This results in happier patients and happier surgeons who aren't getting called as often. If a surgeon can effectively numb the area they are operating on and operate without extending beyond the anesthetized area (or with a willingness to administer more local during the procedure if necessary), it is possible and highly desirable to anesthetize the patient without using any opioids (*vide supra* and see Chapter 4). But even in the situation where a surgeon doesn't maximize the use of local (a predicament in which many anesthesiologists find themselves), the liberal use of lidocaine greatly facilitates minimizing intraoperative drug consumption, especially opioids. The only caveat is to not exceed maximum safe doses of local anesthetics (see Chapter 8 on lidocaine toxicity and Chapters 9 and 10 on local analgesia techniques).

EMESIS—#1 NEMESIS

The single biggest concern expressed by patients undergoing anesthesia for cosmetic surgery (or all surgery, for that matter) is the fear of PONV. Studies have shown that when questioned, patients indicate that the fear of PONV is greater than the fear of postoperative pain and other anesthetic side effects.[63,64] Given the choice, most patients would rather deal with pain than nausea and vomiting. PONV doesn't occur just when the patient is under the anesthesiologist's *direct* care. Patients are at risk for PONV into the postdischarge, postoperative period, especially if the surgeon has prescribed opioids for postoperative pain. In order for the patient to have a PONV-free experience, one must have a rational, organized approach for both prevention and treatment of PONV, should it occur.

Who's at Risk?

Theoretically, *every* patient receiving anesthesia is at risk of PONV. Over the years, characteristics and risk factors have emerged that identify patients who are at a higher risk of experiencing PONV. These are (1) female gender, (2) nonsmokers, (3) previous history of PONV, (4) having a surgical procedure associated with a higher incidence of PONV (e.g., gynecologic, laparoscopic, strabismus, and various cosmetic procedures, especially of the face), (5) history of motion sickness, (6) exposure to volatile anesthetic agents, and (7) exposure to opioids (Table 11-3). Several authors have attempted to assign point values to

Table 11-3. Risk factors for PONV
1. Female gender
2. Nonsmoker
3. Young age
4. Previous history of PONV
5. Emetogenic procedure
6. History of motion sickness
7. Volatile anesthetic agents
8. Opioids

each of these risk factors in an attempt to assess an individual patient's relative risk of experiencing PONV. Although no model is perfect, clearly the more of these risk factors that apply to an individual patient, the higher his or her risk of PONV.[65, 68]

Because the overwhelming majority of the cosmetic surgery patients in Barinholtz's practice are female nonsmokers who will most likely receive opioids intra- and postoperatively (many of whom have a history of PONV and motion sickness), all of these patients are treated as at being high risk for PONV. Because of this proactive, aggressive effort to prevent it, the PONV rate in Barinholtz's practice is less than 1%.

Types of PONV

PONV can be separated into two types, immediate and delayed. Immediate PONV occurs immediately after surgery and during the recovery phase while the patient is still under the direct care of the anesthesia provider. Delayed PONV occurs after the patient has been discharged. This could occur on the way home or up to several days postoperatively. Learn to distinguish between these two and develop strategies for prevention and treatment of both. There are some guiding principles common to both types of PONV.

The first is that prophylaxis is better than treatment. It is *far more desirable to prevent the problem altogether than to have to deal with the consequences.*

The second is that **avoidance of opioids is the single largest factor in preventing PONV.**

Any or all of the strategies discussed herein can successfully deal with PONV 99% of the time. If opioids are somehow avoided, approximating 100% PONV-free outcomes could be achieved with less prophylaxis.

Prevention and Treatment of Immediate PONV

In order to determine if the patient is at risk of immediate PONV, delayed PONV, or both, focus on key elements of the history. Patients with a previous history of PONV need to be questioned carefully as to *when* the PONV occurred. Did it occur in the recovery room, on the way home, or after the patient returned home? Did it occur after taking oral opioids for pain? Did they follow the instructions and make sure to have a full stomach before taking oral opioids? Did it linger for days after surgery? Does the patient have a history of motion sickness (putting them at risk for PONV on the ride home)? The answers to these very specific questions can help the practitioner determine when and where the patient is most at risk for developing PONV and help arrive at a specific plan for both prevention and treatment.

Table 11-4 lists specific factors that put patients at more risk for immediate PONV. A previous history of immediate PONV or an emetogenic procedure automatically makes the patient at higher risk. Adding volatile agents and/or opioids further increases the risk.

The most effective strategy for these patients is to make certain they're well hydrated (follow the ASA guidelines and not only allow but encourage clear liquids up to three hours before surgery), avoid volatile agents, and avoid opioids. Whereas the first two admonitions are easy to accomplish, unfortunately opioids cannot always be avoided. If a cosmetic surgery patient who is considered high risk for immediate PONV receives opioids, he or she should also receive multimodal therapy.[69] Inspired by the works of Scuderi, White, Gan, and Chung, it makes sense that utilizing small doses of different classes of antiemetics to disrupt the nausea/vomiting pathway at different points will yield a higher success rate with a lower incidence of side effects (e.g., dysphoria, somnolence, or tardive dyskinesia) than monotherapy.

Whereas Scuderi et al. describe various "cocktails," the one Barinholtz employs has been utilized clinically in the treatment of more than 3,000 cosmetic surgery patients over the past five years. Low-dose droperidol (0.625 mg for the average adult) and dexamethasone (10 mg for the average adult) shortly after induction, followed by low-dose ondansetron (1 mg for the average adult) at the conclusion of the procedure, are administered.

The Barinholtz "cocktail" has been 99% effective in the prevention and treatment of immediate PONV in his practice and is very cost effective for routine use. In the rare instance of PONV in the PACU, additional ondansetron (1 mg or 4 mg orally dissolving tablet [ODT®]) is generally effective. Another effective approach can be to administer 50 mg IM ephedrine. This is effective even in the normotensive patient. The effect appears to be centrally mediated. Ephedrine "perks" up the patients and is usually effective within ten to fifteen minutes after administration.

Pay close attention to these patients as they begin to move around, stand up, get dressed, and walk. If the therapy is effective and they remain nausea-free during the getting-ready-to-leave phase, the patients can be discharged without further therapy (as long as there are not additional risk factors for delayed PONV). If, however, the patient is still nauseated despite all of the above, further therapy is required.

Nonpharmacologic Therapy

An effective adjunct to pharmacologic therapy is P_6 accupoint stimulation. Based on the principles of acupuncture and backed by impressive clinical results in several recent studies,[70,71] stimulation of the P_6 accupoint has been shown to be very effective in the prevention and treatment of PONV (as well as nausea/vomiting secondary to motion sickness, pregnancy, and chemotherapy). Located on the inside of the wrist, approximately 1 inch below the palmar crease, in the distribution of the median nerve, the P_6 accupoint is easily identifiable. Whereas some authors have chosen to needle the P_6 accupoint or apply pressure in order to stimulate it, the most effective practical approach is electrostimulation. The Reliefband® (Abbott Laboratories) is the only device currently available and approved by the FDA for electrostimulation of the P_6 accupoint for the prevention and treatment of PONV (as well as nausea and vomiting from pregnancy, motion sickness, or chemotherapy).[70,71] Reliefband® see Fig. 11.7 is easy to use, patient controlled, and portable, and Barinholtz has employed it as an adjunct to (or, in some cases, replacement of) pharmacologic agents for PONV for more than five years. In patients with resistant PONV, or in whom pharmocologic agents are contraindicated, or in patients at risk of delayed PONV, Reliefband® has been a very clinically effective as well as cost-effective approach in Barinholtz's practice. Combined with 5-HT3 antagonists (e.g., ondansetron), it has been shown to be remarkably effective.[72] Also, the combination of Reliefband® and ondansetron is easy for

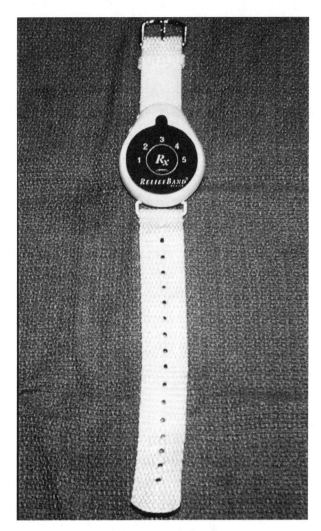

Figure 11-7. Reliefband.

the patient to continue at home for up to several days postoperatively if necessary.

Prevention and Treatment of Delayed PONV

Table 11-4 outlines specific factors that put a patient in the high-risk category for delayed PONV. These are a previous history of delayed PONV, a history of motion sickness, a history of ineffective (or questionable) treatment of immediate PONV, and any prescription for oral opioids for postoperative pain. For patients in this category, have a strategy that is practical for home therapy. The options are pills, orally dissolving tablets (ODTs), suppositories, and P_6 accupoint stimulation (*vide supra*).

Patients do not generally favor suppositories. Pills can be hard to swallow in the face of active PONV. Also, some

Table 11-4. Assessing risk and strategies for prevention and treatment of PONV

	Risk factors	Prevention	Treatment
Immediate PONV	Previous history immediate PONV Emetogenic procedure Exposure to volatile anesthetic Intraoperative and/or postoperative opioids	Make sure patient is well hydrated preoperatively (encourage clear liquids up to 3 hours before surgery) Avoid volatile agent Avoid (or at least minimize) opioid usage Multimodal pharmacologic therapy	Additional pharmacologic agents—consider nonpharmacologic therapy (P_6 accupoint stimulation)
Delayed PONV	Previous history delayed PONV History of motion sickness Prescription for oral opioids for postop pain Ineffective treatment of immediate PONV	Make sure immediate PONV resolved before discharging patient Instruct driver on careful driving (especially in patients with history of motion sickness) Avoid postoperative opioids (employ local anesthetics for postop pain) Reiterate need for full stomach before taking PO opioids	Prescribe PO antiemetic Consider nonpharmacologic therapy

of the drugs historically prescribed in pill form have many undesirable side effects. Prochlorperazine (Compazine®) can cause dysphoria, somnolence, restlessness, and extrapyramidal symptoms like tardive dyskinesia. Tardive dyskinesia is particularly distressing because the highest incidence of this unpleasant side effect appears to occur in elderly women. Traditionally, elderly women comprise a high percentage of rhytidectomy patients. *Primum non nocere* (First, do no harm). Make sure the cure is not worse than the disease.

Antihistamines (e.g., diphenhydramine) are effective but also cause undesired somnolence (of course, the antihistamines are sedative-sparing, don't cross the blood-brain barrier, and are thus ineffective as antiemetic. Barinholtz does, however, occasionally recommend diphenhydramine to patients with PONV who are also trying to get to sleep). The most effective drug treatment with the fewest side effects are the 5-HT_3 antagonists. However, this can become quite expensive. Pharmacies charge approximately $25 (in 2005 dollars) for one 4 mg Zofran ODT.® Patients may need this for many postoperative days. This therapy could cost hundreds of dollars. However, some prescription plans will cover this expense. Employing P_6 accupoint electrostimulation with a Reliefband® may be a more cost-effective solution. A disposable, prescription Reliefband® (which many prescription plans also cover) costs about $100 and will last twenty-four hours per day for up to six days. Utilizing one or both therapies is very effective in almost all patients.

The best way to avoid delayed PONV is to avoid postoperative opioids altogether.

Employing adequate local analgesia intraoperatively and postoperatively (in the form of a continuous local anesthetic infusion with a commercially available, disposable pain pump) is the most effective way to achieve this goal.

PUTTING IT ALL TOGETHER

The principles of TIVA for cosmetic surgery have been discussed. A real case scenario follows. In detail, the preoperative and postoperative care of a prototypical cosmetic surgery patient is examined. This technique is relatively generic in caring for patients having virtually *any* cosmetic procedure, in any operative position.

Preoperative Care—Prior to the Day of Surgery

After assessing a patient's health status and determining whether the patient is an appropriate candidate for elective, outpatient cosmetic surgery, the first step in caring for the patient is to make direct contact. Speak directly with the patient before the day of surgery to assess risk and give preoperative instructions. Address any questions or concerns the patient may have. This five- to ten-minute encounter (almost always by phone) can have a dramatic anxiolytic effect and actually reduce anesthetic requirements. It can also help avoid delays on the day of surgery. Issues generally discussed are concerns about being awake during surgery (a frequently asked question in Barinholtz's practice), putting risk in perspective (driving in a car is riskier than receiving anesthesia), and assuring that issues such as postoperative pain and PONV will be addressed. With the interview, assess the risk of PONV (immediate and/or delayed) and discuss the strategy.

Preoperative Care—Day of Surgery

On the day of surgery and after time is spent making sure preoperative instructions were followed (including NPO instructions and assurance of responsible adult escort), the patient is prepared for surgery. In addition to starting the IV, it is at this time that clonidine (usually 0.2 mg po) is administered. It is important that the patient arrive at least thirty minutes prior to entering the OR to take the clonidine. If clonidine is contraindicated (e.g., because the patient is hypotensive preoperatively), a small amount of benzodiazepine (1–2 mg midazolam IV) may be administered for anxiolysis, if necessary, prior to entering the OR.

Intraoperative Care

Upon entering the OR and after placement of monitors (ECG, NIBP, pulse oximeter, BIS), anesthesia is induced. If a patient did not receive clonidine or preoperative midazolam, a small dose of midazolam can be administered at this time. This is usually followed by a small dose of fentanyl (50–75 ug IV) and a propofol bolus. Propofol is administered and titrated to the BIS while oxygen is being administered blow-by via the modified oropharyngeal airway (lidocaine 1%, 1cc per 10cc of propofol is mixed in with the initial syringe of propofol to reduce burning). When the BIS is between 40 and 50, the patient will tolerate placement of the oropharyngeal airway (usually somewhere between 1 and 2 mg · kg^{-1} of propofol has been administered by this time).

After placement of the oropharyngeal airway and confirmation of a patent airway by end-tidal CO_2 tracing, ketamine (usually 50 mg IV) is administered. Two to three minutes after ketamine administration, the surgeon may inject the local analgesia. In addition to assuring the ketamine has taken effect, BIS is usually maintained in the range of 40–50 with the propofol infusion, and small doses (25 ug increments) of fentanyl are administered and titrated to a respiratory rate of approximately ten breaths per minute (easily monitored by observing the end-tidal CO_2 tracing) *before* the surgeon is allowed to inject the local analgesia. This (i.e., GA) will assure a virtually immobile patient for local injections. Obviously, additional boluses of propofol and/or fentanyl may occasionally need to be administered (guided by BIS and respiratory rate, respectively). If one decides to administer additional ketamine, make sure the total dose doesn't exceed 1 mg · kg^{-1}. Higher doses may be associated with undesirable side effects such as dysphoria, prolonged recovery, and even PONV.

Once the surgery is underway (and appropriate antibiotics have been administered if necessary), the BIS is allowed to come up and is generally maintained at 60 (+/−10) for the remainder of the procedure.

Prophylactic antiemetics are administered. At this point, and for the remainder of the procedure, the propofol infusion is titrated according to the BIS. Usual infusion rates are 75–120 ug · kg^{-1}· min^{-1}, but rates as low as 25 ug · kg^{-1} · min^{-1} or as high as 300 ug · kg^{-1}· min^{-1} are sometimes required. The ability to respond to this patient variation underscores the importance of BIS monitoring. Additional opioids are titrated to achieve or maintain a respiratory rate of ten to fifteen breaths per minute. Close communication with the surgeon and close attention to the surgery must be maintained in order to be able to respond to the more and less stimulating parts of the procedure by adjusting the propofol infusion and opioid boluses accordingly. If muscle relaxation is required for rectus muscle repair, utilize the technique described earlier.

When the surgeon is placing the last stitches (or placing the garment on the patient), the propofol infusion is discontinued. Low-dose ondansetron is administered. The patient is allowed to awaken, which occurs typically within three to five minutes of discontinuation of propofol. With BIS >80, the patient will open his or her eyes and respond to commands.

At this time the patient is transferred to a recliner and taken to the PACU. Propofol is generally consumed at a rate of approximately 50 cc · hr^{-1} for the average patient. Opioid administration varies widely depending on patient characteristics (e.g., history of smoking or drinking), procedure (nature and length), and surgeon's skill with local.

If the procedure is one that historically is associated with significant postoperative pain (i.e., abdominoplasty or subpectoral breast augmentation), the surgeon will frequently utilize a local anesthetic pain pump significantly decreasing, if not eliminating, the need for opioids postoperatively.

Postoperative Care

Once in PACU, patients are observed, postoperative issues (i.e., pain, PONV) are addressed as necessary, and the patients are discharged to go home in the company of a responsible adult escort. Most patients (more than 90%) arrive in PACU with an Aldrette score of 9 or greater, thus putting them in phase recovery. It is the rare patient in Barinholtz's practice that spends more than one hour in recovery.

As part of the postoperative instructions and follow-up, Barinholtz takes on the burden of addressing postanesthetic complications directly. Patients and/or their families are instructed to call the anesthesia provider if there are anesthetic-related issues such as PONV. The surgeons greatly appreciate this. Luckily, by employing these techniques, calls are rare.

CONCLUSION

Office-based anesthesia has come a long way since Dr. Crawford Long successfully administered the first ether anesthetic in 1842. Advances in pharmacology and technology have made anesthesia better and safer than ever. It is now a rare event (especially for healthy people having elective cosmetic surgery) for patients to suffer their demise under the anesthesiologist's care. Improving the quality of the perioperative experience has become a primary focus. In the future, with better drugs, better monitoring technologies, and better delivery systems, further improvements in patient care should evolve toward these ideal anesthetic.

REFERENCES

1. Long CW: An account of the first use of sulphuric ether by inhalation as an anesthetic in surgical operations. *South Med Surg J* 5:705,1849.
2. Heynick F: William T. G. Morton and "The Great Moment," 1944 Paramount Movie, 2003.
3. Wright AJ: Horace Wells, DDS and "Rebel with a Cause," 1815–1848, *ASA Newsletter*, American Society of Anesthesiologists, Park Ridge, IL, 63:6,1999.
4. Kitz RJ, Vandam LD: Scope of Modern Anesthetic Practice, in Miller RD (ed.): *Anesthesia*, 3rd ed., New York, Churchill Livingstone, 1990, p 9.
5. Lagasse RS: Anesthesia Safety: Model or myth? A review of published literature and analysis of current original data. *Anesthesiol* 97:1609,2002.
6. Fragen RJ: Diprivan (Propofol): A historical perspective. *Semin Anesth* 7:1,1988.
7. Rutter DV, Morgan M, Lumley J, Owen R: ICI 35 868 (Diprivan): A new intravenous induction agent. *Anaesthesia* 35:1188,1980.
8. Heath PJ, Kennedy DJ, Ogg TW, et al.: Which intravenous induction agent for day surgery: A comparison of propofol thiopentone, methohexitone and etomidate. *Anaesthesia* 43:365,1988.
9. Doze VA, Westphal LM, White PF: Comparison of propofol with methohexital for outpatient anesthesia. *Anesth Analg* 65:1189,1986.
10. Oxorn DC, Ferris LE, Harrington E, Orser BA: The effects of midazolam on propofol-induced anesthesia: Propofol dose requirements, mood profiles, and perioperative dreams. *Anesth Analg* 85:553,1997.
11. Friedberg BL: Paradoxical increase in pain requirements with midazolam premedication. *Anesth Analg* 99:1268,2004.
12. Cote CJ, Cohen IT, Santhanam S, et al.: A comparison of three doses of a commercially prepared oral midazolam syrup in children. *Anesth Analg* 94:37,2002.
13. Pettinger WA: Drug therapy: Clonidine, a new antihypertensive drug. *N Engl J Med* 293:1179,1975.
14. Mannion S, Hayes I, Loughnane F, et al.: Intravenous but not perineural clonidine prolongs postoperative analgesia after pso as compartment block with 0.5% levobupivacaine for hip fracture surgery. *Anesth Analg* 100:873,2005.
15. Strebel S, Gurzeler JA, Schneider MC, et al.: Small-dose intrathecal clonidine and isobaric bupivacaine for orthopedic surgery: A dose-response study. *Anesth Analg* 99:1231, 2004.
16. Baker A, Klimscha W, Eisenach J, et al.: Intrathecal clonidine for postoperative analgesia in elderly patients: The influence of baricity on hemodynamic and analgesic effects. *Anesth Analg* 99:128,2004.
17. Koch M, Famenne F, Deckers G, et al.: Epidural clonidine or sufentanil for intraoperative and postoperative analgesia. *Anesth Analg* 81:1154,1995.

18. Bernard JM, Kick O, Bonet F: Comparison of intravenous and epidural clonidine for postoperative patient-controlled analgesia. *Anesth Analg* 81:706,1995.
19. Casati A, Magistris L, Fanelli G, et al.: Small-dose clonidine prolongs postoperative analgesia after sciatic-femoral nerve block with 0.75% ropivacaine for foot surgery. *Anesth Analg* 91:388,2000.
20. Joshi W, Reuben S, Kilaru P, et al.: Postoperative analgesia for outpatient arthroscopic knee surgery with intra-articular clonidine and/or morphine. *Anesth Analg* 90:1102,2000.
21. Man D: Premedication with oral clonidine for facial rhytidectomy. *Plast Reconstr Surg* 94:214,1994.
22. Baker TM, Stuzin JM, Baker TJ, et al.: What's new in aesthetic surgery? *Clin Plast Surg* 23:16,1996.
23. Friedberg BL, Sigl JC: Clonidine premedication decreases propofol consumption during bispectral index (BIS) monitored propofol-ketamine technique for office-based surgery. *Dermatol Surg* 26:848,2000.
24. Higuchi H, Adachi Y, Dahan A, et al.: The interaction between propofol and clonidine for loss of consciousness. *Anesth Analg* 94:886,2002.
25. Higuchi H, Adachi Y, Arimura S, et al.: Oral clonidine premedication reduces the awakening concentration of propofol. *Anesth Analg* 94:609,2002.
26. Ishiyama T, Kashimoto S, Oguchi T, et al.: The effects of clonidine premedication on the blood pressure and tachycardiac responses to ephedrine in elderly and young patients during propofol anesthesia. *Anesth Analg* 96:136, 2003.
27. Taittonen MT, Kirvela OA, Aantaa R, et al.: The effect of clonidine or midazolam premedication on perioperative responses during ketamine anesthesia. *Anesth Analg* 87:161, 1998.
28. Arain SR, Ebert TJ: The efficacy, side effects, and recovery characteristics of dexmedotomidine versus propofol when used for intraoperative sedation. *Anesth Analg* 95:461,2002.
29. Mayer D: Personal communication. October 2004.
30. Shapiro F: Personal communication. November 2004.
31. Corssen G, Domino EF: Dissociative anesthesia: Further pharmacologic studies and first clinical experience with the phencyclidine derivative CI-581. *Anesth Analg* 45:29,1966.
32. Guit JBM, Koning HM, Costner ML: Ketamine as analgesia for intravenous anesthesia with propofol (TIVA) anesthesia. *Anaesthesia* 46:24,1991.
33. Badrinath S, Avramov MN, Shadrick M, et al.: The use of ketamine-propofol combination during monitored anesthesia care. *Anesth Analg* 90:858,2000.
34. Friedberg BL: Propofol ketamine anesthesia for cosmetic surgery in the office suite, chapter in Osborne I (ed.), *Anesthesia for Outside the Operating Room. International Anesthesiology Clinics.* Baltimore, Lippincott, Williams & Wilkins, 41(2):39,2003.
35. White PF: The role of nonopoid analgesic techniques in the management of pain after ambulatory surgery. *Anesth Analg* 94:577,2002.
36. Fauno P, Petersen KD, Husted SE: Increased blood loss after preoperative NSAID: Retrospective study of 186 hip arthroplasties. *Acta Orthop Scand* 64:522,1993.

37. Robinson CM, Christie J, Malcolm-Smith N: Non-steroidal anti-inflammatory drugs, perioperative blood loss, and transfusion requirements in elective hip arthroplasty. *J Arthroplasty* 8:607,1993.

38. Splinter WM, Rhine EJ, Roberts DW, et al.: Preoperative ketorolac increases bleeding after tonsillectomy in children. *Can J Anaesth* 43:560,1996.

39. Wierod FS, Frandsen NJ, Jacobsen JD, et al.: Risk of haemorrhage from transurethral prostatectomy in acetylsalicylic acid and NSAID-treated patients. *Scand J Urol Nephrol* 32:120,1998.

40. FitzGerald GA, Patrono C: Drug therapy: The coxibs, selective inhibitors of cyclooxygenase-2. *N Engl J Med* 345:433,2001.

41. Reuben SS, Connelly NR: Postoperative analgesic effects of celecoxib or rofecoxib after spinal fusion surgery. *Anesth Analg* 91:1221,2000.

42. Reuben SS, Bhopatkar S, Maciolek H, et al.: The preemptive analgesic effect of rofecoxib after ambulatory arthroscopic knee surgery. *Anesth Analg* 94:55,2002.

43. Turan A, Emet S, Karamanlioglu B, et al.: Analgesic effects of rofecoxib in ear-nose-throat surgery. *Anesth Analg* 95:1308,2002.

44. Buvanendran A, Kroin JS, Tuman KJ, et al.: Effects of perioperative administration of a selective cyclooxygenase 2 inhibitor on pain management and recovery of function after knee replacement: A randomized controlled trial. *JAMA* 290:2411,2003.

45. Ma H, Tang J, White PF, et al.: Perioperative rofecoxib improves early recovery after outpatient herniorrhaphy. *Anesth Analg* 98:970,2004.

46. Barton SF, Langeland FF, Snabes MD, et al.: Efficacy and safety of intravenous parecoxib sodium in relieving acute postoperative pain following gynecologic laparotomy surgery. *Anesthesiol* 97:306,2002.

47. Joshi GP, Viscusi ER, Gan TJ: Effective treatment of laparoscopic cholecystectomy pain with intravenous followed by oral COX-e specific inhibitor. *Anesth Analg* 98:336,2004.

48. Kim PS, Reicin AS, Villalba L, et al.: Rofecoxib, Merck, and the FDA. *N Engl J Med* 351:2875,2004.

49. Psaty BM, Furberg CD: COX-2 Inhibitors—Lessons in drug safety. *N Engl J Med* 352:1133,2005.

50. Calverly RK: Anesthesia as a specialty: Past, present, and future, in Barash PG, Cullen BF, Stoelting RK (eds.), *Clinical Anesthesia*. Philadelphia, Lippincott, 1989, p 21.

51. Griffith HR, Johnson GE: The use of curare in general anesthesia. *Anesthesiol* 3:418,1942.

52. Calverley RK: Arthur E Guedel (1883–1956), in Repreht J, van Lieburg MJ, Lee JA, and Erdmann W (eds.), *Anaesthesia Essays on Its History*. Berlin, Springer-Verlag, 1985, p 49.

53. Brain AIJ: The laryngeal mask airway: A new concept in airway management. *Br J Anaesth* 55:801,1983.

54. Brain AIJ, McGhee TD, McAteer EJ, et al.: The laryngeal mask airway: Development and preliminary trials of new type of airway. *Anaesthesia* 40:356,1985.

55. ASA Publication: Practice Guidelines for Management of the Difficult Airway (last amended 10/16/02), p 21.

56. Calverley RK: Anesthesia as a specialty: Past, present and future. In Barash, Cullen, Stoelting (eds.), *Clinical Anesthesia*, Philadelphia, Lippincott, 1989, p 25.

57. Bruhn J, Bouillon TW, Ropcke H, et al.: A manual slide rule for target-controlled infusion of propofol: Development and evaluation. *Anesth Analg* 96:142,2003.

58. Suttner S, Boldt J, Schmidt C, et al.: Cost analysis of target-controlled infusion-based anesthesia compared with standard anesthesia regimens. *Anesth Analg* 88:77, 1999.

59. Woolf CJ, Chong MS: Preemptive analgesia: Treating postoperative pain by preventing the establishment of central sensitization. *Anesth Analg* 77:362,1993.

60. Ong KS, Lirk P, Seymour RA: The efficacy of preemptive analgesia for acute postoperative pain management: A meta-analysis. *Anesth Analg* 100:757,2005.

61. McQuay HJ: Pre-emptive analgesia: A systematic review of clinical studies. *Ann Med* 27:249,1995.

62. McQuay HJ: Pre-emptive analgesia. *Br J Anaesth* 69:1,1992.

63. Macario A, Weinger M, Carney S, et al.: Which clinical anesthesia outcomes are important to avoid? The perspective of patients. *Anesth Analg* 89:652,1999.

64. Lee A, Gin T, Lau A, et al.: A comparison of patients' and health care professionals' preferences for symptoms during immediate postoperative recovery and the management of postoperative nausea and vomiting. *Anesth Analg* 100:87,2005.

65. Pierre S, Corno G, Benais H, et al.: A risk score-dependent antiemetic approach effectively reduces postoperative nausea and vomiting—A continuous quality improvement initiative. *Can J Anaesth* 51:320,2004.

66. Apfel CC, Laara E, Koivuranta M, et al.: A simplified risk score for predicting postoperative nausea and vomiting: Conclusions from cross-validations between two centers. *Anesthesiol* 91:693,1999.

67. Apfel CC, Kranke P, Eberhart LH, et al.: Comparison of predictive models for postoperative nausea and vomiting. *Br J Anaesth* 88:234,2002.

68. Apfel C, Korttila K, Abdalla M, et al.: A factorial trial of six interventions for the prevention of postoperative nausea and vomiting. *N Engl J Med* 350:2441,2004.

69. Scuderi P, James R, Harris L, et al.: Multimodal antiemetic management prevents early postoperative vomiting after outpatient laparoscopy. *Anesth Analg* 91:1408, 2000.

70. Gan TJ, Jiao K, Zenn M, et al.: A randomized controlled comparison of electro-accupoint stimulation or ondansetron versus placebo for the prevention of postoperative nausea and vomiting. *Anesth Analg* 99:1070,2004.

71. Zarate E, Mingus M, White PF, et al.: The use of transcutaneous accupoint electrical stimulation for preventing nausea and vomiting after laparoscopic surgery. *Anesth Analg* 92:629,2001.

72. White PF, Hamza M, Recart A, et al.: Optimal timing of acustimulation for antiemetic prophylaxis as an adjunct to ondansetron in patients undergoing plastic surgery. *Anesth Analg* 100:367,2005.

Regional Anesthesia for Cosmetic Surgery

Holly Evans, M.D., F.R.C.P., and Susan M. Steele, M.D.

Table 12-1. Goals of anesthesia for cosmetic surgery

Intraoperative analgesia
Intraoperative anxiolysis ($\pm$ amnesia)
Postoperative analgesia
Absence of postoperative side effects (nausea, vomiting, sedation, urinary retention)
Early return of baseline cognitive abilities
Timely postoperative discharge

INTRODUCTION

Anesthesia for patients undergoing cosmetic surgery must accomplish a number of important goals (Table 12-1). Regional anesthesia, which includes both central neuraxial techniques as well as peripheral nerve blocks, has a commendable safety profile[1] and unique attributes that allow these goals to be met. Nerve blocks provide dense intraoperative anesthesia and analgesia. This minimizes requirements for additional anesthetic, analgesic, or sedative agents; consequently, side effects such as postoperative nausea, vomiting, and sedation can be minimized.[2,5] This enhances patient recovery and discharge and may also improve patient satisfaction.[6,8] Peripheral nerve blocks with long-acting local anesthetic can extend the duration of postoperative analgesia and further minimize opioid use and associated side effects.[2] This chapter describes the use of central neuraxial blocks and peripheral nerve blocks in cosmetic surgical patients. A discussion of appropriate preoperative evaluation, monitoring, sedation, and nerve block technique, as well as postoperative recovery and discharge, is included.

PREOPERATIVE ASSESSMENT

General Assessment

Evaluation of patients contemplating regional anesthesia should include a full history and physical examination as well as investigations or consultations as indicated. A complete history is obtained to document active medical issues, past medical history, prescription and nonprescription medication use, allergies, and personal and family anesthesia history. The physical examination involves assessment of the patient's height, weight, vital signs, and airway. Cardiovascular, respiratory, and neurologic evalu-

ations are performed. In addition, the site where regional anesthesia is to be administered is inspected. Laboratory investigations are performed based on the patient's underlying medical problems and the anticipated surgery. For example, an otherwise healthy thirty-year-old woman having breast augmentation may require no preoperative testing. A sixty-year-old woman with hypertension treated with a diuretic would be appropriately investigated with electrolytes and an electrocardiogram prior to her abdominoplasty. Similarly, consultations with other medical specialists may be required for active medical issues. The physiologic effects of regional anesthesia must be considered in the context of the patient's underlying medical condition(s) (Table 12-2). Subsequently, potential contraindications to regional anesthesia as well as ambulatory surgery must be sought and addressed (see Tables 12-3, 12-4, and 12-5). Ideally, the preoperative anesthesia assessment is performed several days prior to the scheduled procedure to enable such consultation, patient optimization, and rescheduling if required.

The preoperative visit provides an ideal time for patient education. Patients are instructed about fasting guidelines, which medications to take the day of surgery, and the timing of medications and herbal remedies to be discontinued preoperatively (see Ch. 14 & Appendix A). Outpatients should be notified that they require a responsible caregiver to accompany them to and from surgery and to stay with them the night of surgery. In the process of obtaining informed consent for anesthesia, patients should be educated about the expected intra- and postoperative

Table 12-2. Physiologic effects of neuraxial anesthesia

Cardiovascular	Sympathectomy
	Vasodilation
	Hypotension ($\pm$ bradycardia)
Respiratory	With high block:
	Subjective dyspnea
	Impaired active exhalation
	Impaired cough
Gastrointestinal	Increased secretions
	Sphincter relaxation
	Bowel constriction
Endocrine-Metabolic	Inhibition of surgical stress response

Table 12-3. Conditions associated with increased risk of neuraxial anesthesia

Condition	Risk
Increased intracranial pressure	Brain stem herniation
Significant coagulopathy	Spinal or epidural hematoma
Uncorrected hypovolemia	Shock, cardiovascular collapse
Infection overlying needle puncture site	Neuraxial infection
Systemic sepsis	Neuraxial infection
Significant aortic stenosis	Cardiovascular collapse
Unstable neurologic disease	Neurologic deficit
Local anesthetic allergy	Allergic reaction

Table 12-5. Conditions associated with increased risk for ambulatory surgery

Condition	Risk
Malignant hyperthermia	Perioperative MH[a] reaction
Obstructive sleep apnea, obesity	Postoperative airway obstruction Oxygen desaturation
Unstable systemic disease	Exacerbation of symptoms
Absence of reliable caregiver	Insufficient assistance for patient after discharge
Surgery involving significant blood loss	Intravascular volume depletion and fluid shifts
Surgery associated with prolonged recovery	Potential for hospital admission
Surgery associated with severe postoperative pain	Potential for hospital admission for analgesia
Local anesthetic allergy	Allergic reaction

[a]MH = malignant hyperthermia

course as well as the potential side effects and risks of the anesthetic technique(s) contemplated.

Patients having cosmetic surgery are a unique subset.

They often have numerous questions, seek more information than the general surgical population, and have extremely high standards and expectations.

Table 12-4. Conditions associated with increased risk of peripheral nerve blocks

Condition	Risk
Infection overlying needle puncture site	Perineural infection
Significant coagulopathy	Blood loss ± transfusion Hematoma ± nerve compression
Uncorrected hypovolemia	Shock, cardiovascular collapse
Perineural tumor	Tumor seeding and spread
Perineural vascular malformation	Blood loss ± transfusion Hematoma ± nerve compression
Unstable neurologic disease	Neurologic deficit
Previous thoracic surgery	Obliteration of paravertebral space by scar tissue Pneumothorax from paravertebral block
Infection within chest cavity (i.e., empyema)	Paravertebral or neuraxial infection from paravertebral block
Local anesthetic allergy	Allergic reaction

Special Consideration: Coagulation Abnormalities

As discussed, the patient's underlying medical conditions factor into the decision regarding the suitability of regional anesthesia. Altered coagulation is one such condition that deserves special mention as it increases the risk of neuraxial hematoma following spinal or epidural anesthesia. Coagulopathy may result from an intrinsic defect in the patient's coagulation system, from prescribed anticoagulant medication, or from nonprescription drug use like garlic, ginger, or ginko biloba (see Table 14-3 in Chapter 14).

Patients with an intrinsic bleeding diathesis such as hemophilia or thrombocytopenia represent a subset of patients with altered coagulation. Preoperative assessment includes a focused bleeding history and physical examination. Appropriate laboratory evaluation depends on the underlying disorder, and perioperative management usually occurs in conjunction with a hematologist. Individuals with moderate and severe disease would rarely be considered for ambulatory cosmetic surgery because of the increased surgical and anesthetic risk. Patients with mild disease having low-risk surgical procedures may be suitable. However, these patients require a thorough evaluation of their coagulation system and coordination with their hematologist prior to being considered for neuraxial anesthesia. The risk of neuraxial hematoma increases as coagulation parameters fall out of the range of normal. The risk-to-benefit ratio must be considered in the context of this population of patients who are having *entirely* elective procedures.

Patients with altered coagulation as a result of anticoagulants used for thromboprophylaxis represent another subset of anticoagulated patients. Preoperative evalua-

tion is as described previously. The American Society of Regional Anesthesia guidelines for the perioperative management of anticoagulation therapy for patients having spinal or epidural anesthesia are summarized in Table 12-6.[9]

Guidelines regarding the use of peripheral nerve blocks for patients with altered coagulation due to an intrinsic bleeding diathesis or the use of thromboprophylactic

---

Table 12-6. American Society of Regional Anesthesia and Pain Medicine recommendations regarding neuraxial anesthesia in the patient receiving thromboprophylaxis

Thromboprophylactic agent	Recommendation
Antiplatelet Medication	No contraindication with NSAIDs[a]
	Discontinue ticlopidine 14 d in advance
	Discontinue clopidogrel 7 d in advance
	Discontinue GP IIb/IIIa[b] inhibitors 8–48 h in advance
Unfractionated Heparin (Subcutaneous)	No contraindication
	Consider delaying heparin until after block if technical difficulty anticipated
Unfractionated Heparin (Intravenous)	Heparinize 1 h after neuraxial technique
	Remove catheter 2–4 h after last heparin dose
	No mandatory delay if traumatic
Low Molecular Weight Heparin	Twice daily dosing:
	LMWH[c] 24 h after surgery, regardless of technique
	Remove neuraxial catheter 2 h before first LMWH[c] dose
	Single daily dosing (as per the following European guidelines):
	Neuraxial technique 10–12 h after LMWH[c]
	Next dose at least 4 h after needle or catheter placement
	Catheters removed 10–12 h after LMWH[c] and 4 h prior to next dose
	Postpone LMWH[c] 24 h if traumatic
Warfarin	Document normal INR[d] after discontinuation (prior to neuraxial technique)
	Remove catheter when INR[d] ≤ 1.5 (initiation of therapy)
Thrombolytics	No data on safety interval for performance of neuraxial technique or catheter removal
	Follow fibrinogen level
Herbal Therapy	No evidence for mandatory discontinuation prior to neuraxial technique
	Be aware of potential drug interactions

Adapted from Horlocker TT, Wedel DJ, Benzon HP, et al.: Regional anesthesia in the anticoagulated patient: Defining the risks (the second ASRA consensus conference on neuraxial anesthesia and anticoagulation). *Regional Anesthesia & Pain Medicine* 28;172,2003.[9]
[a]NSAIDs = nonsteroidal anti-inflammatory drugs
[b]GP IIb/IIIa = glycoprotein IIb/IIIa inhibitors
[c]LMWH = low molecular weight heparin
[d]INR = international normalized ratio

agents are extrapolated from those described previously.[9] Adherence to these guidelines should be more stringent for peripheral nerve blocks performed near noncompressible vessels (i.e., intercostal or sciatic nerve block) and for those where hematoma formation could result in significant injury to nerves or other surrounding structures (i.e., paravertebral or lumbar plexus block).[10]

MONITORING AND SEDATION

Monitoring

Intravenous access, supplemental oxygen, and appropriate monitors are imperative to the safe practice of regional anesthesia. Nerve blocks can produce significant physiologic changes (see Table 12-2). Furthermore, multisystemic side effects may result from the intravascular absorption of large volumes of local anesthetic. Consequently, monitoring with pulse oximetry, noninvasive blood pressure, and electrocardiogram are required both during block placement and intraoperatively.

Sedation for Block Placement

Sedation may be required during block placement. In this setting, the goal is to relieve apprehension and pain as well as to maintain a communicative patient able to convey information about potential adverse effects of regional anesthesia. For example, description of paresthesias allows needle redirection and prevention of intraneural injection of local anesthetic. And communication about tinnitus and metallic taste allows discontinuation of injection of local anesthetic and prevention of more serious symptoms related to local anesthetic toxicity.

Intravenous agents are typically used for their titratability (see Table 12-7). Benzodiazepines provide anxiolysis and anterograde amnesia. They raise the seizure threshold, which is advantageous when large doses of local anesthetic are used. The benzodiazepine midazolam is frequently used owing to its rapid onset, relatively short half-life, and lack of active metabolites. Analgesia and additional sedation result from supplementation with opioid analgesics. The potent, short-acting agent fentanyl is frequently employed for this purpose. Benzodiazepines and opioids can both be reversed with specific antagonists, and this further enhances their safe application for perioperative sedation. The half-life of reversal agents is sometimes shorter then the drugs being reversal. Dependence on reversal agents provides, the illusion of safety.

Ketamine affords an alternate option for analgesia with a lower incidence of opioid-related side effects such as nausea, vomiting, respiratory depression, and pruritus. The dysphoria associated with ketamine may limit the use of this agent; however, the concurrent use of midazolam can minimize side effects.[11] The alpha2 agonist, clonidine, also offers analgesia with minimal opioid-related side effects, though this agent may cause hypotension and bradycardia as well as prolonged postoperative sedation. Nonpharmacologic anxiolysis is generated from verbal reassurance or music.[12] The importance of this cannot be overemphasized.

Intraoperative Sedation

Intraoperative sedation should enhance patient comfort yet have minimal postoperative effects allowing for timely patient recovery. Sedation can be continued intraoperatively using incremental doses of the agents described herein. Alternatively, an infusion of a short-acting, easily titratable agent can be used (see Table 12-7). Target-controlled infusion devices may be used to minimize drug dose and associated side effects and have also been used to provide patient-controlled sedation.[13]

The pharmacokinetics of propofol make it well suited for sedation by continuous infusion. It has a rapid onset, is easily titratable, and is associated with prompt awakening upon discontinuation of the infusion. The use of propofol has also been effective in reducing the incidence of postoperative nausea and vomiting.[14] The ultrashort-acting potent opioid remifentanil is designed for continuous infusion and provides sedation as well as additional analgesia. Servin et al. compared sedation with an infusion of remifentanil ($0.1\ \mu g \cdot kg^{-1} \cdot min^{-1}$ IV) or propofol ($50\ \mu g \cdot kg^{-1} \cdot min^{-1}$ IV) in patients who received regional anesthesia for their surgical procedure.[15] Servin et al. found that remifentanil provided greater analgesia, less amnesia, and a higher incidence of respiratory depression and postoperative nausea and vomiting (PONV).[15] Dexmedetomidine is a short-acting alpha2 agonist suitable for continuous infusion. It provides improved postoperative analgesia and has opioid-sparing effects compared to propofol. However, it has a slower onset of action, a longer duration of action after discontinuation of infusion, and a greater incidence of postoperative hypotension and sedation.[16]

Table 12-7. Selected intravenous agents used for sedation

Class of agent	Mechanism of action	Systemic effects	Adverse effects	Specific agents and dose
Benzo-diazepines	Bind to GABA[a] A receptor Facilitate central nervous system inhibition of GABA[a]	Sedation Anxiolysis Anterograde amnesia Anticonvulsant Skeletal muscle relaxation	Hypotension Respiratory depression Prolonged sedation in some patients Paradoxical excitement in some patients	Midazolam Incremental doses of 20–30 ug/kg IV up to 0.1 mg · kg^{-1}
Opioids	Opioid receptor (i.e., mu, kappa, delta) agonists Decrease neurotransmitter release	Sedation Analgesia No amnesia	Nausea, vomiting Pruritus Respiratory depression Urinary retention Constipation Muscle rigidity Bradycardia	Fentanyl: Incremental doses of 0.5–1.5 ug · kg^{-1} IV Alfentanil: 5–10 ug · kg^{-1} IV Remifentanil: 0.025–0.2 ug · kg^{-1}
Ketamine	NMDA[b] receptor antagonist May also interact with opioid receptors	Dissociative state Sedation Analgesia Amnesia Pharyngeal and laryngeal reflexes maintained near normal Sympathomimetic effects Bronchodilation	Emergence delirium[c] Psychosis[c] Hallucinations[c] Increases salivary secretions Nystagmus Increases ICP[d] and IOP[e]	0.15–0.5 mg · kg^{-1}
Alpha$_2$ Agonists	Sympathetic alpha$_2$ receptor agonists Decrease neurotransmitter release	Sedation Analgesia Minimal respiratory depression	Hypotension Bradycardia Prolonged sedation (clonidine > dexmetetomidine)	Clonidine 1–2 ug · kg^{-1} IV or 0.2 mg po Dexmedetomidine Bolus: 0.4–1 ug · kg^{-1} IV over 10–20 min Infusion: 0.2–0.7 ug · kg^{-1} · hr^{-1} IV
Propofol	Presumed via interaction with GABA[a] receptor	Sedation Amnesia Antipruritic Anticonvulsant Antiemetic	Pain on intravenous injection Hypotension Respiratory depression, apnea Spontaneous excitatory movements Supports growth of microorganisms	25–100 ug · kg^{-1} · min^{-1} IV

[a]GABA = Gamma-amino-butyric acid
[b]NMDA = N-methyl-D-aspartate
[c]Editor's note: This information is correct only when ketamine is given as a sole IV agent. Friedberg BL : Hypnotic doses of propofol block ketamine induced hallucinations. *Plast Reconstr Surg* 91:196,1993. —BLF
[d]ICP = Intracranial pressure
[e]IOP = Intraocular pressure

Table 12-8. Potential advantages of spinal anesthesia for cosmetic surgery[1,3,7]

Ease of performance
Dense anesthesia
Minimal additional sedation required
Prompt return of awake state
Low incidence of PONV[a]
Reduced physiologic stress response
Reduced thromboembolic complications
Low incidence of local anesthetic toxicity
Cost savings

[a]PONV = postoperative nausea and vomiting

Table 12-9. Selected potential adverse effects of spinal anesthesia[1,9,27,64,77–83]

Self-limiting	Back pain
	Urinary retention
	Transient neurologic symptoms
	Postdural puncture headache
Rare but serious	Epidural abscess
	Spinal or epidural hematoma
	Meningitis
	Cauda equina syndrome
	Isolated nerve injury
	Total spinal anesthesia
	Bradycardia and cardiac arrest

SPINAL ANESTHESIA

Indications and advantages

Spinal anesthesia provides rapid onset, bilateral surgical anesthesia for cosmetic procedures of the abdomen and lower extremities. Potential advantages are outlined in Table 12-8.

Equipment

Two classes of spinal needles are available. *Cutting* needles, such as the Quincke or Greene, have a beveled distal tip with an end orifice. *Pencil-point* needles, such as the Whitacre or Sprotte, have a blunt distal tip and an orifice on the side of the distal needle shaft. Pencil-point needles provide an enhanced tactile feel as the needle is advanced through the various tissues. Spinal needles in current use have an inner stylet that prevents plugging of the needle with skin or fat and subsequent deposition into the epidural or subarachnoid space. Both classes of needles are available in a range of diameters and lengths. The gauge describes the outer diameter of the needle. A larger gauge represents a smaller diameter needle (i.e., a 29 ga needle has a smaller diameter than a 22 ga needle). The use of pencil-point and small-gauge needles is associated with a lower incidence of postdural puncture headache (PDPH).[17] Small gauge needles can be more technically difficult to use as they are more prone to deflection and often have slower return of cerebrospinal fluid.

Local anesthetics and adjuvants

The selection of local anesthetic for spinal anesthesia is based on the desired block onset, duration, and spread, as well as the drug's side-effect profile.

Lidocaine and mepivacaine both have a rapid onset and short to intermediate duration of action.[18,19] Lidocaine has been associated with transient neurologic symptoms, which has significantly curtailed its use, particularly in the outpatient population.[20,26] In addition, there is some evidence that this complication may also occur with mepivacaine.[27] Procaine is another short-acting agent. However, its use has been limited by frequent block failure.[28]

A preparation of chloroprocaine without the preservative methylparaben or the antioxidant bisulfite has recently been used for spinal anesthesia.[29,34] In a crossover study of volunteers, intrathecal chloroprocaine (40 mg) was compared to lidocaine (40 mg).[29] Investigators found that both provided adequate anesthesia. However, the chloroprocaine group had faster resolution of sensory block by twenty-three minutes as well as earlier time to ambulation and voiding by thirty minutes. Transient neurologic symptoms occurred in 87.5% in the lidocaine group and none in the chloroprocaine group. In a study of similar design, spinal anesthesia with chloroprocaine (40 mg) was compared to low-dose bupivacaine (7.5 mg).[35] Both agents had a similar peak block height and time to peak block; however, complete regression of sensory and motor block, ambulation and voiding occurred over one hour later in the bupivacaine group. Despite the beneficial profile described, the addition of epinephrine to hyperbaric chloroprocaine has been associated with transient neurologic symptoms and nonspecific, transient, flu-like symptoms.[30] Transient neurologic symptoms are rare with bupivacaine and levobupivacaine.[36] These agents have a long duration of action, which can potentially delay recovery and discharge of ambulatory patients.[37] A reduction in dose has been used in an attempt to shorten the duration of action; however, this can potentially lead to block failure.[37] Intrathecal ropivacaine also has a long duration of action.[38–42] However, some studies have shown earlier recovery of sensory and motor function when compared to bupivacaine, which may be advantageous to outpatients.[42]

The naturally occurring lumbar lordosis and thoracic kyphosis affect the spread of both hypo- and hyperbaric solutions. A hyperbaric solution injected into a lumbar interspace (near the peak of the lumbar lordosis) gravitates cephalad to the thoracic kyphosis and caudally to the sacral nerve roots in a patient in the supine position (Fig. 12-1). A mid-thoracic block may also result from a hypobaric solution if the patient remains sitting for several minutes after injection. Unilateral spinal anesthesia can be achieved with either hypo- or hyperbaric solutions administered to patients in the lateral decubitus position.

The effect of spinal local anesthetics can be impacted by the addition of adjuvant medications. Intrathecally administered opioids are commonly used adjuvants that act by binding to opiate receptors in the spinal cord.[43] They enhance the quality of spinal anesthesia and increase the duration of sensory anesthesia. As a result, the dose of spinal local anesthetic can be reduced, facilitating recovery and outpatient discharge. Ben-David et al. illustrated this in a population of patients who received 5 mg hyperbaric spinal bupivacaine.[44] The incidence of inadequate block was 24% in the group who received bupivacaine alone, whereas there were no failed blocks in the group who received 10 ug intrathecal fentanyl with bupivacaine. Pruritus is a known side effect of intrathecal opioids and is usually mild and self-limiting.[45] The highly lipophilic agent fentanyl (10–25 ug) is well suited for ambulatory

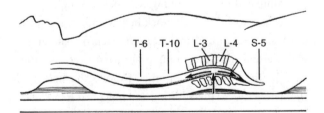

Figure 12-1. Distribution of hyperbaric local anesthetic solution in the intrathecal space after injection at L3–4 (at the apex of the lumbar lordosis) in a patient turned immediately supine. Note higher concentrations in midthoracic and sacral regions as the local anesthetic solution runs "down hill." Reproduced with permission from Neuraxial Blocks by Stevens RA, in *Regional Anesthesia and Analgesia*, edited by Brown DL; WB Saunders; 1996.

anesthesia for cosmetic surgery as it has a rapid onset and short duration of action.[44,46,48] Hydrophilic opioids, such as morphine (0.1–0.3 mg), have a longer duration of effect and more extensive rostral spread within the neuraxis. As a result, intrathecal morphine can provide prolonged postoperative analgesia to inpatients.

The risk of delayed respiratory depression contraindicates the use of intrathecal morphine for outpatients.

The alpha₂ agonist clonidine increases the quality and duration of sensory and motor block when administered intrathecally.[34] Side effects such as hypotension, bradycardia, and sedation are common with intrathecal doses between 75 and 225 ug, and this may limit the use of this agent in outpatients.[49] A number of investigators have studied a lower dose of intrathecal clonidine (15 ug) and have shown enhanced block quality with limited systemic side effects.[34,50]

Vasoconstrictors such as epinephrine (0.2–0.3 mg) and phenylephrine (2–5 mg) can increase the density and duration of lidocaine spinal block.[51,56] Prolonged motor block and urinary retention may limit more widespread use of these agents. In addition, phenylephrine has been associated with the development of transient neurologic symptoms.[54,56]

Adverse effects

If spinal anesthesia is planned for outpatient cosmetic surgery, appropriate patient selection based on a thorough preoperative assessment and meticulous technique can significantly minimize the risk. Nevertheless, potential risks do exist (see Table 12-9). Patients must be informed about these risks and should be provided with appropriate contact information in the event that problems arise.

Back pain is estimated to occur in **11%** of surgical patients twenty-four to thirty-six hours after spinal anesthesia.[57] (Any additional discomfort, beyond the surgical, in the cosmetic surgical patient may be cause for complaint. Therefore, the possibility of back pain must be disclosed to adjust the patient's expectations as well as to obtain an informed consent.) Back pain may result from needle trauma, from intrinsic effects of the local anesthetic, or from ligamentous strain. Urinary retention is related to inhibition of detrusor muscle activity from S3 nerve root block. Risk factors include male gender, age greater than sixty years, surgery duration greater than 120 minutes, and systemic analgesia.[58,59]

Transient neurologic symptoms involve pain or dyses-
thesia in the legs or buttocks that occurs within twenty-
four hours of spinal anesthesia.[60,61] Risk factors include
the use of lidocaine, possibly mepivacaine, ambulatory
surgery, and the lithotomy position. Treatment is symptomatic and spontaneous recovery typically occurs within
days.

A postdural puncture headache (PDPH) is a fronto-
occipital headache that occurs in a sitting or standing
position and is immediately improved upon assuming a
supine position.[62] The incidence is greater with cutting
and large bore spinal needles, a transversely directed needle bevel, young age, and female sex.[63,64] Treatment is initially conservative with fluid hydration, analgesics, and
possibly caffeine.[65] An epidural blood patch can be considered, although spontaneous resolution generally occurs
in one to two weeks.

Serious neurologic injury related to spinal anesthesia
is extremely rare.[66,69] Nonetheless, any new neurologic
deficit should be promptly assessed in the event that a
potentially reversible etiology exists. An epidural abscess
presents with progressive sensory or motor deficits, bowel
or bladder dysfunction, fever, or back pain.[70,72] A neuraxial hematoma may present similarly.[70] Magnetic resonance imaging can establish the diagnosis of either condition. Following diagnosis, immediate surgical evacuation
of the abscess or hematoma may be required. Subsequently,
abscesses are also managed with antiobiotics.[73] Menin-
gitis is suspected if the patient presents with headache,
fever, nuchal rigidity, or a new neurological deficit.[73,75]
Cerebrospinal fluid analysis can yield the diagnosis, and
systemic antibiotic therapy is begun early. Cauda equina
syndrome presents with pain in the lower back or legs,
lower extremity sensorimotor deficit, and bowel or bladder dysfunction.[70,75] Risk factors include the use of 5%
hyperbaric lidocaine and continuous spinal anesthesia
with microcatheters. Emergent investigation and treatment are necessary. The diagnosis and management of
other neurologic complications (i.e., isolated nerve injury)
can be greatly facilitated with the assistance of a consultant
neurologist.

Total spinal anesthesia results from excessive cephalad spread of the spinal block. Apnea, bradycardia,
profound hypotension, and cardiac arrest can result.[76]
Prompt recognition and initiation of supportive therapy
is crucial.

Table 12-10. Selected potential adverse effects
of epidural anesthesia[1,64,73,77,82,105,106]

Self-limiting	Back pain
	Urinary retention
	Postdural puncture headache
Rare but serious	Local anesthetic toxicity
	Total spinal anesthesia
	Cardiac arrest
	Isolated nerve injury
	Cauda equina syndrome
	Epidural abscess
	Meningitis
	Epidural hematoma
	Retained catheter

EPIDURAL ANESTHESIA

Indications and advantages

Epidural anesthesia achieves bilateral surgical anesthesia
with similar advantages to spinal anesthesia (Table 12-10).
In addition, epidurals provide the option for extended
postoperative analgesia for patients admitted to hospital.
Thoracic epidurals have applications for cosmetic procedures involving the breast and thorax, whereas thoracolumbar epidurals are more suited to abdominal, lower
extremity, and buttock surgery.

Equipment

In order to facilitate catheter placement, epidural needles
have a curved distal tip (i.e., Tuohy or Hustead) and a larger
diameter (i.e., 16–18 ga) than spinal needles. Multiorificed,
polyamide epidural catheters have a closed end and three
orifices at the distal tip. This design enhances even distribution of local anesthetic. The loss-of-resistance syringe
is a 3 or 5 ml size and is made of glass or plastic.

Local anesthetics and adjuvants

The selection of local anesthetic for epidural anesthesia is
based on the desired block onset and duration as well as
the drug's side-effect profile. The mass of the local anesthetic administered also affects onset time and duration
as well as depth of anesthesia and the extent of cranio-
caudal spread.[77,79] In addition, the volume of injectate
affects the extent of the block.[79] Other factors such as pregnancy and age may also be important.[80,82] When dosed
with concentrated local anesthetic, the epidural catheter

provides surgical anesthesia. Chloroprocaine has a fast onset and short duration of action.[83,85] A number of studies have investigated the use of epidural chloroprocaine for ambulatory surgical procedures and have found onset of maximal block in 16 minutes, a time to ambulation of 78 minutes, and *outpatient discharge as soon as 130 minutes after completion of surgery.*[83,85] This agent has historically been associated with back pain following epidural administration of large and repeated doses.[86,87] In addition, there are reports of persistent neurologic deficits and adhesive arachnoiditis following accidental intrathecal administration.[88] Preservatives and antioxidants in older preparations were likely causal. Recent data supporting the safe intrathecal use of preservative-free chloroprocaine may lead to more frequent epidural use of this agent.

Lidocaine and mepivacaine both have a rapid onset and short to intermediate duration of action.[89] Bupivacaine, levobupivacaine, and ropivacaine have a long onset and duration. These agents would not be suitable for ambulatory procedures; however, they are effective in providing extended postoperative analgesia for patients admitted to hospital. When a bolus dose of concentrated long-acting local anesthetic is administered epidurally, ropivacaine is selected preferentially in order to minimize the risk of cardiovascular toxicity associated with bupivacaine.[90] In addition, ropivacaine provides a greater separation of sensory and motor block.

Adjuvant medications can be used to enhance epidural anesthesia. Epidural opioids can improve block quality, though they may be associated with postoperative nausea and vomiting, pruritus, or urinary retention. Short-acting agents such as fentanyl are preferentially chosen for ambulatory patients. Long-acting epidural morphine is reserved for inpatients because of the risk of delayed respiratory depression. Clonidine (100–200 ug epidurally) enhances the duration of epidural anesthesia.[91] However, side effects such as hypotension, bradycardia, and sedation may impede safe outpatient recovery and discharge.[92] Vasoconstrictors such as epinephrine (2.5–5 ug · ml^{-1}) can enhance the quality of the block, prolong the duration of short-acting local anesthetics, and decrease the risk of local anesthetic toxicity.[93] Bicarbonate (0.1 mEq · ml^{-1}) increases speed of onset of chloroprocaine, lidocaine, and mepivacaine.[94,96]

A continuous epidural can be used to provide postoperative analgesia.[97] The combination of low-dose opioid (i.e., fentanyl 5 ug · ml^{-1}) and dilute ropivacaine, levobupivacaine, or bupivacaine (i.e., 0.1–0.2%) is used to provide sensory anesthesia with minimal opioid- or local-anesthetic–related side effects. For example, this combination minimizes the motor block and hypotension that result from higher concentrations of local anesthetic and reduces the pruritus typically seen with larger doses of neuraxial opioids.

Adverse effects

Epidural anesthesia shares many of the potential side effects and complications described for spinal anesthesia (see Table 12-9).

Back pain occurs in up to **31%** at twenty-four to thirty-six hours after surgery and is more common than with spinal anesthesia (i.e., > 11%). Urinary retention can occur as discussed previously. PDPH can result from unintentional dural puncture with an epidural needle. Presentation and treatment have been previously outlined.

Epidural anesthesia is associated with the risk of systemic local anesthetic toxicity. This may result from systemic absorption of a large volume of local anesthetic administered epidurally or from inadvertent intravascular injection. Prompt recognition of the symptoms of local anesthetic toxicity is required in order to initiate timely treatment (see Table 12-11). Total spinal block and

---

Table 12-11. Signs and symptoms of local anesthetic toxicity

1. Disorientation, restlessness
2. Tremor
3. Metallic taste
4. Perioral paresthesias
5. Tinnitus
6. Auditory hallucinations
7. Muscle spasms
8. Tonic/clonic seizures
9. Coma
10. Respiratory arrest
11. Cardiac arrest, ventricular fibrillation
12. Death

Editor's note: Signs 1–6 may be seen only in patients receiving regional anesthesia with minimal or no additional sedation. In particular, seizure threshold will be elevated in patients receiving either benzodiazepine or propofol. A-V dissociation and hypotension may precede #11, cardiac arrest. —BLF

subsequent cardiac arrest can occur following acciden-tal intrathecal injection of a large volume of local anes-thetic intended for the epidural space. This was described in the context of spinal anesthesia along with isolated nerve injury, cauda equina syndrome, epidural abscess, menin-gitis, and epidural hematoma. Finally, catheter shearing with retention of catheter fragments in vivo has been reported.[98,99] To minimize this risk, avoid withdrawing the catheter through the epidural needle.

PERIPHERAL NERVE BLOCKS

Paravertebral Nerve Blocks
Anatomy
The thoracic paravertebral space is a wedge-shaped space present on either side of the vertebral column[100,101] (see Fig. 12-2). It is bound anterolaterally by the parietal pleura and medially by the posterolateral aspect of the vertebral body, the intervertebral disks, the interverte-bral foramina, and its contents. The superior costotrans-verse ligaments represent the posterior boundary of the space. These ligaments extend from the superior aspect

of each rib to the inferior aspect of the transverse process above.

The endothoracic fascia exists within the paraverte-bral space between the parietal pleura and the superior costotransverse ligament.[102] This deep thoracic fascia is attached anteriorly to the periosteum of the sternum and the perichondrium of the costal cartilages (see Fig. 12-3). Posteriorly, it fuses with the periosteum of the verte-bral bodies and is continuous with the prevertebral fascia (see Fig. 12-4). The endothoracic fascia divides the par-avertebral space into an anterior extrapleural paravertebral compartment and a posterior subendothoracic paraver-tebral compartment.[103] The anterior section contains the sympathetic trunk and loose connective tissue called the subserous fascia. The posterior segment contains the sympathetic rami communicantes, the spinal/intercostal nerves with their associated dorsal ramus, and the seg-mental spinal blood vessels. The spinal nerves are in fact groups of small nerve rootlets surrounded by fatty tissue. There is no encompassing fascial sheath, which enhances the nerve's susceptibility to local anesthetic blockade in this location.

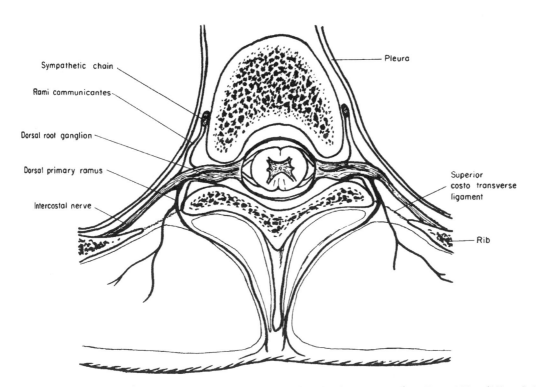

Figure 12-2. Transverse section at level of intervertebral foramen. Reproduced with permission from Eason MJ and Wyatt R, in *Anaes-thesia* 34:638,1979.[108]

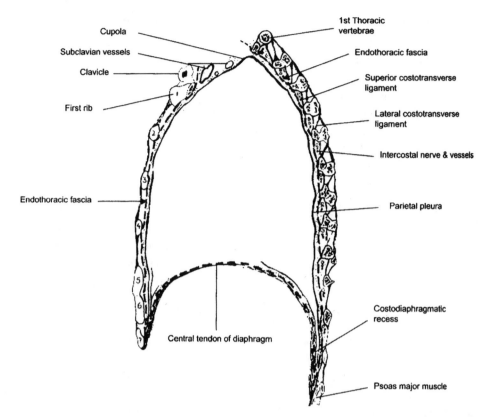

Figure 12-3. Paravertebral saggital section of the thorax portraying the extent of the endothoracic fascia. Reproduced with permission from Karmakar MK, in *Regional Anesthesia & Pain Medicine* 25(3):325–7;2000.[110]

Each thoracic paravertebral space communicates with adjacent spaces superiorly and inferiorly across the heads and necks of the ribs. This communication occurs predominantly in the anterior extrapleural compartment, whereas the posterior subendothoracic compartment is more segmental. The thoracic paravertebral space is continuous with the intercostal space laterally and the epidural space medially via the intervertebral foramen[101] (see Fig. 12-5). Communication with the contralateral paravertebral space can occur either through the epidural space or the prevertebral space.[102]

The thoracic paravertebral space is limited caudally by the origin of the psoas muscle. Nevertheless, the endothoracic fascia continues below the diaphragm as the fascia transversalis, and continuity between the thoracic and lumbar paravertebral spaces occurs via the medial and lateral arcuate ligaments.[103]

Indications and advantages
Paravertebral nerve block involves injection of local anesthetic close to the spinal nerves as they emerge from the intervertebral foramen and pass through the paravertebral space. Unilateral or bilateral segmental block can be performed. Long-acting local anesthetics provide intraoperative anesthesia and up to twenty-three hours of postoperative analgesia.[104] Thoracic paravertebral blocks are useful for cosmetic surgical procedures of the breast and/or chest wall (see Chapter 10). Thoracolumbar paravertebral nerve blocks are suitable for lower abdominal surgery such as abdominoplasty (Table 12-12).

Klein et al. studied the efficacy of thoracic paravertebral nerve blocks for breast augmentation or reconstruction. They randomized sixty patients to T1-7 paravertebral blocks with bupivacaine or general anesthesia. The group that received the nerve blocks had decreased opioid requirements in the postanesthesia care unit (0.8 ± 2.0 mg vs 3.6 ± 4.0 mg of morphine equivalent; p = 0.001), lower verbal analog pain scores for the first seventy-two hours postoperatively ($p < 0.05$), and reduced nausea scores at twenty-four hours (p = 0.04) compared to the general anesthesia group. Similar beneficial effects were noted in comparable studies involving breast surgery and

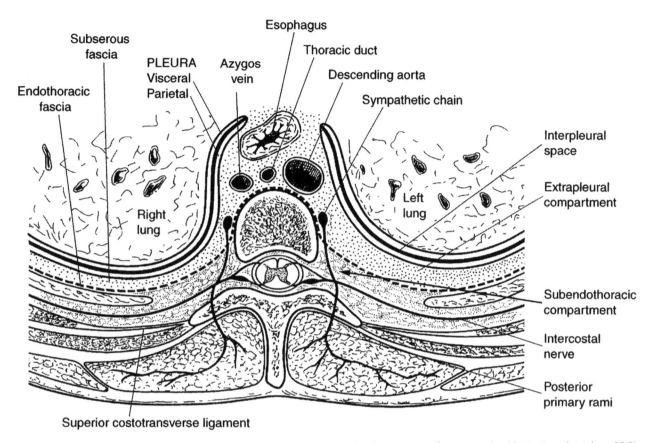

Figure 12-4. Anatomy of the thoracic paravertebral space. Reproduced with permission from Karmakar MK, in *Anesthesiology* 95(3): 771–80,2001.[109]

lower abdominal procedures.[105] Table 12-13 summarizes these advantages.

Technique

An intravenous is placed, monitors are attached, and resuscitation equipment is made available. Light sedation may be provided. The patient can be placed lateral decubitus or prone, though identification of landmarks is greatly facilitated in the sitting position.

The neck is flexed forward, the back is rounded, and the shoulders are maximally relaxed. Levels to be blocked are chosen based on the nature of the surgical procedure (Table 12-14). The superior aspect of the spinous process is identified and a mark is placed 2.5 cm lateral to it (Fig. 12-6). Because of the extreme angulation of the thoracic spinous processes, this mark overlies the transverse process of the vertebra below. For example, the T5 spinous process is at the same horizontal level as the T6 transverse process. The spinous processes project more

horizontally in the lumbar spine. As a result, the palpable lumbar spinous process is usually in line with the transverse processes of the same vertebra. The most prominent spinous process in the neck corresponds to C7, the lower border of the scapula is T7, and the intercristal line marks L4. The skin is cleaned with disinfectant and subcutaneous infiltration of local anesthetic is given at all needle entry sites.

A number of ways to identify the paravertebral space have been described. The paravertebral space can be located when a change in resistance (or "pop") is felt as a Tuohy needle passes through the costotransverse ligament[106] (Fig. 12-7). A 10 cm, 22 ga Tuohy needle is attached to extension tubing and a 20 ml syringe containing local anesthetic. The needle is inserted perpendicular to the skin 2.5 cm lateral to the midpoint of the superior border of the spinous process. The needle is advanced to contact the transverse process and the depth is noted. The transverse processes in the high thoracic spine (T1,2)

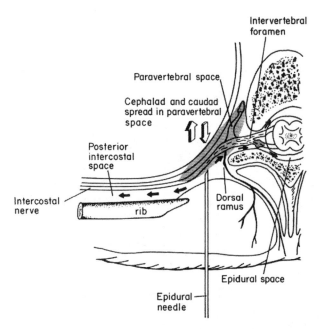

Figure 12-5. The paravertebral space is contiguous with the intercostal and epidural spaces. Thus, local anesthetic may spread laterally to the intercostal space, cephalad and caudad in the paravertebral space, and medially to the epidural space. Reproduced with permission from Continuous Thoracic Paravertebral Block by Chan VWS and Ferrante FM, in *Postoperative Pain Management*, edited by Ferrante FM and VadeBoncoeur TR; Churchhill-Livingstone; 1993.

Table 12-13. Potential advantages of paravertebral blocks[2,4,5]
Dense, long-lasting analgesia
Profound segmental sympathectomy
Reduced postoperative opioid requirements
Reduced PONV[a]
Low incidence of hemodynamic perturbations
Early postoperative ambulation
Low incidence of urinary retention
Decreased hospital length of stay

[a]PONV = postoperative nausea and vomitting

and the low lumbar spine (L4,5) are deeper than those in the midthoracic spine (T5–10); precise depth depends on patient size. The needle tip is withdrawn to the subcutaneous tissue and subsequently redirected caudal to the transverse process. Recall that in the thoracolumbar spine, nerve roots exit below their associated transverse process. The needle is advanced and a change in resistance is appreciated 1 cm past the depth of the transverse process as the superior costotransverse ligament is penetrated. A cautious approach is warranted because bone contacted deep to the transverse process may represent the rib. The needle should not be advanced deep to the rib because of the risk of pleural puncture and pneumothorax. In the lumbar area, the technique is slightly modified. After locating the transverse process, the needle is advanced only 0.5 cm deeper because the transverse processes are much thinner. In addition, no loss of resistance is appreciated because of the absence of the costotransverse ligament.

An alternate localization technique involves the use of loss of resistance to air or saline.[101] The loss of resistance upon entering the paravertebral space is more subtle and subjective compared to that observed upon entering the epidural space.[107]

Table 12-12. Paravertebral blocks for cosmetic surgery: application and suitability		
Surgical Procedure	Paravertebral Block Level	Supplemental Anesthesia
Breast (augmentation, reduction, mastopexy)	T2–6 ± T1, T7 Unilateral or bilateral according to surgical procedure	Superficial cervical plexus Medial and lateral pectoral nerve blocks for analgesia during pectoral dissection
Truncal liposuction	According to location of surgery	
Abdominoplasty	T9,10,11,12,L1 Bilateral	± T7,8 depending on cephalad extent of undermining
Truncal scar revision	According to location of surgery	

Table 12-14. Selected potential adverse effects of paravertebral blocks and their incidence[4,114]

	Adverse Effect
Self-limiting	Failed block
	Vascular puncture
	Injection-site hematoma
	Pain at injection site
	Epidural spread
	Postdural puncture headache
	Brachial plexus block
	Horner's syndrome
Rare but serious	Pneumothorax
	Pulmonary hemorrhage
	Local anesthetic toxicity
	Nerve injury
	Intrathecal injection, total spinal anesthesia
	Septic complications

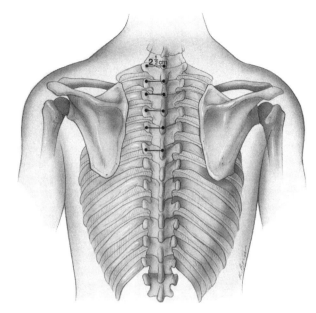

Figure 12-6. Superficial skin markings for left breast surgery. Reproduced with permission from Greengrass R and Steele S, in *Techniques in Regional Anesthesia & Pain Management* 2(1): 8–12, January 1998.

Others have used nerve stimulation to identify the spinal nerve roots in the paravertebral space. A 21 or 22 ga short-bevel insulated stimulating needle is advanced to contact transverse process. The needle is subsequently redirected while connected to a nerve stimulator providing a current output greater than 1.5 mA. Paraspinal muscle contraction occurs initially as the needle passes through these muscles. On further needle advancement, intercostal or abdominal muscle contractions are observed depending on the dermatomal level of the block. The stimulating current is decreased to 0.5–0.6 mA while appropriate muscle contraction is maintained. Isolated posterior spinal muscle contraction is not accepted as this may represent either direct muscle stimulation or stimulation of the posterior ramus of the spinal nerve root after it diverges from the spinal nerve. An additional option involves pressure measurement to confirm paravertebral needle placement.[108] When the needle tip is in the erector spinae muscle, measured pressure is higher during inspiration than expiration. Within the paravertebral space, there is a sudden lowering of pressures and a pressure inversion occurs. Expiratory becomes higher than inspiratory pressure.

A further method to identify the paravertebral space involves the injection of contrast material. Contrast may distribute linearly as it spreads superiorly and inferiorly; this is presumed to occur within the anterior compartment. Alternatively, there may be cloud-like dispersal of

contrast dye within one or two spinal segments; this is thought to occur when the needle is in the posterior compartment.[109]

Some advocate a technique whereby after contact with the transverse process, the needle is redirected superior to it[108,109] (Fig. 12-7). Using this approach, it is possible to inadvertently contact rib first and walk off superiorly into the pleura and lung. In addition, this technique blocks the nerve root and dermatomal segment above the transverse process contacted. The authors prefer redirecting the needle caudad to the transverse process.[110] If rib is contacted first, caudal redirection will bring the needle into contact with the transverse process at a shallower depth. Consequently, more accurate estimation of the depth of the paravertebral space is made and the risk of pneumothorax is minimized.

When the needle is properly sited, an assistant aspirates the syringe for blood, cerebrospinal fluid, and air. If air is detected, it is likely that penetration of the pleura and lung has occurred. The needle should be removed and patient stability ensured. Similar steps are taken if blood or cerebrospinal fluid is detected. When the paravertebral space is correctly identified, there is no resistance to injection of local anesthetic. Smaller volumes of local anesthetic (3–5 ml per level) are used for thoracic paravertebral

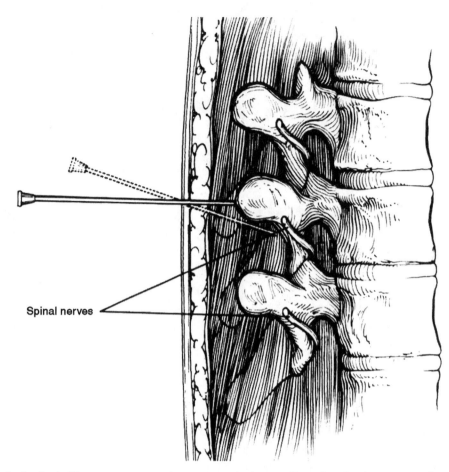

Spinal nerves

Figure 12-7. Needle "walked off" transverse process into paravertebral space. Reproduced with permission from Greengrass R and Steele S, in *Techniques in Regional Anesthesia & Pain Management* 2(1),8–12, January 1998.

blocks, whereas larger volumes (5–7 ml per level) are used in the lumbar area. Doses may need to be reduced when multiple and/or bilateral levels are blocked. Patients will often experience a pressure paresthesia upon injection of local anesthetic. Block adequacy is evaluated in a number of ways. Sensory anesthesia and motor block are sought in the appropriate dermatomes. For example, successful upper thoracic paravertebral block is associated with loss of sensation over the breast and upper chest wall. In addition, motor block of the intercostal muscles occurs and can be confirmed by inspection and palpation of limited hemithorax expansion. Vasodilation and warmth in the corresponding distribution provides evidence of a successful sympathetic block.

Using the majority of the techniques described, it is difficult to determine whether the needle tip exists in the anterior extrapleural paravertebral compartment or the posterior subendothoracic paravertebral compartment of the thoracic paravertebral space. As discussed previously, the pattern of spread of contrast dye may help with this differentiation. Adequate block will result following multilevel injection into either compartment; however, more extensive craniocaudad spread occurs when the needle is in the anterior compartment (mean 4.5 dermatomal levels) compared to when it exists in the posterior compartment (mean 2.3 dermatomal levels).[111] These results reflect more complete cephalocaudad continuity between anterior segments. Consequently, it is here that a single-level injection of a larger volume of local anesthetic or placement of a continuous catheter should occur.

Continuous paravertebral block can provide extended postoperative analgesia. This technique can be used both in patients admitted to hospital as well as outpatients.[110]

A large-bore Tuohy needle is first used to identify the paravertebral space. Subsequently, a flexible catheter with a single distal orifice is threaded 1–2 cm into the space.

Equipment

The equipment required depends on the technique used to identify the paravertebral space. As described previously, commonly used equipment consists of a 10 cm 22 ga Tuohy needle with wings and centimeter gradations. This is attached to extension tubing and a 20 ml syringe containing local anesthetic. If loss of resistance is utilized, a loss of resistance syringe is also needed. When a nerve-stimulation technique is used, a 10 cm 21–22 ga insulated short-bevel needle and a nerve stimulator are required. And when pressure measurement is undertaken, a three-way stopcock, pressure tubing, and a pressure transducer are employed. A sterile skin marker and ruler should also be included.

Local anesthetics and adjuvants

The local anesthetic agent selected is based on the desired onset and duration of the nerve block. Block onset occurs within ten minutes and surgical anesthesia within forty minutes following injection of short-acting local anesthetic.[112] Analgesia lasts up to twenty-three hours when long-acting local anesthetic is used.[106] Epinephrine is frequently added to enhance block quality and limit systemic toxicity. The proximity of the paravertebral space to the intercostal space raises concern about significant systemic absorption of local anesthetic following paravertebral block. However, plasma local anesthetic levels have been below toxic range when standard doses are used.[113] In addition, systemic absorption is similar when a single-level injection of 20 ml is given at T3-4 compared to when injections of 4 ml each are given over five levels between T2 and T6 (total 20 ml).[113]

Adverse effects

The adverse effects of paravertebral blocks are summarized in Table 12-15. Vascular puncture, injection site hematoma, and pain at the site of needle puncture are usually mild, self-limiting, and respond to symptomatic treatment. Epidural spread may be due to excessively medial needle placement. A more extensive block than expected may result and hypotension may occur.[114] Brachial plexus block or Horner's syndrome may result

Table 12-15. Comparison between paravertebral and intercostal nerve blocks

Paravertebral nerve blocks	Intercostal nerve blocks
Segmental sensory and motor block	Segmental sensory and motor block
Posterior ramus blocked	Posterior ramus not reliably blocked
Sympathetic block	Sympathetic chain not reliably blocked
Some LA spread to adjacent levels	Minimal LA spread to adjacent levels
Continuous catheter can provide multilevel analgesia	Continuous catheter usually provides only single-level analgesia
Risk of pneumothorax	Risk of pneumothorax
Risk of vascular puncture	Risk of vascular puncture
Risk of epidural spread, dural puncture	Lower risk of epidural spread, dural puncture
Less systemic LA absorption	Significant LA systemic absorption

from cephalad extension of injected local anesthetic. The features of Horner's syndrome include ptosis, miosis, and anhydrosis and result from block of the sympathetic stellate ganglion.

Pleural puncture following paravertebral block is rare. Pneumothorax results infrequently and is suspected if a pleural "pop" is felt during needle advancement, if air is aspirated into the syringe attached to the block needle, or if the patient develops an irritating cough or a sharp pain in chest or shoulder. Resulting pneumothoraces are often small enough to warrant conservative management.[100] However, when a chest tube is indicated and hospital admission is required, this significantly impacts the patient's postoperative recovery. A case report describes pulmonary hemorrhage as a complication following paravertebral block in a patient who had previous thoracic surgery.[115] In addition, this patient population may have pleural scarring affecting paravertebral anatomy, and this can increase the risk of pneumothorax. Local anesthetic toxicity (Table 12-11) can result from the use of large volumes of local anesthetic or from accidental intravascular injection. Precalculation of the maximum allowable dose of local anesthetic and meticulous aspiration technique to detect intravascular needle location should minimize this risk. Nerve injury is rare, though a case report describes a patient who developed chronic segmental thoracic pain following paravertebral nerve block. Intrathecal injection, dural puncture, and postdural puncture headache may result from overly medial needle placement or from penetration of a dural cuff that extends into the paravertebral space.[116] Significant resuscitation may be required depending on the dose of local anesthetic injected intrathecally and the resulting symptoms.

Intercostal Nerve Blocks
Anatomy
The intercostal space is continuous with the lateral aspect of the paravertebral space. Upon exiting the paravertebral space, the spinal nerve becomes the intercostal nerve. Medial to the angle of the rib, the intercostal nerve is found between the pleura and the fascia of the internal intercostal muscle. The angle of the rib is located 6 to 8 cm from midline. At this point, the intercostal nerve continues its course between the internal and the innermost intercostal muscles. The nerve lies in close proximity to the segmental intercostal vessels, but its relation to the subcostal groove is variable.[117] Each intercostal nerve has four branches (Fig. 12-8). The gray ramus communicans passes anteriorly to the sympathetic ganglion, and the posterior ramus passes posteriorly to supply the skin and muscle in the paravertebral area. These branches are more reliably anesthetized with paravertebral than intercostal nerve blocks. The intercostal nerve also gives rise to lateral and anterior cutaneous branches.

Indications and advantages
An intercostal nerve block is indicated for analgesia following breast or chest-wall procedures and is predominantly used when paravertebral or epidural blocks are not indicated. The differences between paravertebral and intercostal blocks are outlined in Table 12-15.

Technique
An intravenous is placed, monitors are attached, and resuscitation equipment is made available. Light sedation may be provided. The patient is typically placed prone, although the lateral decubitus, sitting, or supine positions can also be used. In the prone position, a pillow is placed under the upper abdomen to promote thoracic spine flexion and to widen the intercostal spaces. The patient's arms hang over the edge of the bed to displace the scapulae laterally (see Fig. 12-8).

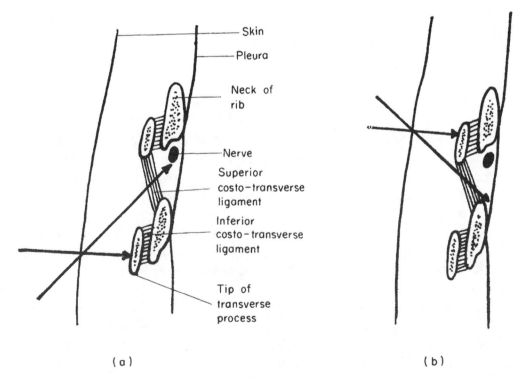

(a)   (b)

Figure 12-8. Longitudinal section to show direction of needle: (a) above, (b) below: transverse process or rib. Reproduced with permission from Eason MJ and Wyatt R, in *Anaesthesia* 34(7):638–42,1979.[108]

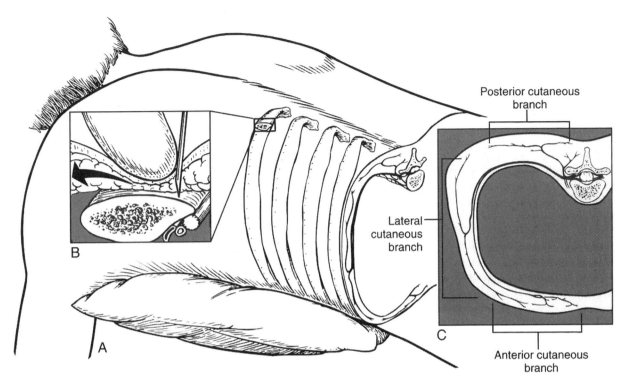

Figure 12-9. (A) Intercostal nerve block: patient positioning. (B) The index finger displaces the skin up over the rib. The needle is inserted at the tip of the finger and rests on the rib. The needle is walked off the lower rib edge and inserted 3 to 5 mm. (C) An intercostal nerve and its branches. Reproduced with permission from Nerve Blocks by Wedel DJ, in *Anesthesia*, 5th edition, edited by Miller RD; Churchhill-Livingstone; 2000.

A paraspinal line is drawn 5 to 9 cm lateral to the midline where the posterior angulation of the ribs is most easily palpable. In order to avoid the scapula, the line diverges medially in the upper thoracic segments. This location is chosen for the nerve block as it is proximal to the divergence of the lateral cutaneous branch. The inferior border of each rib is marked along the length of the paraspinal line. The appropriate levels to be blocked are identified according to the surgical procedure. The skin is cleaned with disinfectant and sterile drapes are placed. The anesthesiologist stands to the patient's side. A subcutaneous skin wheal is placed at the mark representing the inferior border of the angle of the rib at each level to be blocked. The left hand is used to move the skin wheal so that it overlies the rib. The right hand holds a 3–4 cm 22 ga short bevel needle attached to a 10 ml syringe and advances it onto the rib (Fig. 12-9). The left hand grasps the needle while the right hand holds the syringe. The needle is subsequently walked in a caudal direction past the inferior border of the rib and advanced 3–5 mm past the depth at which the rib was contacted. A subtle change in resistance if often felt as the needle passes through the internal intercostal muscle.

After negative aspiration for blood, 3–5 ml of local anesthetic is injected and the nerve block is repeated at each of the desired levels. The most caudal rib to be anesthetized is blocked first. Subsequent nerve blocks gradually proceed in a cephalad direction.

Equipment

A 3–4 cm 22 ga short bevel needle and a 10 ml syringe are required.

Local anesthetics and adjuvants

There may be significant systemic absorption of local anesthetic following intercostal nerve block. Therefore, the dose of local anesthetic used should be carefully calculated. Ropivacaine offers long-acting anesthesia with an acceptable safely profile. Epinephrine can be added to further reduce the risk of toxicity.

Adverse effects

Pneumothorax is rare (0.42%), despite the close proximity of the lung and pleura.[118] The risk of local anesthetic toxicity is related to the large volumes of local anesthetic used to obtain an adequate block and to the significant systemic absorption that occurs in this highly vascular area.

RECOVERY AND DISCHARGE

Recovery

Patients require a period of monitoring postoperatively because both surgery and anesthesia can be associated with significant physiologic changes. Standard monitors such as pulse oximeter, noninvasive blood pressure, and electrocardiogram are used. In addition, the vigilance of a nurse with resuscitation skills is of critical importance. A physician with advanced cardiac life-support skills should be immediately available.

A plan is required for analgesia as block resolution occurs. This transition is managed in the postanesthesia care unit following spinal or epidural anesthesia. For both groups, multimodal analgesia is ideal. This involves the used of regular, scheduled doses of acetaminophen and nonsteroidal anti-inflammatory medication in addition to oral opioid tablets.

Discharge

Many cosmetic surgical procedures are performed on an ambulatory basis. Traditional outpatient discharge criteria include adequate analgesia; absence of side effects such as nausea, vomiting, and sedation; as well as the ability to ambulate, void, and tolerate fluid intake.

Recent literature has challenged the requirements to drink and void prior to discharge.[119,120] In a randomized trial, Jin et al. documented the feasibility of discharging patients prior to fluid intake.[119] They found no difference in the incidence of postoperative nausea and vomiting when they compared a group of patients who drank prior to discharge versus a group who did not drink. Patients with a history of urinary retention, men, those who have had spinal anesthesia, and those who have had anal, urogenital, and hernia surgery are known to be at high risk of postoperative urinary retention. Mulroy and colleagues have shown the viability of discharging ambulatory patients who have received short-acting spinal or epidural anesthesia without requiring them to void.[120] In their study, they used bladder ultrasound to estimate the volume of urine prior to determining suitability of

discharge. Forty-six patients had less than 400 ml urine and were discharged home without voiding. They were instructed to return to hospital if they had not voided within eight hours; however, all were able to void spontaneously. Twenty-three patients had urine volume greater than 400 ml. Most (97.7%) voided spontaneously during the subsequent sixty minutes in which they were detained in hospital; however, three patients required catheterization. The quantification of urine volume with bladder ultrasound and a defined protocol certainly led to their success and excellent results. The use of this protocol in cosmetic surgical patients who have received regional anesthesia remains unexplored.

Finally, all patients should receive appropriate contact numbers should complications arise following discharge, and contingency plans should be in place for those patients who do not meet discharge criteria and who require admission to an inpatient facility.

SUMMARY

Regional anesthesia has broad application for cosmetic surgical procedures. Neuraxial techniques provide rapid-onset, dense anesthesia with minimal postoperative sedation, nausea, and vomiting. Spinal anesthesia, in particular, has been tailored for day-case procedures by the use of low doses of local anesthetics, short-acting agents, dose-sparing adjuvants such as opioids, and small-gauge, pencil-point needles. As a result, side effects have been minimized and there is timely recovery of motor strength as well as ability to ambulate and to void.

Paravertebral nerve blocks uniquely offer dense intraoperative anesthesia and prolonged postoperative analgesia with rare side effects. This technique is surprisingly underutilized given its benefits. With appropriately selected patients, surgical procedures, and nerve block techniques, regional anesthesia can facilitate successful cosmetic surgery and result in positive patient outcome with high patient satisfaction.

REFERENCES

1. Auroy Y, Benhamou D, Bargues L, et al.: Major complications of regional anesthesia in France: The SOS Regional Anesthesia Hotline Service. *Anesthesiol* 97:1274,2002.
2. Naja MZ, Ziade MF, Lonnqvist PA: Nerve-stimulator guided paravertebral blockade vs. general anaesthesia for

breast surgery: A prospective randomized trial. *Eur J Anaesthesiol* 20:897,2003.

3. Borgeat A, Ekatodramis G, Schenker CA: Postoperative nausea and vomiting in regional anesthesia: A review. *Anesthesiol* 98:530,2003.

4. Pusch F, Freitag H, Weinstabl C, et al.: Single injection paravertebral block compared to general anaesthesia in breast surgery. *Acta Anaesthesiol Scand* 43:770,1999.

5. Klein SM, Bergh A, Steele SM, et al.: Thoracic paravertebral block for breast surgery. *Anesth Analg* 90:1402,2000.

6. Gebhard RE, Al-Samsam T, Greger J, et al.: Distal nerve blocks at the wrist for outpatient carpal tunnel surgery offer intraoperative cardiovascular stability and reduce discharge time. *Anesth Analg* 95:351,2002.

7. Song D, Greilich NB, White PF, et al.: Recovery profiles and costs of anesthesia for outpatient unilateral inguinal herniorrhaphy. *Anesth Analg* 91:876,2000.

8. Williams BA, Kentor ML, Vogt MT, et al.: Femoral-sciatic nerve blocks for complex outpatient knee surgery are associated with less postoperative pain before same-day discharge: A review of 1,200 consecutive cases from the period 1996–1999. *Anesthesiol* 98:1206,2003.

9. Horlocker TT, Wedel DJ, Benzon HP, et al.: Regional anesthesia in the anticoagulated patient: Defining the risks (the second ASRA consensus conference on neuraxial anesthesia and anticoagulation). *Reg Anesth Pain Med* 28:172, 2003.

10. Klein SM, D'Ercole F, Greengrass RA, et al.: Enoxaparin associated with psoas hematoma and lumbar plexopathy after lumbar plexus block. *Anesthesiol* 87:1576,1997.

11. Deng XM, Xiao WJ, Luo MP, et al.: The use of midazolam and small-dose ketamine for sedation and analgesia during local anesthesia. *Anesth Analg* 93:1174,2001.

12. Koch ME, Kain ZN, Ayoub C, et al.: The sedative and analgesia sparing effect of music. *Anesthesiol* 89;300,1998.

13. Milne SE, Kenny GN: Future applications for TCI systems. *Anaesthesia* 53(S1):56,1998.

14. Apfel CC, Korttila K, Abdalla M, et al.: A factorial trial of six interventions for the prevention of postoperative nausea and vomiting. *N Engl J Med* 350:2441,2004.

15. Servin FS, Raeder JC, Merle JC, et al.: Remifentanil sedation compared with propofol during regional anaesthesia. *Acta Anaesthesiol Scand* 46:309,2002.

16. Arain SR, Ebert TJ: The efficacy, side effects, and recovery characteristics of dexmedotomidine versus propofol when used for intraoperative sedation. *Anesth Analg* 95:461, 2002.

17. Halpern S, Preston R: Postdural puncture headache and spinal needle design. Meta-analyses. *Anesthesiol* 81:1376, 1994.

18. Pawlowski J, Sukhani R, Pappas AL, et al.: The anesthetic and recovery profile of two doses (60 and 80 mg) of plain mepivacaine for ambulatory spinal anesthesia. *Anesth Analg* 91:580,2000.

19. Zayas VM, Liguori GA, Chisholm MF, et al.: Dose response relationships for isobaric spinal mepivacaine using the combined spinal epidural technique. *Anesth Analg* 89:1167, 1999.

20. Zaric D, Christiansen C, Pace NL, et al.: Transient neurologic symptoms (TNS) following spinal anaesthesia with lidocaine versus other local anaesthetics. *Cochrane Database Syst Rev* 2:CD003006,2003.

21. Pollock JE: Transient neurologic symptoms: Etiology, risk factors, and management. *Reg Anesth Pain Med* 27:581,2002.

22. Salazar F, Bogdanovich A, Adalia R, et al.: Transient neurologic symptoms after spinal anaesthesia using isobaric 2% mepivacaine and isobaric 2% lidocaine. *Acta Anaesthesiol Scand* 45:240,2001.

23. Johnson ME: Potential neurotoxicity of spinal anesthesia with lidocaine. *Mayo Clin Proc* 75:921,2000.

24. Freedman JM, Li DK, Drasner K, et al.: Transient neurologic symptoms after spinal anesthesia: An epidemiologic study of 1,863 patients. *Anesthesiol* 89:633,1998.

25. Liguori GA, Zayas VM, Chisholm MF: Transient neurologic symptoms after spinal anesthesia with mepivacaine and lidocaine. *Anesthesiol* 88:619,1998.

26. Hampl KF, Schneider MC, Ummenhofer W, et al.: Transient neurologic symptoms after spinal anesthesia. *Anesth Analg* 81:1148,1995.

26. Liguori GA, Zayas VM: Repeated episodes of transient radiating back and leg pain following spinal anesthesia with 1.5% mepivacaine and 2% lidocaine. *Reg Anesth Pain Med* 23:511,1998.

27. Le Truong HH, Girard M, Drolet P, et al.: Spinal anesthesia: a comparison of procaine and lidocaine. *Can J Anaesth* 48:470,2001.

28. Kouri ME, Kopacz DJ: Spinal 2-chloroprocaine: A comparison with lidocaine in volunteers. *Anesth Analg* 98:75,2004.

29. Smith KN, Kopacz DJ, McDonald SB: Spinal 2-chloroprocaine: A dose-ranging study and the effect of added epinephrine. *Anesth Anal* 98:81,2004.

30. Vath JS, Kopacz DJ: Spinal 2-chloroprocaine: The effect of added fentanyl. *Anesth Analg* 98:89,2004.

31. Warren DT, Kopacz DJ: Spinal 2-chloroprocaine: The effect of added dextrose. *Anesth Analg* 98:95,2004.

32. Yoos JR, Kopacz DJ: Spinal 2-chloroprocaine for surgery: An initial 10-month experience. *Anesth Analg* 100:553,2005.

33. Davis BR, Kopacz DJ: Spinal 2-chloroprocaine: The effect of added clonidine. *Anesth Analg* 100:559,2005.

34. Yoos JR, Kopacz DJ: Spinal 2-chloroprocaine: a comparison with small-dose bupivacaine in volunteers. *Anesth Analg* 100:566,2005.

35. Gonter AF, Kopacz DJ: Spinal 2-chloroprocaine: A comparison with procaine in volunteers. *Anesth Analg* 100:573, 2005.

36. Glaser C, Marhofer P, Zimpfer G, et al.: Levobupivacaine versus racemic bupivacaine for spinal anesthesia. *Anesth Analg* 94(1):194,2002.

37. Liu SS, Ware PD, Allen HW, et al.: Dose-response characteristics of spinal bupivacaine in volunteers. Clinical implications for ambulatory anesthesia. *Anesthesiol* 85:729,1996.

38. Wille M: Intrathecal use of ropivacaine: A review. *Acta Anaesthesiol Belg* 55:251,2004.

39. Wahedi W, Nolte H, Klein P: Ropivacaine for spinal anesthesia. A dose-finding study. *Anaesthesist* 45:737,1996.

40. Kallio H, Snall EV, Kero MP, et al.: A comparison of intrathecal plain solutions containing ropivacaine 20 or 15 mg versus bupivacaine 10 mg. *Anesth Analg* 99:713,2004.

41. McNamee DA, McClelland AM, Scott S, et al.: Spinal anaesthesia: Comparison of plain ropivacaine 5 mg · ml⁻¹ with bupivacaine 5 mg · ml⁻¹ for major orthopaedic surgery. *Br J Anaesth* 89:702,2002.

42. Gautier PE, De Kock M, Van Steenberge A, et al.: Intrathecal ropivacaine for ambulatory surgery. A comparison between intrathecal bupivacaine and intrathecal ropivacaine for knee arthroscopy. *Anesthesiol* 91:1239,1999.

43. Cousins MJ, Mather LE: Intrathecal and epidural administration of opioids. *Anesthesiol* 61:276,1984.

44. Ben-David B, Solomon E, Levin H, et al.: Intrathecal fentanyl with small-dose dilute bupivacaine: Better anesthesia without prolonging recovery. *Anesth Analg* 85:560, 1997.

45. Ballantyne JC, Loach AB, Carr DB: Itching after epidural and spinal opiates. *Pain* 33:149,1988.

46. Goel S, Bhardwaj N, Grover VK: Intrathecal fentanyl added to intrathecal bupivacaine for day case surgery: A randomized study. *Eur J Anaesthesiol* 20:294,2003.

47. Gupta A, Axelsson K, Thorn SE, et al.: Low-dose bupivacaine plus fentanyl for spinal anesthesia during ambulatory inguinal herniorrhaphy: A comparison between 6 mg and 50.5 mg of bupivacaine. *Acta Anaesthesiol Scand* 47:13, 2003.

48. Liu S, Chiu AA, Carpenter RL, et al.: Fentanyl prolongs lidocaine spinal anesthesia without prolonging recovery. *Anesth Analg* 80:730,1995.

49. Eisenach JC, De Kock M, Klimscha W: Alpha2 adrenergic agonists for regional anesthesia. A clinical review of clonidine (1984–1995). *Anesthesiol* 85:655,1996.

50. De Kock M, Gautier P, Fanard L, et al.: Intrathecal ropivacaine and clonidine for ambulatory knee arthroscopy: A dose-response study. *Anesthesiol* 94:574,2001.

51. Kito K, Kato H, Shibata M, et al.: The effect of varied doses of epinephrine on duration of lidocaine spinal anesthesia in the thoracic and lumbosacral dermatomes. *Anesth Analg* 86:1018,1998.

52. Moore JM, Liu SS, Pollock JE, et al.: The effect of epinephrine on small-dose hyperbaric bupivacaine spinal anesthesia: Clinical implications for ambulatory surgery. *Anesth Analg* 86:973,1998.

53. Chiu AA, Liu S, Carpenter RL, et al.: The effects of epinephrine on lidocaine spinal anesthesia: A cross-over study. *Anesth Analg* 80:735,1995.

54. Sakura S, Sumi M, Sakaguchi Y, et al.: The addition of phenylephrine contributes to the development of transient neurologic symptoms after spinal anesthesia with 0.5% tetracaine. *Anesthesiol* 87:771,1997.

55. Vaida GT, Moss P, Capan LM, et al.: Prolongation of lidocaine spinal anesthesia with phenylephrine. *Anesth Analg* 65:781,1986.

56. Leicht CH, Carlson SA: Prolongation of lidocaine spinal anesthesia with epinephrine and phenylephrine. *Anesth Analg* 65:365,1986.

57. Seeberger MD, Lang ML, Drewe J, et al.: Comparison of spinal and epidural anesthesia for patients younger than 50 years of age. *Anesth Analg* 78:667,1994.

58. Petros JG, Rimm EB, Robillard RJ: Factors influencing urinary tract retention after elective open cholecystectomy. *Surg Gyn Obstet* 174:497,1992.

59. Lamonerie L, Marret E, Deleuze A, Lembert N, Dupont M, Bonnet F. Prevalence of postoperative bladder distension and urinary retention detected by ultrasound measurement. *Br J Anaesth* 92:544,2004.

60. Hodgson PS, Neal JM, Pollock JE, et al.: The neurotoxicity of drugs given intrathecally (spinal). *Anesth Analg* 88:797, 1999.

61. Pollock JE, Neal JM, Stephenson CA, et al.: Prospective study of the incidence of transient radicular irritation in patients undergoing spinal anesthesia. *Anesthesiol* 84:1361, 1996.

62. Lybecker H, Moller JT, May O, et al.: Incidence and prediction of postdural puncture headache. A prospective study of 1021 spinal anesthesias. *Anesth Analg* 70:389, 1990.

63. Norris MC, Leighton BL, DeSimone CA: Needle bevel direction and headache after inadvertent dural puncture. *Anesthesiol* 70:729,1989.

64. Aguilera Celorrio L, Martinez-Garbizu I, Saez de Equilaz Izaola JL, et al.: Influence of needle bevel, age and sex on the appearance of post-puncture headaches. *Rev Esp Anestesiol Reanim* 36:16,1989.

65. Camann WR, Murray RS, Mushlin PS, et al.: Effects of oral caffeine on postdural puncture headache. A double-blind, placebo-controlled trial. *Anesth Analg* 70:181, 1990.

66. Auroy Y, Narchi P, Messiah A, et al.: Serious complications related to regional anesthesia: Results of a prospective survey in France. *Anesthesiol* 87:479,1997.

67. Moore DC, Bridenbaugh LD: Spinal (subarachnoid) block. A review of 11,574 cases. *JAMA* 195:907,1966.

68. Dripps RD, Vandam LD: Long-term follow-up of patients who received 10,098 spinal anesthetics: Failure to discover major neurological sequelae. *JAMA* 156:1486,1954.

69. Vandam LD, Dripps RD: A long-term follow-up of 10,098 spinal anesthetics. II. Incidence and analysis of minor sensory neurological defects. *Surg* 38:463,1955.

70. Moen V, Dahlgren N, Irestedt L: Severe neurological complications after central neuraxial blockades in Sweden 1990–1999. *Anesthesiol* 101:950,2004.

71. Wedel DJ, Horlocker TT: Risks of regional anesthesia – Infectious, septic. *Reg Anesth* 21(6S):57,1996.

72. Loarie DJ, Fairley HB: Epidural abscess following spinal anesthesia. *Anesth Analg* 57:351,1978.

73. Kilpatrick ME, Girgis NI: Meningitis—A complication of spinal anesthesia. *Anesth Analg* 62:513,1983.

74. Burke D, Wildsmith JA: Meningitis after spinal anaesthesia. *Br J Anaesth* 78:635,1997.

75. Aromaa U, Lahdensuu M, Cozanitis DA: Severe complications associated with epidural and spinal anaesthesias in Finland 1987–1993. A study based on patient insurance claims. *Acta Anaesthesiol Scand* 41:445, 1997.

76. Caplan RA, Ward RJ, Posner K, et al.: Unexpected cardiac arrest during spinal anesthesia: A closed claims analysis of predisposing factors. *Anesthesiol* 68:5,1988.

77. Scott DB, McClure JH, Giasi RM, et al.: Effects of concentration of local anaesthetic drugs in extradural block. *Br J Anaesth* 52:1033,1980.

78. Park WY, Hagins FM, Rivat EL, et al.: Age and epidural dose response in adult men. *Anesthesiol* 56(4):318,1982.

79. Liu SS, Ware PD, Rajendran S: Effects of concentration and volume of 2-chloroprocaine on epidural anesthesia in volunteers. *Anesthesiol* 86:1288,1997.

80. Arakawa M: Does pregnancy increase the efficacy of lumbar epidural anesthesia? *Internat J Obstr Anesth* 13:86, 2004.

81. Fagraeus L, Urban BJ, Bromage PR: Spread of epidural analgesia in early pregnancy. *Anesthesiol* 58:184,1983.

82. Nydahl PA, Philipson L, Axelsson K, et al.: Epidural anesthesia with 0.5% bupivacaine: Influence of age on sensory and motor blockade. *Anesth Analg* 73:780,1991.

83. Neal JM, Deck JJ, Kopacz DJ, et al.: Hospital discharge after ambulatory knee arthroscopy: A comparison of epidural 2-chloroprocaine versus lidocaine. *Reg Anesth Pain Med* 26:35,2001.

84. Allen RW, Fee JP, Moore J: A preliminary assessment of epidural chloroprocaine for day procedures. *Anaesthesia* 48:773,1993.

85. Kopacz DJ, Mulroy MF: Chloroprocaine and lidocaine decrease hospital stay and admission rate after outpatient epidural anesthesia. *Reg Anesth* 15:19,1990.

86. Stevens RA, Urmey WF, Urquhart BL, et al.: Back pain after epidural anesthesia with chloroprocaine. *Anesthesiol* 78:492,1993.

87. Stevens RA, Chester WL, Artuso JD, et al.: Back pain after epidural anesthesia with chloroprocaine in volunteers: Preliminary report. *Reg Anesth* 16:199,1991.

88. Reisner LS, Hochman BN, Plumer MH: Persistent neurologic deficit and adhesive arachnoiditis following intrathecal 2-chloroprocaine injection. *Anesth Analg* 59:452, 1980.

89. Terai T, Yukioka H, Fujimori M: A double-blind comparison of lidocaine and mepivacaine during epidural anaesthesia. *Acta Anaesthesiol Scand* 37:607,1993.

90. Groban L, Deal DD, Vernon JC, et al.: Cardiac resuscitation after incremental overdosage with lidocaine, bupivacaine, levobupivacaine, and ropivacaine in anesthetized dogs. *Anesth Analg* 92:37,2001.

91. Klimscha W, Chiari A, Krafft P, et al.: Hemodynamic and analgesic effects of clonidine added repetitively to continuous epidural and spinal blocks. *Anesth Analg* 80:322, 1995.

92. Nishikawa T, Dohi S: Clinical evaluation of clonidine added to lidocaine solution for epidural anesthesia. *Anesthesiol* 73:853,1990.

93. Bromage PR, Burfoot MF, Crowell DE, et al.: Quality of epidural blockade. I. Influence of physical factors. *Br J Anaesth* 36:342,1964.

94. Stevens RA, Chester WL, Grueter JA, et al.: The effect of pH adjustment of 0.5% bupivacaine on the latency of epidural anesthesia. *Reg Anesth* 14:236,1989.

95. DiFazio CA, Carron H, Grosslight KR, et al.: Comparison of pH-adjusted lidocaine solutions for epidural anesthesia. *Anesth Analg* 65:760,1986.

96. Capogna G, Celleno D, Tagariello V: The effect of pH adjustment of 2% mepivacaine on epidural anesthesia. *Reg Anesth* 14:121,1989.

97. Block BM, Liu SS, Rowlingson AJ, et al.: Efficacy of postoperative epidural analgesia: A meta-analysis. *JAMA* 290:2455,2003.

98. Staats PS, Stinson MS, Lee RR: Lumbar stenosis complicating retained epidural catheter tip. *Anesthesiol* 83:1115, 1995.

99. Sakuma N, Hori M, Suzuki H, et al.: A sheared off and sequestered epidural catheter: A case report. *Masui-Jap J Anesthesiol* 53:198,2004.

100. Eason MJ, Wyatt R: Paravertebral thoracic block—A reappraisal. *Anaesthesia* 34:638,1979.

101. Karmakar MK: Thoracic paravertebral block. *Anesthesiol* 95:771,2001.

102. Karmakar MK, Chung DC: Variability of a thoracic paravertebral block. Are we ignoring the endothoracic fascia? *Reg Anesth Pain Med* 25(3):325,2000.

103. Saito T, Den S, Tanuma K, et al.: Anatomical bases for paravertebral anesthetic block: Fluid communication between the thoracic and lumbar paravertebral regions. *Surg & Radiol Anat* 21:359,1999.

104. Weltz CR, Greengrass RA, Lyerly HK: Ambulatory surgical management of breast carcinoma using paravertebral block. *Ann Surg* 222:19,1995.

105. Naja MZ, el Hassan MJ, Oweidat M, et al.: Paravertebral blockade vs general anesthesia or spinal anesthesia for inguinal hernia repair. *Middle East J Anesthesiol* 16:201,2001.

106. Greengrass R, Buckenmaier CC: Paravertebral anaesthesia/analgesia for ambulatory surgery. *Best Pract Res Clin Anaesthesiol* 16:271,2002.

107. Naja Z, Lonnqvist PA: Somatic paravertebral nerve blockade. Incidence of failed block and complications. *Anaesthesia* 56:1184,2001.

108. Richardson J, Cheema SP, Hawkins J, et al.: Thoracic paravertebral space location. A new method using pressure measurement. *Anaesthesia* 51:137,1996.

109. Naja MZ, Ziade MF, El Rajab M, et al.: Varying anatomical injection points within the thoracic paravertebral space: Effect on spread of solution and nerve blockade. *Anaesthesia* 59:459,2004.

110. Buckenmaier CC, 3rd, Klein SM, Nielsen KC, et al.: Continuous paravertebral catheter and outpatient infusion for breast surgery. *Anesth Analg* 97:715,2003.

111. Saito T, Den S, Cheema SP, et al.: A single-injection, multisegmental paravertebral block-extension of somatosensory and sympathetic block in volunteers. *Acta Anaesthesiol Scand* 45:30,2001.

112. Lemay E, Guay J, Cote C, et al.: The number of injections does not influence local anesthetic absorption after paravertebral blockade. *Can J Anaesth* 50:562,2003.

113. Richardson J, Sabanathan S: Thoracic paravertebral analgesia. *Acta Anaesthesiol Scand* 39:1005,1995.

114. Thomas PW, Sanders DJ, Berrisford RG: Pulmonary haemorrhage after percutaneous paravertebral block. *Br J Anaesth* 83:668,1999.

115. Bigler D, Dirkes W, Hansen R, et al.: Effects of thoracic paravertebral block with bupivacaine versus combined thoracic epidural block with bupivacaine and morphine on pain and pulmonary function after cholecystectomy. *Acta Anaesthesiol Scand* 33:561,1989.

116. Lekhak B, Bartley C, Conacher ID, et al.: Total spinal anaesthesia in association with insertion of a paravertebral catheter. *Br J Anaesth* 86:280,2001.

117. Hardy PA: Anatomical variation in the position of the proximal intercostal nerve. *Br J Anaesth* 61(3):338,1988.

118. Moore DC, Bridenbaugh LD: Pneumothorax: Its incidence following intercostal nerve block. *JAMA* 182:1005, 1962.

119. Jin FL, Norris AM, Chung F: Should adult patients drink before discharge from ambulatory surgery? *Anesth Analg.* 87:306,1998.

120. Mulroy MF, Salinas FV, Larkin KL, et al.: Ambulatory surgery patients may be discharged before voiding after short-acting spinal and epidural anesthesia. *Anesthesiol* 97:315,2002.

13 | General Inhalation Anesthesia for Cosmetic Surgery

Meena Desai, M.D.

INTRODUCTION

The ultimate in consumer-driven medical care is the business of cosmetic surgery. These are purely elective procedures performed for the convenience and wishes of the buyer patient and at the convenience of the patient. Traditional ideology of surgical care is maximized as service is optimized. The maximization of service should never, however, compromise the prevailing medical, surgical, or anesthetic standard of care. Meeting the standard of care is the minimum requirement of the cosmetic surgical practice.

Much has been written regarding the safety of general anesthesia in the office.[1–4] One should have a structure and plan for the administration of care that adheres to known standards. The care offered to entice the consumer to an individual practice and practitioner is multifaceted. Several studies have found that the friendliness and courtesy of the staff were top predictors of patient satisfaction.[5] The rendering of anesthetic care must be cognizant of the consumerism of plastic surgery and be sensitive of delivering their care with a practice philosophy suited to the surgical practice. Care is often beyond expectations as patients and their idiosyncratic requests are willingly accommodated.

In this chapter, some of the specific particulars of general anesthetic care are provided as they relate to individual procedures. There are also some methods of care that cater to the consumerism milieu.

Many patients respond to the branding of names in relationship to the care that is rendered. Hospital-based care may be analogized as the "Cadillac," whereas the plastic surgical care that is provided in an ASC or office-based cosmetic surgical suite may be analogized as the "Rolls Royce." Attempts are made to preempt postoperative nausea and vomiting (PONV) instead of addressing it after it occurs. Comforters are provided for blankets, linens have lace, neck pillows have aromatherapy, heat, and so forth. This is the "spa" surgical experience.

Keeping abreast of the cosmetic surgery literature provides some assurance that one is collaborating with a surgeon that also has the highest regard for the standard of care. This may vary from state to state. Florida, for example, currently has modeled its office regulations around those of the AAAASF, namely, level: local only, level II, intravenous (sedation), and level III (general anesthesia).

Additionally, surgical societies may have consensus statements and practice standards that are changing and are prudent to regard. Some practices may have outside or independent peer review as a gauge of practice quality. Alternatively, the surgeon who is part of a hospital staff is subject to peer review from that avenue. Postprocedure care and patient satisfaction are vital to a surgical practice. In association with the surgical practice, check anesthetic parameters of patient care and satisfaction as well.

Screen one's surgeons as carefully as one would one's anesthesia colleagues. Verify their licenses and credentials. Check their references and run a query via the AMA data bank or the National Practitioner data bank. What is the surgeon's rate of infection? How many "redos" or "touch-ups" does the practice do?

What is the admission rate to the acute care center or hospital postprocedure? In how many litigious encounters is your surgeon involved? Do not hesitate to "credential" them within your practice much as one do one's own staff and reciprocally provide the same information to your surgeon. Encourage one's staff to keep all of your practice credentialing files up to date. If one is in a state that has no local or state guidelines, then it is incumbent on one to develop them. The office-based guidelines approved by the American Society of Anesthesiologists (ASA)[6] are an excellent template for the development of one's own internal guidelines.

PATIENT SELECTION FOR THE COSMETIC SURGICAL SUITE

An invaluable service that can be monitored by the anesthesia group is appropriate patient selection for the facility. Desai's group screens every patient well in advance of the date of the procedure. The screening process begins as soon as the patient is scheduled. Testing is procedure and history specific. Algorithms may be developed and implemented to make the flow of the preanesthesia interviews and laboratory screening succinct.

Desai's screening criteria are constantly updated and revised as the literature and experience warrants. Preexisting medical conditions can be predictors of adverse events in the ambulatory setting.[7–10] The American College of Cardiology and the American Heart Association have updated guidelines for Perioperative Cardiovascular Evaluation for Noncardiac Surgery[11] that are useful for appropriate patient evaluation and selection. The *British Journal of Anaesthesia* also has an excellent review that helps one judge perioperative cardiac risk.[12]

Many surgeons' practices track patients with postoperative follow-up calls.

Satisfaction with the anesthesia services may not always be a part of this interview. Therefore, the anesthesia practice should also follow up to ensure a high level of patient satisfaction, specifically with their anesthesia care. These

---

Table 13-1. Selection list of patients undergoing general anesthesia criteria that suggest a patient may be unsuitable for a procedure in the office suite

1. Unstable angina
2. History of myocardial injury within three to six months
3. Severe cardiomyopathy
4. Uncontrolled hypertension
5. End stage renal disease on dialysis
6. Sickle-cell anemia
7. Patient on major organ transplant list
8. Active multiple sclerosis
9. Severe chronic obstructive pulmonary disease (COPD)
10. Abnormal airway (difficult intubation and mask ventilation[9]
11. Malignant hyperthermia
12. Acute illegal substance abuse
13. Morbid obesity: body mass index[10]
14. Dementia
15. Psychological instability: rage/anger problems
16. Myasthenia gravis
17. Recent CVA within three months
18. Obstructive sleep apnea[11]
19. Patients with implanted electrical devices (i.e., AICD)

---

calls and the tracking of postoperative information can be utilized to maintain a very high standard of practice and a very high standard of patient satisfaction.

GENERAL ANESTHETIC CONCERNS FOR STANDARD AESTHETIC PROCEDURES

In the fast-paced, efficiency driven environment, it behooves one to employ the best use of time to ensure patient satisfaction and safety in a mode that is also cost conscious. An ideal general anesthetic technique should provide smooth and rapid induction, optimal operating conditions, and a rapid recovery with minimal or no side effects. One would like to tailor the anesthetic technique to promote fast-tracking.

Several comparisons have been done to facilitate the selection of the inhalation agents desflurane, isoflurane, or sevoflurane.[13–17] Although one may have varied results with each agent and each anesthesiologist, the differences in time can be minor. The use of a Bispectral Index (BIS) monitor correlates increasing sedation and loss of consciousness. BIS can facilitate the titration of the anesthetic to ensure a rapid emergence.[19–24] Studies in the past however, have not been clear on the impact of the monitor on real cost saving,[25] nor is it proven to reduce the risk of awareness.[26] Recent studies show cost savings range between 21–39% with BIS monitoring.[27,28] N.B. The B-Aware trial[29] also recently demonstrated a statistically significant 82% reduction in intraoperative awareness under anesthesia, whereas the SAFE2 Trial[30] recently demonstrated a similarly significant 77% reduction in intraoperative awareness under anesthesia.

The ongoing discussion of the use of nitrous oxide in the balanced inhalational anesthetic technique has proponents and antagonists.[17,31] In Desai's experience delivering the "Rolls Royce" of care, the use of nitrous oxide has been eliminated as it may increase the incidence of PONV in some patients. The choice of opioids has also been studied.[32,33] The short-acting remifentanil (Ultiva®) versus fentanyl should be reviewed within any given practice. Remifentanil is clearly more costly. Its very short-acting profile may not leave the homebound postsurgical patient with adequate analgesia. Additionally, it has been shown to have a higher frequency of hypotension in equivalent doses. Inasmuch as many cosmetic surgical procedures involve postoperative pain, Desai preferentially administers fentanyl. Fentanyl allows for a comfortable patient and facilitates timely discharge. Changes in clinical practice that are geared toward well-titrated, short-acting agents can substantially affect how a patient feels and can shorten the time to discharge.[34]

Rhytidectomy or Facelift

The purpose of the facelift is to decrease skin wrinkling and rejuvenate the appearance of the face with the removal of excess skin and the suspension of facial fascia and tissues.

Most patients seeking rhytidectomy are over the age of forty-five. This is a procedure for which the anesthetic technique has a great deal of variation. Much of it is dependent on the choice of anesthesia by the surgeon as well as the skills of the surgeon with that choice of anesthesia. The concepts to consider in general anesthesia and facelifts follow.

Preoperative considerations

These patients are often elderly and require proper screening. A thorough examination of comorbid conditions is important to ensure they are maximally optimized for elective surgery. These procedures are often four or more hours and may have a significant impact on the patient. A thorough review of all herbal and other medications also should be noted, as many may impact on clotting, and care should be taken to stop all herbals for at least two weeks (see Chapter 14 and Appendix A). Premedication with clonidine is useful for sedation as well as for helping with hemodynamic control.

Intraoperative considerations

The endotracheal tube is inserted and secured in a few different ways. The surgeon must work around the tube and the anesthesiologist must be able to see that it is stable and connected during the case. Each surgeon will have a preferred method of securing the tube and one must adapt to it. Endotracheal tubes, either oral or oral RAE®, may be secured with sterile bio-occlusive dressing onto the chin or tied to the canine or front teeth with wire or dental floss. Some anesthesiologists prefer to use a laryngeal mask airway (LMA) to deliver inhalational anesthesia. In any case, it is important not to distort the face when securing any airway device. Doing so is a powerful subliminal message of the anesthesiologist's indifference to the surgeon's task! Indifference is anathema to cooperation.

The eyes will be protected with gel or eye shields during the case. The control of blood pressure during the procedure is key. Maintain the pressure 20–30% lower than baseline during the resection and then bring it back up close to baseline prior to closing. Restoring normotension allows the surgeon to observe additional oozing prior to closing when the patient reaches their normotensive range.

Keep fluid load to a minimum as bleeding is minimal. There are no appreciable third-space losses with rhytidectomy. Administer maintenance fluid only, as excess fluid administration can contribute significantly to facial edema. Some surgeons will request dexamethasone to help minimize edema. Doses from 4–10 mg have been safely used.

Emergence considerations

Extubate the patient without coughing and bucking as both acts increase venous return and bleeding. Most surgeons want complete dressings applied on or before awakening. Many will hold pressure to minimize postextubation bleeding. The head dressing is circumferential of the face and neck. One needs to make sure the dressing is not too constricting around the neck. Elevate the head as soon as it is feasible as it helps with postprocedure swelling.

Postprocedure considerations

As local anesthetic is used for facelifts, there is not much postoperative pain in the immediate recovery area. PONV is a great concern, and a multimodal regimen plan may have better outcomes. Some surgeons prefer to observe the patient in recovery for a period of time in excess of that required for discharge according to Aldrete scores.

Browlift

This procedure serves to lift "excess" skin over the eye as aging and gravity pull the eye and eyebrow down from the supraorbital rim.

This procedure also is used to remove excess skin and wrinkling on the brow. There are a few common types of browlifts that are incisional. There is the full coronal incisional browlift and the side oblique incisional browlift. The incisions are within the hairline for the full coronal lift, and the undermining of tissues is done under direct visualization. The oblique incisional lift places the incision at the start of the hairline oblique to the brow. There is some blood loss with the scalp incision and dissection as control is gained after incision. There is not the same concern over the use of muscle relaxants for browlift as applies to rhytidectomy. One may elect to intubate and paralyze the patient. Considerations about coughing on extubation and increase in blood pressure are similar to those for rhytidectomy. Often pressure is applied to the dressings upon extubation.

Endoscopic browlift

The browlift procedure lends itself well to the endoscopic approach. The approach involves three to five minimal incisions and is dissected endoscopically. The repair and suspension may be held together with installed screw hardware in the frontal mid-scalp well within the hairline. This approach may involve a longer operative time as compared to the incisional lift but does leave less scarring for the patient.

Breast Augmentation

Preoperative considerations

Breast augmentation is an extremely popular procedure. Although many of the patients are in the forty-and-

younger age groups, all ages of patients may present themselves (see Chapter 15).

The preoperative interview is the ideal time to address postprocedure pain-management strategy and expectations. The nature of pain post–breast implantation should be discussed. The quality of the pain is that of pressure and heaviness. As a weight has been added to their chest and many will have a firm circumferential pressure dressing, this sensation, of pressure and heaviness, is acutely experienced with each breath. The expectation should be that pain is to be expected, however, it should be tolerable. The stretching of skin in a very short time period is often felt as a deep ache in the shoulders and back. Submuscular dissection and implant placement will also involve postprocedure deep muscular pain. Submuscular implant placement produces spasm as well as pain. Postoperative oral diazepam can be very helpful in relieving pain secondary to spasm.

Intraoperative considerations

One of the key factors for a good surgical result is to have total control of the bleeding and oozing in the breast pocket. Blood in the pocket is known to increase the incidence of capsule contracture and breast immobility. The placement of the implants also requires position changes intraprocedurally from supine to sitting.

Airway circuits and IV lines of sufficient length should enable a smooth and timely transition from supine to sitting during the procedure.

The position of the arms is at the discretion of the surgeon. Whether the arm placement is at the patient's side or out on arm boards, check pressure points and abduction angles. Also, ensure the arms will transition safely from supine to sitting as placement of implants is confirmed. Consider the effects of position as pertains to vascular tone and blood pressure and be prepared to treat accordingly as one may change supine to sitting positions frequently. Awareness of serious surgical complications would encompass pneumothorax and uncontrolled bleeding from the thoracic vessels. A plan for transfer and admission to an acute-care facility should be in place in the event that complications cannot be definitively addressed in the office surgical suite setting.

Emergence considerations

As in much of plastic and cosmetic surgery, the preference of the surgeon is key. Many will want *all* dressings on prior to extubation. Dressings will involve wound covering as well as bras and elastic bands or bandages that are positioned to mold the placement of the implant in the pocket. If the surgeon would prefer all dressings in place, one must maintain an adequate level of anesthesia that keeps the patient still as they are sat up. The ideal awakening would involve extubation without coughing as increases in venous pressures may increase the chance of bleeding and oozing in the pocket.

Postprocedure considerations

Pain management solutions may include continuous infusion pumps (i.e., On-Q,® or others) and intercostal and incisional blocks.

Endoscopic breast implants

Most breast implants are still placed using the traditional inframammary approach. Alternative approaches are used by some surgeons as a marketing tool in their practices. For example, the larger incision of the inframammary approach is excellent for silicone implants. As often as not, the peri-areaolar approach is used for inflatable saline implants.

Endoscopic breast implants allow for a smaller incision and dissection under direct endoscopic view. The approaches may be either transaxillary or transumbilical for the placement of breast implants. The anesthetic concerns remain similar to the other various approaches of breast implant placement.

Mastopexy

Mastopexy may be performed alone or in conjunction with augmentation. Reduction mammoplasty will have similar position change concerns as breast size, shape, and contour are manipulated.

Intraoperative considerations

The duration of the case is directly related to the extent of the mastopexy and its repair. As cosmetic surgery is assessed with appearance, each incision is painstakingly closed by hand. Blood loss and fluid-balance concerns in reduction mammoplasty are dependent on the extent of the resection, the amount of tissue, and the extent of the flaps in question. Some surgeons may apply nitropaste 0.5–1.0 inch to the nipple areola complex to increase blood flow to the flap. The effects of the nitropaste are usually subclinical. However, attention must be paid to the potential effects on the patient's vital signs.

Liposuction

Contouring lipoplasty is a very common plastic surgery procedure. This procedure is not a weight-loss procedure but is a body-contouring procedure. Almost any area of the body is amenable to liposculpture. The most common method to perform liposuction is the tumescent technique. This technique involves the instillation of saline mixed with a dilute solution of lidocaine (0.05–0.1%) and epinephrine (1:1,000,000) into the areas of lipoplasty (see Chapter 8).

The lidocaine in the mixture is a method of analgesia, and the epinephrine component is to aid hemostasis. The tumescent technique takes advantage of the tissue-binding capacity of lidocaine with this dilute concentration, where there is the slow uptake of lidocaine into the bloodstream with serum level peaking as late as 10–14 hours after the infusion. The surgeon keeps a precise tally of the infusion amount of each tumesced site, and specific attention is given to tumescent input and aspirate output.

The most common method of suction is the use of a power suction canister. The suction cannulae vary in the number and placement of the suction ports and have a varied diameter depending on the effect desired. Fibrous areas of the body are difficult to suction and also are less conducive to the even spread of the tumescent fluid. These difficult fibrous areas may be suctioned using an ultrasonic suction that will "liquefy" the fat before the area is resuctioned with the standard liposuction machine to remove the liquefied fat. The ultrasonic liposuction adds another element of complexity (viz., timing its use) as there is an association of seroma formation with increased time usage. Additionally, heat injury is a concern with this technology, and particular care must be taken to watch and protect the skin.

Much has been discussed in the plastic surgical literature over the amount of liposuction volume. The consensus would lead the prudent plastic and cosmetic surgeon to suction volumes less than 5,000 cc of aspirate. The removal of larger volumes may require overnight stays and additional postprocedure monitoring of fluid balance, blood loss, and pain management.

Preoperative concerns

Liposuction is a potentially serious surgery and is of a moderately invasive nature.

The mortality rate is 19 in 1,000, where the most common cause of death is from thromboembolism.[35]

Thromboembolic concerns need to be addressed to minimize risk. Particular attention should be paid to herbal and other medications that may elevate this risk (see Chapter 14 and Appendix A). Oral contraceptives (and smoking) will increase this risk, and these issues must be discussed by the practice with the patient. Preoperative education should include discussions on early ambulation and exercises to ward against venous pooling. The character of liposuction pain is often that of incisions, and patients may experience some interior orthostatic symptoms (described as "burning") in the first twelve to twenty-four hours. The discomfort after twenty-four hours will be that of a deep ache that is accentuated when the muscles under the suctioned fat are being used. The patient may continue to ooze fluid from the first twenty-four hours. The patient should have immediate home help for that time.

Intraoperative concerns

The most immediate anesthetic concern is the fluid management of this patient, along with adequate analgesia.

Much of the tumescent fluid is absorbed by the patient,[36] even though it appears that much is aspirated out with the fat. With the use of epinephrine, the blood loss is limited.[37,38] One can observe the amount of hemoglobin staining or "redness" of the aspirate. Using the "wet" technique of liposuction, one can keep the fluid requirements to a minimum, "maintenance only"[37] level. Amounts of liposuction greater than 4,000 cc should be replaced with 0.25 ml intravenous crystalloid per ml of aspirate removed over 4,000.[38] Other intraoperative complications must be considered in the diagnostic differential if difficulties arise. These complications include viscus perforation, pulmonary edema, vascular perforation, fat embolism, local anesthetic toxicity, and hypothermia.[37] Positioning and repositioning the patient from side-to-side and supine-to-prone is frequently done as one infuses the tumescent solution to all the sites. The surgeon allows it to work and then repositions for suctioning. This is an intraoperative challenge as one must be careful to position safely and continuously be aware of body alignment and all pres-

sure points. The anesthesiologist must also ensure that all monitoring cables and intravenous tubing will allow for ease of movement during repositioning. The anesthesiologist must prepare ahead with padding and positioning devices because they are often managing much of the "moves" on their own. It is most helpful to have all the devices handy as one also has to be careful with the instrumented airway. Attention to the patient's temperature is in order because hypothermia is a real risk.[36] The patient has many exposed areas to the loss of convective heat. The infiltration of tumescent fluid produces losses of body heat. Often the skin is wet because the surgeon checks for evenness of liposculpture. There is additional heat loss through evaporation. Methods to increase patient temperature need to involve Bair® huggers and keeping OR temperatures higher than normal. The procedure concludes with feathering the edges of the fat deposit that involves the suction cannula, providing a transition between the suctioned and residual fat to provide a natural contour. This feathering will trespass into less anesthetized areas because the tumescent solution will not have been infused there. There is often transient pain at the end of procedure. This is best addressed with short-acting hypnotics to manage hyperdynamic changes, which will resolve suddenly at the end of the procedure. The liposuction garment is a snug elastic garment applied immediately at the end of the procedure to control fluid sequestration. The compression of the potential "third space" created by the suction of the fat is largely eliminated by the use of compression garments. Failure to appreciate this issue has led some anesthesia providers to administer overzealous fluid replacement. Inappropriate fluid management can lead to dilutional anemia, dilution of platelets, and other clotting factors, sometimes with fatal outcomes. The garment is worn for several weeks to smooth the skin and promote retraction to the newly sculpted areas.

Postprocedure considerations

Despite the use of lidocaine tumescent, there can be pain in the "feathered" areas. One must ensure that the patient is comfortable as they are assessed in PACU. Our practice utilizes nalbuphine (Nubain®) in doses of 5–10 mg IVP in PACU. In doses exceeding 10 mg, there is often an increased element of sedation that will delay discharge. Warming the patient with a Bair® hugger in the PACU is also very useful after liposuction.

Rhinoplasty

Rhinoplasty is a common procedure that involves contouring the nose. Repairs can be simple or quite involved, as many aspects may need to be manipulated to achieve the desired result.

Intraoperative concerns

Rhinoplasty is a procedure well suited to general anesthesia with an instrumented airway. The endotracheal tube is positioned over the mandible and the oral RAE® tube with its curve may be quite helpful in its profile. An armored or flexible style LMA will also do well for administering inhalation anesthesia. The tube may be easily taped to the patient's chin to keep it out of the surgeon's field of vision. The flexible tube's advantage is the additional ballotment of the esophagus, reducing the amount of blood that can drip down into the stomach. Blood in the stomach is a well-recognized cause of PONV following rhinoplasty. Insertion of the flexible LMA is facilitated by lubricating an uncuffed #5 endotracheal tube and using it as a stylet to stiffen the outer tube.

Extensive repair with osteotomies may involve bleeding, which may compromise the airway and put the patient at a higher risk for aspiration. The use of an endotracheal tube with throat packing may help in controlling how much blood goes down the esophagus and into the stomach. Attention must be paid to see that the throat packs are removed. Unfortunately, even when dampened with saline, the throat packs are still very abrasive to the esophageal mucosa. Since the patient will likely have a sore throat complaint from the endotracheal tube, they may have difficulty understanding why swallowing is painful as well. Limiting the cuff inflation of the LMA to the least effective amount will lower the incidence of sore throat complaints compared with the endotracheal tube throat pack combination. Cosmetic surgery patients will complain if the IV insertion hurt. They will not fail to complain about a sore throat. "Rolls Royce" anesthesia care means eliminating any and all avoidable patient complaints.

Emergence concerns

The application of the surgical splint and dressing at the completion of the rhinoplasty is an art and varies with every surgeon. Awaken the patient after the dressing is in place and the splint has stiffened and contoured. The awakening is a challenge because the patient should not cough, which will increase bleeding, and yet must be awake to guard against aspiration. In addition, because one cannot exert proper mask pressure with a "new nose" without potentially injuring the repair, the patient must be awake at extubation to eliminate the propensity for laryngospasm.

Postprocedure concerns

The patient is generally comfortable because local has been used during the procedure. Nausea and vomiting may be a problem and will need to be addressed.

Abdominoplasty

This is a procedure that is designed to remove excess skin and skin laxity and to remove fat with the abdominal skin flap. Liposuction does not address the issue of excess skin, and abdominoplasty is the definitive procedure to solve this problem. Most abdominoplasty patients are past child-bearing age and many are moderately overweight. The number of men undergoing this procedure is also steadily increasing.[39] The procedure is moderately invasive, and patients will need a thorough workup preoperatively. The procedure is extraperitoneal and often accompanied by liposuction.

Liposuction may be done to the hips and flanks. Aggressive liposuction of the flap is to be avoided because it compromises the blood supply to the flap and increases the chance of flap necrosis.

Preoperative considerations

Abdominoplasty patients are particularly at increased risk for thromboembolic events. Teaching must be done to advise patients of this particular risk, to inform them of their postoperative role in the recognition of the symptoms of this complication, and to instruct them in their role in decreasing the incidence of this complication. Many patients also describe muscular back pain, back muscle spasm, and tightness in the first twenty-four hours. These discomforts can be best addressed with local heat, ice therapy, and comfortable positioning.

Intraoperative concerns

Abdominoplasties can be performed with general anesthesia, oral endotracheal intubation, and muscle paralysis. After the imbrication of the rectus muscle sheath Muscle paralysis is not required for sufficient conditions to imbricate the rectus muscle sheath. Less is more is completed, the patient will be positioned in a flex position with the back up and the knees bent. The back is raised and the patient is flexed at approximately 30–40 degrees. This flexion allows the abdominal flap to be closed under tension. The patient is kept in this position throughout the remainder of the procedure and in the PACU. Drains are usually placed and removed in seven to ten days. If pain-infusion systems are to be used, they are placed and primed at this time.[40]

Emergence concerns

Because the sutures are closed under tension, one should try and extubate without coughing. Coughing can increase intra-abdominal pressure, which can impact on the repair.

Postprocedure concerns

The greatest immediate concern is to ensure the patient is comfortable with tolerable pain. Adequate opioid analgesia intraoperatively is key.

Many practices are now utilizing local pain-infusion pumps that will deliver local anesthetic to the site over a number of days. Home instructions need to stress the necessity of moving about after surgery and the importance of leg and feet exercises that can be done to deter venous pooling.

Laser Facial Resurfacing

Laser facial resurfacing serves to reduce fine-line wrinkles and to even out skin coloration. It can also be useful to lessen facial scarring owing to previous injury. This is particularly applicable to acne scarring. The laser seeks to damage a skin layer that with healing will come in with stronger connective tissue and "tighten" the face. The insult generated by the laser is similar in quality to a second-degree burn. The procedure itself is quite painful and does require adequate analgesia. The duration of the procedure may change from fifteen to forty-five minutes depending on the area to be covered and the number of passes to be made.

Intraoperative concerns

Protect the eyes with shield protectors during the procedure. A major concern is that of fire in and around the patient. Precaution should be taken to use a laser-resistant endotracheal tube. The patients should be insulated with water-soaked drapes and gauze. Water-soaked gauze should be applied to the endothracheal tube and placed over the eyes. Critical attention must be paid to ensure the laser beam does not come into contact with the endotracheal tube. The endotracheal tube provides the least leakage of oxygen to the areas and is therefore the best option versus another airway device choice. One must also keep the inspired oxygen concentration to a minimum in case of airway fire.

Postprocedure concerns

Adequate analgesia is key after this procedure. When adequate intraoperative analgesia was supplied for laser facial resurfacing, only 12 percent of patients required postoperative analgesia and the PONV rate was zero.[41] In comparison, when intraoperative analgesia was inadequate, 70 percent of patients required postoperative analgesia and the PONV rate was 35 percent![42] The patient often remarks that the face feels like it is on fire. Occlusive ointment applied topically shields the face and does alleviate some pain. Cool compresses and cold-water-soaked gauze also aid in decreasing the pain. Narcotic analgesia given intraoperatively may need to be supplemented in the PACU.

Blepharoplasty

Blepharoplasty and cosmetic eye surgery is performed to improve the appearance of the eye. The patient usually wishes to alter excess skin wrinkling and puffiness due to excess fat deposition. General anesthesia is provided at the request of the patient or surgeon. Most often these cases are done with IV sedation; however, some patients may not be able to tolerate four quadrant blephroplasty or may wish to have general anesthesia.

Emergence concerns

The most critical time is that of emergence and extubation. One must attempt to ensure that the patient is extubated without coughing and bucking. Patients are less likely to cough or buck on an LMA compared to an endotracheal tube because any increase in venous and arterial pressure is deleterious to the surgical result and may lead to uncontrolled bleeding. Keeping the head elevated at least 30 degrees will aid in reducing the venous pressure impacting on the surgical site.

PRACTICAL CONSIDERATION OF CLINICAL ISSUES

Fast Tracking and Discharge Criteria

The length of postoperative stay among ambulatory surgical patients is mainly determined by the type of surgery and adverse events such as excessive pain, PONV, dizziness, drowsiness, and unexpected cardiovascular events.[43] An approach that incorporates concepts to avoid pitfalls and increase the feasibility of fast tracking is well reviewed.[44,45] One should utilize a modified Aldrete score for bypassing the intensive PACU and also develop and use Postanesthesia Discharge Scoring System (PADS) criteria for determining home readiness.[46] New ideas in ambulatory postprocedure care also allow for oral fluids in selected patients but not as routine for all discharge protocols. The issue of voiding before discharge can also be individualized, as it may not be necessary in those patients at low risk for urinary retention.[47]

Pain medication in recovery

Oftentimes the general surgical cosmetic suite has one OR and one acute recovery bay. The nursing staff, though qualified, is limited, and the efficient flow of patients is dependent on minimal to no delays in the discharge area. The greatest concerns of patients in the PACU relate to pain management[48,49] and PONV issues.

Pain management

Excepting rhytidectomies, most cosmetic surgical procedures involve some postprocedure pain. The adequate dosing of an analgesic intraoperatively may be the key to prompt discharge in the PACU. The patient that awakens with a tolerable comfort level will fare better fulfilling the discharge and home-readiness protocols of the center. Desai's practice largely uses intraoperative fentanyl because it provides cost-effective analgesia and allows for timely discharge with comfort. The patient may resume oral medications at home as soon as they begin to feel pain. Rescue analgesia is primarily done after the patient is assessed and a pain score value is determined. For pain score values 7 or less, treatment with nalbuphine is instituted in rapid incremental doses of 5, 7.5, or 10 mg. Nalbuphine, a mixed agonist/antagonist opioid, has a good analgesic profile and a respiratory ceiling. The patient is still monitored after the intravenous dose before being

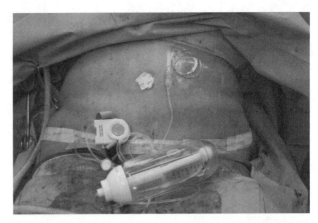

Figure 13-1. Abdominoplasty patient shown at the conclusion of the procedure with pain pump.

safely discharged home. Dosing greater than 10 mg does often lead to unwanted side effects, such as drowsiness, that may delay discharge. For pain score values 8 or greater, dose with up to two incremental doses of 25 ug of fentanyl intravenously in the PACU.

Many surgeons are also employing continuous infusion pain-management techniques that involve local anesthetic pumps. These pumps may be patient-controlled as well as continuous infusion via indwelling soaker catheters. They are most commonly used for abdominal surgeries and breast surgeries (see Figures 13-1, 13-2, and 13-3). The catheters are placed prior to closing, and the initial dosing of local anesthetic is delivered prior to awakening. They are typically kept in place for three to five days and then removed at a postprocedure office visit. Many surgeons may also place local anesthesia on incision sites to

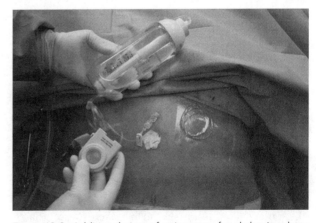

Figure 13-2. Additional view of pain pump for abdominoplasty patient.

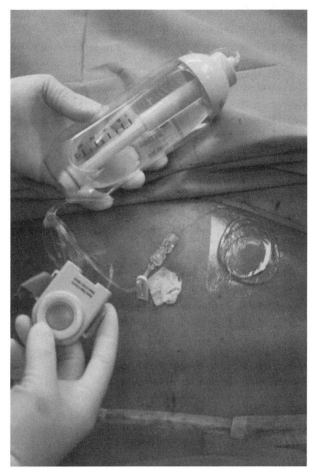

Figure 13-3. Close-up view of pain pump for abdominoplasty patient.

decrease postoperative discomfort. Others may also use intercostals or other local field blocks. Many plastic and cosmetic surgeons are averse to using nonsteroidal anti-inflammatory medications (NSAIDs) because they do not wish to do anything that may increase the risk of bleeding. Intravenous ketorolac (Toradol,®) has an increased bleeding and oozing profile that has made cosmetic surgeons less amenable to its use. The recent controversies of the COX-2 inhibitors have led many patients and plastic surgeons away from their use.

PONV

The other main concern for patients is nausea and vomiting after the procedure. For many in this satin-gloved service, even the feeling of nausea is distasteful. Many recent analyses have developed a model for predicting high- and low-risk anesthesia groups for PONV.[50,51] At this level of

consumerism, one must attend to all aspects of the surgical experience by considering all patients as a PONV risk. Many patients will consider paying out of pocket for the avoidance of this complication.[53]

A simplified PONV risk score includes the female gender, history of motion sickness or PONV, nonsmoker, and the use of postoperative opioids as being predictive of risk.[54,55] Although high-dose opioids are implicated in increasing nausea, it has been shown that usual opioid doses used in the course of outpatient surgery do not promote an increased incidence of PONV.[56]

The use of reversal agents are also implicated in increasing the incidence of PONV; however, their use is guided by clinical necessity.[57,58] Consider the guidelines or consensus statements regarding PONV.[51] A multimodal approach may be a successful regime.[59,60] The timing of antiemetic dosing has been shown to affect its efficacy. It appears that 5-HT$_3$ blockers, such as ondansteron, may be best administered immediately before the end of surgery for the greatest efficacy.[61,62] The use of a second dose of a 5-HT$_3$ blocker has been shown to have a diminished efficacy as a rescue drug.[52,62]

Prophylactic intravenous administration of dexamethasone immediately after induction rather than at the end of anesthesia was most effective in preventing PONV.[63] A single prophylactic dose of dexamethasone has not been shown to have any clinically relevant toxicity in otherwise healthy patients. The combination of dexamethasone and a 5-HT$_3$ receptor antagonist may be a more efficacious combination that either one administered alone.[64,65]

The use of a multidrug regime can reduce the nausea and vomiting propensity of an inhalational general anesthetic. Mandatory po fluid intake is unnecessary as a discharge criterion.[66] Patients also need to be counseled as to how to deal with the car ride home, especially if they have a propensity toward motion sickness. They should be advised to recline the chair, close their eyes, and sit quietly. Additionally, they should be told to avoid sudden movements, which can increase the incidence of motion sickness.

MALIGNANT HYPERTHERMIA (MH) PROTOCOL

In Desai's practice, extreme diligence is used obtaining in-depth patient history as soon as the case is booked. The collection of patient anesthetic history often precedes the procedure by two weeks. Under no circumstances should a patient with a personal or a family history of MH undergo a triggering anesthetic in an office-based setting.

The level of staffing, materials, and testing required in case of an attack of malignant hyperthermia would not be adequate in most office locations. One keeps an office location that performs triggering anesthetics equipped with dantrolene, iced fluids, bicarbonate, mannitol, insulin, and so forth as advised by the many societies (i.e., JACHO, MHAUS, AAAASF, and AAAHC) to ensure the initiation of timely treatment. Guidelines and policies are available on the MHAUS web site.[67] One should routinely have practice drills for how to deal with this as well as other emergencies in the office cosmetic suite setting. Preparedness may be lifesaving.

THROMBOEMBOLISM

Thromboembolism is a dreaded complication of surgery. Deep venous thrombosis and pulmonary embolus can cause significant morbidity and even death. Certain guidelines have been published that can significantly reduce the incidence of this complication.[68] The plastic and cosmetic surgeon walks a fine line between postoperative bleeding and thromboembolism. Abdominoplasty has one of the highest rates of deep venous thrombosis and pulmonary embolus in plastic surgery.[69]

Recent investigations into deaths in Florida have shown a significant association of pulmonary embolus as cause of death. Thromboembolic risk increases when abdominoplasty is combined with other aesthetic procedures.[70] The association of pulmonary embolus and abdominoplasty may be related to the reduction of ease of superficial venous drainage from the pelvis and legs. Adding suction-assisted lipectomy to abdominoplasty does not increase the risk of deep venous thrombosis or pulmonary embolus.[70] The American Society of Plastic Surgery has formulated a task force on Deep Venous Thrombosis Prophylaxis and has established some guidelines.[68] It is recommended that patients be stratified according to their risk of deep venous thrombosis and pulmonary embolus. The low-risk group represents patients who have known risk factors, require surgical procedures of thirty minutes or less, and are under the age of forty (see Table 13-2). A moderate risk exists for patients who are greater than forty years of age, require procedures longer than thirty minutes, or are tak-

---

Table 13-2. Risk factors for deep venous thrombosis and pulmonary embolism[68]

1. Virchow's triad (stasis, hypercoaguability, vascular injury)
2. Immobilization (e.g., from surgery or a fracture)
3. Malignancy
4. Thrombophlebitis
5. Pregnancy, and for six to twelve weeks postpartum
6. Extremity trauma
7. Hormone replacement therapy or oral contraceptives
8. Smoking
9. Obesity (body mass index >30)
10. Recent myocardial infarction or cerebrovascular accident
11. Previous history of deep vein thrombosis (pulmonary embolism)
12. History of radiation therapy (especially pelvic)
13. Antiphospholipid antibody syndrome
14. Homocystinemia
15. Polycythemia
16. Other hypercoaguable states
    a. Abnormal protein C or S
    b. Factor V Leiden
    c. Abnormal factors XIII, IX, X

---

ing oral contraception or undergoing hormone replacement therapy. Although general anesthesia for less than thirty minutes does not cause significant venous pooling, a linear increase in the risk of deep venous thrombosis occurs with *general anesthesia* times of greater than one hour.[71] High-risk patients are those who have additional risk factors from the moderate-risk group such as malignancy, immobilization, obesity, and hypercoagulable states.

Recommendations according to risk stratification

LOW-RISK PATIENTS. Position the patient comfortably on the operating table with slight knee flexion and a pillow to enhance popliteal venous return. Avoid external pressure on the legs or constricting garments.

MODERATE-RISK PATIENTS. Observe the same comfortable positioning and the use of intermittent pneumatic compression garments worn before, during, and after general anesthesia until the patient is fully awake. If possible, these patients should stop taking risky medications at least one week before surgery, although it is unclear in the literature if the risk for deep venous thrombosis and pulmonary embolus normalizes within this time.[68]

HIGH-RISK PATIENTS. Observe the same measures as the lower-risk categories plus a preoperative consultation from hematology. Consider low-molecular-weight heparin two hours before surgery and until the patient is ambulatory. Prophylactic anticoagulation, however, is considered optional in procedures with a high risk for hematoma. The majority of aesthetic procedures fall into this category.

Intermittent pneumatic compression devices (IPCD) are mechanical devices that increase the pulsatile flow in the veins by preventing stagnation and enhancing endogenous fibrinolytic activity. However, there is no clear-cut evidence that ICPDs influence venous stasis in the pelvic veins, the source of the majority of lethal thromboemboli.

These mechanics reduce levels of tissue plasminogen activator inhibitor and decrease stagnation. There are two types of devices for use: foot pumps that encircle the ankle and compress the venous plexus in the feet, and sequential compression devices that encircle the leg and compress the veins in the calf and thigh.[69] Most important, these devices should be applied and activated prior to the induction of anesthesia and continued until the patient is fully awake. The addition of elastic stockings to intermittent pneumatic compression stockings should be considered for the patient that is a moderate risk, unless their use is precluded by other disease states.[70]

Additionally, patients must be made aware of the signs and symptoms that may indicate venous stasis and pulmonary embolus. Early intervention may decrease morbidity and mortality. "When possible, procedures longer than three or four hours should be performed with local anesthesia and intravenous sedation because general anesthesia is associated with deep venous thrombosis at much higher rates under prolonged operative conditions."[71] Lofsky, the anesthesiologist member of the board of governors of the Doctors' Company (a medical liability carrier), writes that "Newer techniques for intravenous sedation that include the use of propofol drips, often in combination with other drugs, have made it possible to perform lengthy or extensive surgeries without general anesthesia and without the loss of the patient's airway protective reflexes."[72,73] "For the anesthetic itself, overall experiences indicate that the least amount of anesthetic that can be used is the best dose. Local and monitored anesthesia care (MAC) is preferable to regional. Regional techniques are preferable to general anesthesia."[74]

CONCLUSION

The challenge of the office-based, cosmetic surgery suite remains as anesthetic agents and techniques continue to evolve. The satisfaction of the patient and the work atmosphere continue to provide positive reinforcement as anesthesiologists continue to address the challenges in this specialized setting.

REFERENCES

1. Hoefflin SM, Bornstein JB, Gordon M: General anesthesia in office-based plastic surgical facility: A report on more than 23,000 cases. *Plast Reconstr Surg* 107:243,2001.
2. Byrd HS, Barton FE, Orenstein HH, et al.: Safety and efficacy in an accredited outpatient plastic surgery facility. *Plast Reconstr Surg* 112:636,2003.
3. Iverson RE: ASPS task force on patient safety in office-based surgery facilities. *Plast Reconstr Surg* 110:1337,2002.
4. Iverson RE, Lynch DJ: ASPS task force: Patient safety in office-based surgery facilities. *Plast Reconstr Surg* 110:1785, 2002.
5. Deutshn, Wu CL: Patient outcomes following ambulatory anesthesia. *Anesthesiol Clin N Amer* 21:403,2003.
6. ASA Guidelines.
7. Chung F, Merzei G, Tong D: Pre-existing medical conditions as predictors of adverse events. *Brit J Anaesth* 83:262, 1999.
8. Natof HE: Pre-existing medical problems: Ambulatory surgery. *Illinois Med J* 166:101,1984.
9. Langeron O, Massou E, Huraux C, et al.: Prediction of difficult mask ventilation. *Anesthesiol* 92:1229,2000.
10. deJong RH: Body mass index: Risk predictor for cosmetic day surgery. *Plast Reconstr Surg* 108:556,2001.
11. Loadsman JA, Hilman DR: Anesthesia and sleep apnea. *Br J Anesth* 86:254,2001.
12. Eagle KA, Berger PB, Calkins H, et al.: ACC/AHA guideline update for preoperative cardiovascular evaluation: Executive summary report of the American College of Cardiology/American Heart Association Task Froce on Practical Guidelines. *Circulation* 105:1257,2002.
13. Chassot PG, Delabays A, Spahn DR: Preoperative evaluation of patients with, or at risk of, coronary artery disease undergoing non-cardiac surgery. *Br J Anaesth* 89:747, 2002.
14. Boldt J, Jaun N: Economic consideration of the use of new anesthetics: A comparison of propofol, sevoflurane. *Anesth Analg* 86:504,1998.

15. Montes FR, Trillos JE, Rincon IE, et al.: Comparison of total intravenous anesthesia and sevoflurane-fentanyl anesthesia for outpatient otorhinolaryngeal surgery. *J Clin Anesth* 14: 324,2002.

16. Larsen B, Seitz A, Larsen R: Recovery of cognitive function after remifentanil-propofol anesthesia. *Anesth Analg* 90:168,2000.

17. Lebenborm-Mansour MH, Pandit SK, Kothary SP, et al.: Desflurane vs. propofol anesthesia: A comparative analysis. *Anesth Analg* 76:936,1993.

18. Joshi GP: Inhalational techniques in ambulatory anesthesia. *Anesthesiol Clin N Am* 21:263,2003.

19. Gan TJ, Glass PS, Windsor A, et al.: Bispectral index monitoring allows faster emergence and improved recovery. BIS utility study group. *Anesthesiol* 87:808,1997.

20. Song D, Joshi G, White PF: Titration of volatile anesthetics using Bispectral index. *Anesthesiol* 87:842,1997.

21. Kalkman CH, Drummond JC: Monitors of depth of anesthesia (editorial). *Anesthesiol* 96:784,2002.

22. Drover DR, Lemmens HJ, Pierce ET, et al.: Patient state index: Titration of delivery and recovery from propofol. *Anesthesiol* 97:82,2002.

23. Song D: Titration of volatile anesthetics using bispectral index facilitates recovery. *Anesthesiol* 87:842,1997.

24. Pavlin DJ, Hong JY, Friund PR, et al.: The effect of bispectral index monitoring on endtidal gas concentration. *Anesth Analg* 93:613,2001.

25. Yli-Hankala A, Vakkuri A, Annila P, et al.: EEG bispectral index monitoring in sevoflurane or propofol. *Acta Anesthesiol Scand* 43:545,1999.

26. O'Connor MF, Daves SM, Tung A, et al.: BIS monitoring to prevent awareness during general anesthesia. *Anesthesiol* 94:520,2001.

27. Mak S, Crowley J: The utility of the Bispectral Index vs. standard practice anesthetic care: A meta analysis of randomized trials comparing drug reduction and recovery time. Poster presentation at the 2002 annual meeting of SAMBA.

28. Rosow C, Manberg PJ: Bispectral Index monitoring: Monitoring during critical events. *Anesthesiol Clin N Am* 19:947,2001.

29. Myles PS, Leslie K: Bispectral index monitoring to prevent awareness during anaesthesia: The B-Aware randomised controlled Trial. *The Lancet* 363:1757,2004.

30. Ekman A, Lindholm ML, Lennmarken C, et al.: Reduction in the incidence of awareness using BIS monitoring. *Acta Anaesthesiol Scand* 48:20,2004.

31. Tang J, Chen L, White PF, et al.: Use of propofol for office-based anesthesia. *J Clin Anesth* 11:226,1999.

32. Song D, Whitten C, White P: Use of remifentanil during anesthetic induction. *Anesth Analg* 88:734,1999.

33. Joshi GP, Warner DS, Twersky RS, et al.: A comparison of remifentanil and fentanyl adverse effect profile. *J Clin Anesth* 14:494,2002.

34. Apfelbaum JL, Walawander CA, Grascla TH, et al.: Eliminating intensive postoperative care in same day surgery patients using short acting anesthetics. *Anesthesiol* 97:66, 2002.

35. Grazer FM, deJong RH: Fatal outcomes from liposuction: Census survey of cosmetic surgeons. *Plast Reconstr Surg* 105:436,2000.

36. Kenkel JM, Lipschitz AH, Luby M, et al.: Hemodynamic physiology and thermoregulation in liposuction. *Plast Reconstr Surg* 114:503,2004.

37. deJong RH, Grazer FM: Perioperative management of cosmetic liposuction. *Plast Reconstr Surg* 107:1039,2001.

38. Trott SA, Beran SJ, Rohrich RJ, et al.: Safety consideration and fluid resuscitation in liposuction: An analysis of 53 patients. *Plast Reconstr Surg* 102:2220,1998.

39. Steele SM, Nielsen KC, Klein SM (eds.): *Ambulatory Anesthesia Perioperative Analgesia*. New York, McGraw Hill, 2005.

40. Casac L, Jewell M: Non-narcotic acute pain relief after aesthetic surgery. *Aesth Surg J* 22:493,2002.

41. Friedberg BL: Facial laser resurfacing with propofol-ketamine technique: Room air, spontaneous ventilation (RASV) anesthesia. *Dermatol Surg* 25:569,1999.

42. Blakely KR, Klein KW, White PF, et al.: A total intravenous technique for outpatient facial laser resurfacing. *Anesth Analg* 87:827,1998.

43. Chung F, Mezei G: Factors contributing to a prolonged stay after ambulatory surgery. *Anesth Analg* 89:1352,1999.

44. Joshi GP: Fast tracking in outpatient surgery. *Curr Opin Anesthesiol* 14:635,2001.

45. Marshall SI, Chung F: Discharge criteria and complication after ambulatory surgery. *Anesth Analg* 88:508,1999.

46. Joshi GP, Twersky R: Fast tracking in ambulatory surgery. *Ambul Surg* 8:185,2000.

47. Joshi GP: New concepts in recovery after ambulatory surgery. *Ambul Surg* 10:167,2003.

48. McHugh GA, Thoms GM: The management of pain following day case surgery. *Anaesthesia* 57:270,2002.

49. Pavlin DJ, Chen C, Penaloza DA: Pain as a complicating recovery and discharge after ambulatory surgery. *Anesth Analg* 95:627,2002.

50. Marcus JR, Few JW, Chao JD, et al.: Prevention of emesis. *Plast Reconstr Surg* 109:2487,2002.

51. Gan TJ, Meyer T, Apfel CC, et al.: Consensus guidelines for managing postoperative nausea and vomiting. *Anesth Analg* 97:62,2003.

52. Gupta AM, Wu CL, Elkassabany N, et al.: Does the routing prophylactic use of antiemetics affect the incidence of postdischarge nausea? *Anesthesiol* 99:488,2003.

53. Gan TJ, Sloan F, de L Dear G, et al.: How much are patients willing to pay to avoid postoperative vomiting? *Anesth Analg* 92:393,2001.

54. Apfel CC: A simplified risk score for predicting postoperative nausea. *Anesthesiol* 91:693,1999.

55. Cohen MM, Duncan PG, Debor DP, et al.: The postoperative interview: Assessing risk factors for nausea and vomiting. *Analg* 78:7,1994.

56. Cepeda MS, Gonzalez F, Granados V, et al.: Incidence of nausea and vomiting in outpatients undergoing general anesthesia. *J Clin Anesth* 8:324,1996.

57. Geldner G, Wulf H: Muscle relaxants suitable for day case surgery. *Eur J Anaesthesiol* 18(S23):43,2001.

58. Tramer MR, Fuchs-Buder T: Omitting antagonism of neuromuscular block: Effect on postop nausea. *Br J of Anaesth* 82:379,1999.

59. Habib AS, Gan TJ: Combination antiemetics: What is the evidence? *Int Anesthesiol Clin* 41:119,2003.

60. White PF, Hamza MA, Recart A, et al.: Optimal timing of acustimulation for emetic prohylaxis as an adjunct to ondansetron in patients undergoing plastic surgery. *Anesth Analg* 100:367,2005.

61. Tang J, Wang B, White P, et al.: The effect of timing of ondasetron administration on its efficacy, cost-effectiveness. *Anesth Analg* 86:274,1998.

62. Barbosa MV, Nahas FX, Ferreira LM: Ondansetron for the prevention of postoperative nausea and vomiting: Which is the best dosage for aesthetic surgery patients? *Aesth Plast Surg* 28:33,2004.

63. Wang JJ, Ho ST, Tzen JI, et al.: The effect of timing of dexamethasone administration on it efficacy. *Anesth Analg* 91:136,2000.

64. Henzi I, Walder B, Tramer M: Dexamethasone for the prevention of postoperative nausea and vomiting. *Anesth Analg* 90:186,2000.

65. Fuji Y, Tanaka H, Toyooka H: The effects of dexamethasone on posantiemetics in female patients. *Anesth Analg* 85:913,1997.

66. Jin FL, Norris A: Should adult patients drink fluids before discharge from ambulatory surgery? *Can J Anesth* 87:306, 1998.

67. MHAUS: www.mhaus.org.

68. Most D, Koslow J, Heller J: Thromboembolisn in plastic surgery. *Plast Reconst Surg* 115:20,2005.

69. Jewell M: Prevention of DVT in aesthetic surgery. *Aesth Surg J* 2:161,2001.

70. Reinisch JF, Bresnick SD, Walker JW, et al.: Deep venous thrombosis and pulmonary embolus after facelift. *Plast Reconstr Surg* 107:157,2001.

71. McDevitt NB: American Society of Plastic and Reconstructive Surgeons – DVT prophylaxis. *Plast Reconstr Surg* 104:1923,1999.

72. Lofsky AS: Deep venous thrombosis and pulmonary embolism in plastic surgery office procedures. *The Doctors' Company Newsletter.* Napa, CA, 2005 ww.thedoctors.com/risk/specialty/anesthesiology/J4254.asp

73. Friedberg BL: Propofol-ketamine technique, dissociative anesthesia for office surgery: A five year review of 1,264 cases. *Aesth Plast Surg* 23:70,1999.

74. Laurito CE: Anesthesia provided at alternative sites, in Barasch PG, Cullen BF, Stoelting RK (eds.), *Clinical Anesthesia,* 4th ed., Philadelphia, Lippincott, Williams & Wilkins, 2001; p1343.

14 | Preanesthetic Assessment of the Cosmetic Surgery Patient

Norman Levin, M.D.

INTRODUCTION

Over the past two decades, outpatient cosmetic surgical procedures have grown at an exponential rate, progressing from simple procedures in a physician's office surgical suite to a broad spectrum of procedures in offices and freestanding ambulatory surgery centers in addition to the hospital setting. This number continues to grow as more office surgery suites and ambulatory surgical centers continue to open. This rapid growth in ambulatory surgery would not have been possible without the changing role of the anesthesiologist and the development of better and shorter acting anesthetic medications.

The preanesthetic evaluation of the surgical patient is the first duty of an anesthesiologist to a patient. Klafta and Rozien identified six interrelated goals of the preanesthetic evaluation.[1] The first is to assess health and ensure physical readiness for anesthesia-requiring procedures. The second is to devise a mutually agreeable anesthetic plan and to educate the patient about it. The third is to reduce the psychological and physiological consequences of anxiety. The fourth is to plan postoperative care and pain therapy. The fifth is to coordinate patient care in a way that decreases total cost and improves outcomes. The sixth is to obtain informed consent for anesthesia (Table 14-1).

Table 14-1. Six preanesthetic goals

1. Assess health and physical readiness for surgery
2. Devise an anesthetic plan and inform patient thereof
3. Reduce anxiety
4. Plan postoperative care and pain management
5. Coordinate patient care
6. Obtain informed consent for anesthesia

The preanesthetic evaluation provides one of the most formidable challenges for anesthesiologists and represents a focused assessment to address issues relevant to the safe administration of anesthesia. The preanesthetic evaluation gives the anesthesiologist the opportunity to meet, comfort, and allay any anxiety that the patient might have concerning the surgical procedure. The preanesthetic evaluation is also an opportunity to assess the health of the patient, to educate the patient concerning anesthesia, and to obtain pertinent information concerning the patient's medical history and an informed consent.

In the past, only "healthy" patients were acceptable candidates for ambulatory (or office-based) surgery. However, in cosmetic surgery over the years, the number of patients with more severe medical problems has increased through the utilization of different anesthetic techniques. The preanesthetic assessment of the cosmetic patient is of utmost importance and should not be different than that of any patient undergoing other types of surgical procedures in any setting, whether it be in ambulatory surgical centers, office surgical suites, or hospital surgical suites. However, with the continued growth of ambulatory surgery centers and office-based surgical procedures, this has placed the anesthesiologist in a position of being the most involved in the direct medical care of the patient.

Previously unacceptable, high-risk patients, many of whom comprise cosmetic patients, are now being done in outpatient surgical centers. As a result, a new role has been created for the anesthesiologist. That is why the preanesthetic assessment is very important and most beneficial in identifying medical problems, previous anesthetic problems, family history of anesthetic problems, medications and/or herbal supplements patients might be taking, and the hour at which food or liquids were taken.

During the preanesthesia evaluation, information should be reviewed from multiple sources, including the patient's medical records, other physician evaluations and physical examinations, and medical and laboratory tests, in addition to the patient's interview.

Because of the importance of the preanesthetic assessment, this chapter reviews many of the aspects involved in the anesthetic management of the patient undergoing cosmetic surgery. Many cosmetic surgeons utilize the services of other medical specialties, such as internal medicine, for the medical workup and the appropriate laboratory tests. In addition to the internist giving clearance for surgery, it must be emphasized that the anesthesiologist is ultimately responsible for the pre- and postoperative management of that patient.

PAST MEDICAL HISTORY

Obtain information concerning the patient's past medical history. Although the ASA patient-physical-status classification is widely accepted, it is only a gross predictor of the overall outcome and not a predictor of anesthetic risk (Table 14-2). In the past, the majority of patients undergoing cosmetic surgery were healthy individuals (ASA physical status 1 or 2). However, over the years, the number of patients with various severe medical problems (ASA physical status 3) has increased, and these patients have undergone outpatient cosmetic surgery with safety. This has been possible because of newer and better medications for medical conditions, in addition to faster-acting anesthetic agents and the improvement of anesthesia monitoring equipment. Natof concluded that ASA physical status 3 patients, whose systemic diseases were well controlled preoperatively, were at no higher risk for postoperative complications than ASA 1 or 2 patients.[2] Many cosmetic patients come to surgery with numerous medical conditions, but only the most common ones are discussed in this chapter.

Table 14-2. ASA patient physical status

ASA 1	A normal healthy patient
ASA 2	A patient with a mild systemic disease
ASA 3	A patient with a severe systemic disease that limits activity
ASA 4	A patient with severe systemic disease that is a constant threat to life
ASA 5	A moribund patient who is not expected to survive without the operation
ASA 6	A declared brain-dead patient whose organs are being removed for donor purposes

Hypertension

A large number of patients undergoing cosmetic surgery have a history of hypertension and are on blood pressure medications. These patients should continue their medications until and including the day of surgery. Diuretics should not be taken before surgery to limit the possibility of intraoperative enuresis.

At what level of blood pressure in hypertensive patients would it be acceptable to proceed with surgery? According to Dix, there is little evidence to support canceling surgery in patients who present for surgery with systolic blood pressures between 140 and 179 mm Hg and diastolic blood pressures between 90 and 109 mm Hg.[3]

Patients with systolic blood pressures between 180 and 210 mm Hg are **three** *times more likely to suffer postoperative myocardial ischemia than those with a preoperative blood pressure of 120 mm Hg.*[4]

There are some patients who come to the operating room without a history of hypertension, yet the anesthesiologist finds hypertension to be present. Anxiety concerning the procedure can cause the blood pressure to be elevated. Some of these patients could have a cardiac abnormality. Approximately 10% of the general population has an increased incidence of altered left-ventricular structure and function when mildly stressed.[5]

An increase in blood pressure can also occur when epinephrine is injected by the surgeon for surgical hemostasis.

An elevated blood pressure can occur in patients undergoing general anesthesia, especially during the induction of anesthesia and intubation with an endotracheal tube. Compared with direct laryngoscopy, a lower incidence of hypertension in hypertensive patients can be achieved during laryngeal intubation when utilizing a lightwand device or a laryngeal mask airway (LMA) Fastrack™.[6] There is an increasing recognition that systolic blood pressure is as important or more important than diastolic blood pressure in elderly patients. Older patients with systolic hypertension are at increased risk for stroke and cardiac events.[7] Control the patient's blood pressure during the preanesthesia period or immediately prior to the induction of anesthesia or before the injection of epinephrine by the surgeon.

Beta-blockers are used as the first line of antihypertensive drugs for the treatment of hypertension. Beta-blockade in the perioperative period decreases perioperative cardiac morbidity and mortality. There are many cases in which beta-blocker use can be justified, but certainly on any patient with hypertension in the perioperative period. If there are no strong contraindications, atenolol, metoprolol, or labetolol could be considered in such a patient.[8, 9] Patients at risk of cardiovascular morbidity are increasingly receiving perioperative beta-blocker therapy.[10] For those patients in whom beta-blockers might be contraindicated (i.e., asthmatics), hydralazine or a nitrate should be considered. Patients will tolerate pressure elevator but not heart rate elevation. It is mandatory to avoid tachycardia.

Cardiac Disease

Many older patients coming for cosmetic surgery have an abnormal cardiac history and are under good control with pharmacological management. There are many commonly seen dysrhythmias such as sinus tachycardia, sinus bradycardia, and ventricular and atrial premature beats.

Bradycardia is frequently seen in patients who might be athletically active or on medications accounting for their slow heart rate. In other patients, tachycardia might be a new problem needing further study and treatment prior to surgery.

Alternatively, tachycardia might be due only to anxiety with the release of endogenous catecholamines. Sedatives or cardiac medications might be necessary to control the dysrhythmia prior to commencing with the surgical procedure. As previously mentioned, most cosmetic surgeons use epinephrine for hemostasis, and this can cause the dysrhythmia to become more exaggerated and severe.

Patients with a history of myocardial infarction (MI) should not have a cosmetic surgery for at least six months following the occurrence. Multiple studies have demonstrated an increased incidence of reinfarction if the MI was within six months of surgery.[11–13] Patients with unstable acute coronary syndromes, such as unstable angina or decompensated congestive heart failure of ischemic origin, are at high risk of developing further decompensation, myocardial necrosis, and death during the perioperative period. Patients with unstable acute coronary syndromes should **not** be considered for cosmetic (or any) surgery, unless absolutely necessary.[14]

Based on observations of the surgery on thousands of patients, the author notes that neither increasing age nor the presence of **stable** preexisting disease has any effect on the incidence of postoperative complications in the surgical outpatient setting.

Diabetes Mellitus

There are many patients coming for cosmetic surgery with a history of diabetes mellitus. Diabetes mellitus (DM) is the most commonly encountered endocrinopathy and is a progressive disease of glucose dysregulation. This carbohydrate intolerance frequently results in significant acute and long-term systemic sequelae. The goal of the anesthesiologist is to maintain the patient in a physiological state to mimic normal metabolism.

Avoid hypoglycemia. Administer exogenous glucose, if necessary. Prevent excessive hyperglycemia, ketoacidosis, and electrolyte disturbances. Administer exogenous insulin when needed. The well-controlled, diet-treated patient with NIDDM (non–insulin-dependent diabetes mellitus) does not require any type of special treatment. Patients on oral hypoglycemic drugs should continue their medication until the evening before surgery. Patients with well-controlled insulin-dependent diabetes mellitus (IDDM) may not need any adjustment in their usual subcutaneous insulin dosage. In all diabetic patients, an Accu-chek® or some other method of blood sugar determination should be performed during the immediate preoperative evaluation, and insulin medication, where appropriate, should be administered.

Most IDDM patients check their blood sugars on a regular basis. Many internists like to control their patient's insulin dosage for surgery and suggest an amount of insulin to be taken on the day of surgery. If the patient's physician does not recommend an insulin regimen, the anesthesiologist should suggest one. A commonly used approach is to reduce the intermediate preparation of insulin by one fourth (25%) to one half (50%) the usual daily dosage the morning of surgery. If regular insulin is part of the morning schedule, the intermediate-acting insulin dose may be increased by 0.5 unit for each unit of regular insulin.

When a patient receives insulin and is not eating, an intravenous of glucose solution should be started in the preoperative period to minimize the chance of hypoglycemia during or after surgery.

Herbal Supplements

Obtain information during the preanesthesia evaluation about the use of herbal medications that are often found in herbal dietary supplements, diet pills, muscle builders, and so-called power drinks (see Appendix A). The use of over-the-counter herbal medications during the perioperative period is an area of both enormous consumer enthusiasm and physician concern.[15] Several studies have suggested that patients undergoing surgery appear to use herbal medications significantly more frequently than the general population.[16, 17] Many cosmetic surgical patients have not only a concern for their appearance but also a great concern for their health. As a result, they often take herbal medications to improve their physical well-being. Kaye and colleagues reported that nearly a third of the patients in an ambulatory surgical setting admitted to using herbal medications, and over 70% of those patients failed to disclose their herbal medicine use during their routine preoperative assessment.[17]

The danger to patients is that morbidity and mortality with herbal medications may be more likely in the perioperative period because of the polypharmacy and physiologic alterations that occur during that time.[18] Adverse reactions that may be caused by supplements include prolonged bleeding, interference with anesthesia, cardiovascular disturbances, and interactions with pharmaceuticals (Table 14-3). Also, it may be extremely difficult to differentiate cause and effect related to surgery versus the use of herbal medications when dealing with postoperative complications such as myocardial infarction, stroke, coagulation disorders, prolonged effects of anesthetics, and interference with medications necessary for patient care.

The five most popular herbal products in the United States are (1) Gingko Biloba, (2) St. John's Wort, (3) Ginseng, (4) Garlic, and (5) Echinacea. Gingko Biloba can inhibit platelet function, causing intraoperative bleeding (see Chapter 12 for the particular risk with neuraxial blockade). St. John's Wort has multiple drug interactions and is contraindicated with MAOIs and SSRIs. Ginseng can interact with cardiac and hypoglycemic agents. Garlic can inhibit platelet function, causing increased bleeding. Echinacea can cause immunosuppression and a potential for hepatotoxicity.[19, 20] Ephedra (ma huang) is contained in many supplements. Ephedra is dangerous because it *indirectly* causes release of endogenous catecholamines. Increased catecholamines contribute to perioperative instability with hypertension, tachycardia, dysrhythmia, and potentially myocardial infarction. Anesthesiologists must inquire specifically as to the use of herbal medications from their patients.

Table 14-3. Supplements contraindicated in the perioperative period

Supplement	Common Use(s)	Adverse Effects
Echinacea	Simulates immune system, used in common cold and bronchitis	Can cause hepatotoxicity, may decrease effectiveness of corticosteroids
Ephedra (ma huang)	CNS stimulant, diet aid, bronchodilator, nasal decongestant	Death, tachycardia, hypertension, myocardial infarction
Garlic	Blood pressure and lipid lowering, antithrombotic, antiviral	Affects platelet aggregation, avoid with anticoagulants
Ginger	Antispasmodic, antiemetic	Can prolong bleeding time, contraindicated with anticoagulants
Ginkgo Biloba	Enhances blood flow, alleviates vertigo and tinnitus	Can increase bleeding time, contraindicated in patients on anticoagulants
Ginseng	Improves physical and cognitive enhancer, antioxidant	May interact with cardiac and hypoglycemic medication, contraindicated with anticoagulants
Goldenseal	Anti-inflammatory, diuretic	May worsen edema and hypertension
Kava kava	Anxiolytic, sedative, analgesic	May potentiate barbiturates, antidepressants, and general anesthesia
Licorice	Gastric and duodenal ulcers and bronchitis	May cause hypertension, hypokalemia, and edema
Melatonin	Insomnia, jet lag	May potentiate barbiturates and general anesthetics
St. John's Wort	Antidepressant	Multiple drug interactions, contraindicated with MAOIs and SSRIs

When asked about medications for medical reasons, many patients feel that herbals are completely safe and do not consider them to be drugs.

The ASA recommends that supplements producing adverse effects be avoided for at least two weeks prior to surgery and one week after surgery.

PAST ANESTHETIC HISTORY

A review of the patient's past anesthetic and surgical history is important. The review can make the anesthesiologist aware of prior anesthetic problems and/or complications that the patient or a family member might have experienced. This will enable the physician to develop a better anesthetic plan for the care, comfort, and safety of the patient.

Malignant Hyperthermia (MH)

Although extremely rare, malignant hyperthermia is a potentially fatal complication of anesthesia. During

the preoperative evaluation, the anesthesiologist should obtain from the patient or a family member information concerning previous anesthetic problems. This is especially important for those patients who have experienced or are susceptible to MH. In those individuals, preparations for safe administration of anesthesia are necessary to avoid a catastrophic outcome. A treatment plan for MH should be available in every anesthetizing location. MH-triggering agents (i.e., halothane, enflurane, isoflurane, desflurane, sevoflurane, and succinylcholine) should not be used on patients susceptible to MH or their undiagnosed relatives.

All facilities, including ambulatory surgery centers and offices, where MH-triggering anesthetics are administered should stock dantrolene sodium for injection.

With the avoidance of the MH-triggering agents, preanesthesia treatment with dantrolene is not recommended for most MH-susceptible patients. Neither propofol nor ketanine are triggering agents.

PREGNANCY

Occasionally patients who are not aware of being pregnant are scheduled for cosmetic surgery. Mandatory pregnancy testing on all females during their reproductive years (between ages twelve and fifty years) is a controversial issue. Spontaneous abortion and teratogenic effects may occur during the first trimester of pregnancy.[21]

Teratogenic effects of anesthetics are probably minimal to nonexistent and have never been conclusively demonstrated in humans.

The drugs that were of most concern included nitrous oxide and the benzodiazepines.[22,23] In animal studies, nitrous oxide, if not combined with a halogenated (sympatholytic) agent, may cause vasoconstriction of the uterine vessels with a decrease in uterine blood flow. No adverse effect of nitrous oxide has been demonstrated in human pregnancy. The maintenance of uterine perfusion and maternal oxygenation to preserve fetal oxygenation are the keys to any anesthetic during pregnancy, with the avoidance of maternal hypoxia and hypotension being essential.

If, during the presurgical workup, a *positive pregnancy* test occurs, *delay the surgery* until after the delivery. Delay may avoid any suspicion of anesthetic involvement causing either the spontaneous abortion or fetal abnormalities that might occur.

PHYSICAL EXAMINATION

One of the major responsibilities of the anesthesiologist is to physically evaluate the cosmetic surgical patient immediately before surgery concerning the risk of anesthesia and of the procedure to be performed. At a minimum, a focused preanesthetic physical examination should include an assessment of the airway, lungs, and heart with documentation of the vital signs.

The importance of the preanesthesia airway examination of the cosmetic surgical patient cannot be understated. It is not important whether the proposed anesthetic administered to the patient is local with intravenous sedation, total intravenous anesthesia (TIVA), or general anesthesia. The unexpected need for airway support, whether by endotracheal intubation, LMA, or other means, should be evaluated in advance for the possibility of being a difficult airway. If an emergency arises and the need for endotracheal intubation should become necessary, it is impera-

tive to determine which patient might present as a difficult intubation.

The failure of the anesthesiologist to monitor and maintain a patent airway, when involved with the patient undergoing cosmetic surgery, is one of the most common causes of anesthesia-related morbidity and mortality (see Chapter 18).

Keeping the airway patent and protected is an important function of the anesthesiologist. Mallampati suggested that the size of the base of the tongue is an important factor in determining the degree of difficulty of direct laryngoscopy.[24] A relatively simple grading system that involves the preoperative ability to visualize the faucial pillars, soft palate, and base of uvula was designed as a means of predicting the degree of difficulty in laryngeal exposure. Khan modified Mallampati's classification utilizing the upper-lip bite test as an acceptable option for predicting difficult intubation as a simple, single test.[25]

PREOPERATIVE TESTS

Preoperative Tests Should Not Be Routinely Ordered

The ASA Task Force on Preanesthesia Evaluation concluded that routine preoperative tests do not make an important contribution to the process of preoperative assessment and management of the patient by the anesthesiologist.[27] It is the patient's underlying condition and the likelihood that the results will affect the anesthetic plan that should guide the choice of preprocedure laboratory tests, chest x-ray, and EKG. Preoperative tests may be ordered on a selective basis for optimizing perioperative management. Most cosmetic surgical patients come to surgery having had a workup by an internist or other physician giving medical clearance for the surgery. Often a request is made to the anesthesiologist for specific tests or studies. The ASA Task Force on Preanesthesia Evaluation concluded that there should not be rules for ordering preoperative tests but only for selected clinical situations.[26] Depending on the patient's clinical situation, the following studies might act as a guide in preoperative testing.

Electrocardiogram (EKG)

Patients with a known history of cardiovascular disease should have an EKG. *The ASA Task Force feels that age alone is not an indication for an EKG.* However, many others feel that having a baseline EKG for patients over forty years of age might be beneficial.

Laboratory Tests

For active healthy patients, laboratory tests might not be necessary for males below fifty years of age. For females in this age range, only hemoglobin (or hematocrit) should be necessary. Patients with chronic diseases (e.g., hypertension, diabetes) should have the appropriate additional laboratory studies (e.g., electrolytes, glucose) as indicated for a medical condition. Also, patients with an unexplained hemoglobin less than $10 \text{ gm} \cdot \text{dl}^{-1}$ should undergo further evaluation prior to elective cosmetic surgery. Testing should rule out other diseases (e.g., liver disease, anemia, bleeding, and other hematological disorders) that could influence perioperative mortality and morbidity.

Chest Radiographs

Unless the patient has clinically acute pulmonary symptoms, routine chest x-rays are not necessary.

PREOPERATIVE PREPARATION

Anxiety

The preoperative assessment and communication with the patient is essential in obtaining information. Many presurgical patients are very anxious in spite of a telephone conversation with the anesthesiologist the night before surgery.[27] However, Levin has found that a call to the patient the night before surgery has the effect of allaying anxiety and decreasing the need for preoperative sedative medications. In the past, it has been shown that the preoperative visit by the anesthesiologist is more effective than preoperative barbiturate medication in reducing perioperative anxiety.[28] A significant amount of anxiety is present at least six days prior to surgery in *unprepared* patients.[29] High levels of anxiety are often associated with other adverse outcomes, such as an increased incidence of emesis. Frequently, cosmetic surgical patients who need anxiolytics are not given preoperative medications because of concern for prolonged recovery and discharge from the facility. However, midazolam, with a relatively short half-life and the lack of significant side effects produces excellent amnesic and anxiolytic properties without any delay in discharge from the facility (see Chapter 7). Oxorn found a threefold incidence of patients

requesting postoperative analgesia in a group that received preoperative midazolam compared to a group that did not.[29a]

Prevention of Postoperative Nausea and Vomiting (PONV)

As part of the preoperative evaluation, it is important to identify patients in whom PONV occurred following a previous surgical procedure or are at a high risk for developing such a complication. PONV is often a limiting factor in the early discharge of ambulatory surgery patients, in addition to being a leading cause of unanticipated hospital admission.[30,31]

Typically, the administration of opioids, as part of a preanesthetic regimen or during the course of an anesthetic, is known to increase the incidence of PONV. General anesthesia carries a higher risk of PONV than regional anesthesia, major conduction anesthesia (subarachnoid or epidural block), intravenous anesthesia, or monitored anesthesia care. Perhaps the most controversial aspect of general anesthesia is the independent risk associated with the administration of nitrous oxide.

Many patients prefer the avoidance of PONV than the avoidance of postoperative pain.[32]

Not all patients should receive PONV prophylaxis. However, patients at small risk for PONV are unlikely to benefit from prophylaxis and would be put at unnecessary risk from the potential side effects of antiemetics. Thus, prophylaxis should be reserved for those patients at moderate to high risk for PONV. Individuals with four primary risk factors for PONV were reported by Apfel et al.[33] as patients receiving balanced inhalation anesthesia: female sex, nonsmoking status, history of PONV, and opioid use. The incidence of PONV with the presence of none, one, two, three, or all four of these risk factors was approximately 10%, 20%, 40%, 60%, and 80%, respectively. Reduce the risk of PONV whenever clinically practical. Patients receiving general anesthesia had an elevenfold increase in risk for PONV compared with those receiving regional anesthesia.[34]

Propofol, administered for the induction and maintenance of anesthesia, effectively reduced early PONV incidence.[35] Oxygen supplementation restricted to the intraoperative period also halved the risk of PONV.[36] Hydration can also reduce the incidence of PONV.[37] Avoiding nitrous oxide and volatile inhaled anesthetics and minimizing intraoperative and postoperative opioid use reduced the incidence of PONV.[33,38-43] Scuderi et al.[44] tested the efficacy of a multimodal approach to reducing PONV. Their multimodal approach consisted of preoperative anxiolysis, aggressive hydration, oxygen, prophylactic antiemetics (droperidol and dexamethasone at the induction with ondansetron at the end of surgery), total IV anesthesia with propofol and remifentanil, and ketorolac. No nitrous oxide or neuromuscular blockade was used. Patients who received multimodal therapy had a 98% complete response rate, compared with a 76% response rate among patients receiving antiemetic monotherapy and a 59% response rate among those receiving routine anesthetic plus saline placebo.

The introduction of serotonin antagonists (specifically the 5-HT$_3$ subgroup) in the early 1990s offered considerable promise for the management of PONV. Ondansetron, dolasetron, and granisetron are the drugs approved for PONV prophylaxis. Prophylactic administration of this class of medication has been shown to decrease the incidence of PONV in various patient populations. Comparisons of ondansetron and dolasetron for PONV prophylaxis suggest that there are no clinically or statistically significant differences between these medications.[45]

Recently, combinations of antiemetics administered prophylactically appear to be more effective than either antiemetic alone. For instance, the combination of ondansetron and droperidol is more effective than either of the two medications alone.[46] The same is true for the combination of ondansetron and dexamethasone.[47] Dimenhyrinate (Dramamine®) 50 mg IM or IV may also be a useful antiemetic, especially for patients prone to motion sickness. The timing of administration of antiemetics is very important. Some medications work best when given preoperatively, and others work best when given intra- or postoperatively. Dexamethasone administered at prophylactic doses of 2.5–5 mg has been found to effectively prevent nausea and vomiting[48,49] and is most effective when administered before the induction of anesthesia as it peaks one to two hours after administration.[50]

Serotonin Receptor Antagonists are most effective when given at the end of surgery.[51,52] For ondansetron, the optimal dose for prophylaxis seems to be 4 mg administered intravenously at the end of surgery, prior to emergence from anesthesia. The optimal dose of dolasetron appears to be 12.5 mg and the timing of administration for prophylaxis appears to be less important than for ondansetron. For droperidol, the optimal dose is 0.625–1.25 mg and mostly effective when given at the end of surgery. Droperidol in doses of either 0.625 mg or 1.25 mg compares favorably with ondansetron 4 mg in outpatients. In fact, the higher dose of droperidol (i.e., 1.25 mg) is more effective than ondansetron in preventing nausea.[53]

In December 2001, the FDA issued a "black box" warning for droperidol in response to patient deaths associated with cardiac rhythm abnormalities.

Metoclopramide stimulates gastric emptying and is administered at the end of surgery. Metoclopramide's usefulness is uncertain except in patients where gastric stasis is an issue. Prochlorperazine (Compazine®) is as effective as ondansetron but can cause extrapyramidal symptoms. Transdermal scopolamine (Transderm-Scop®) has an onset of action of four hours. Thus, it should be applied far enough in advance to ensure it has time to start working, but it can cause visual disturbances and dry mouth. The various side effects caused by some of these medications – sedation, dysphoria, cardiac effects, and extrapyramidal reactions – have been a concern for clinicians, particularly when treating outpatients.

Prevention of Aspiration Pneumonitis

Many patients with gastrointestinal disorders, such as decreased lower esophageal sphincter tone, hiatal hernia, and gastroesophageal reflux, are at risk for aspiration of gastric contents into the lungs. When patients are anesthetized, aspiration can occur with active vomiting or passive regurgitation, most commonly during the induction of anesthesia, when the airway is unprotected. Patients must be informed of the presurgery fasting requirements either by the anesthesiologist or the surgeon, who must also explain the possible complications if not followed. During the immediate preanesthesia assessment, obtain information concerning the hour at which food or drink was ingested. For patients not at risk for aspiration, the "ASA Practice Guidelines for Preoperative Fasting" recommends that patients may ingest clear liquids until two hours prior to surgery and should avoid solids or nonhuman milk for six or more hours prior to surgery.[54]

There is controversy concerning the administration of prophylactic medication for prevention of pulmonary injury from aspiration of gastric contents. Decreasing the volume and pH of the gastric contents can reduce the risk of pulmonary aspiration. The prophylactic use of medications in all patients to prevent pulmonary aspiration can be associated with unwanted side effects. However, patients with predisposing factors for this complication may be candidates for prophylactic treatment.

Medications used to prevent aspiration pneumonitis include H_2-receptor antagonists, a dopamine antagonist, and nonparticulate oral antacids. The H_2-receptor antagonists cimetidine and ranitidine are effective in decreasing gastric-acid secretion and raising the pH. However, neither cimetidine nor ranitidine influence the acid already present in the stomach. Ranitidine should be given two hours prior to surgery because it peaks in two hours.[55] Metoclopramide, a dopamine antagonist, reduces gastric volume by stimulating gastric emptying without any effect on the pH and increases lower esophageal sphincter tone.[56] Sodium citrate (0.3M, 30 ml) and Bicitra,® both nonparticulate oral antacids, are effective in raising pH, but can increase gastric volume. Used in conjunction with metoclopropamide and when prophylaxis is desired, the onset of action is immediate.[57]

Particulate antacids should not be used, as they can worsen the pulmonary damage if aspirated.

However, according to the "ASA Practice Guidelines for Preoperative Fasting," the use of these medications to decrease the risks of pulmonary aspiration in those patients who are not at an increased risk for this complication is not recommended.[54]

SUMMARY

The preanesthetic evaluation of the cosmetic patient is one of the most important functions for the anesthesiologist. The number of patients with a variety of severe medical conditions undergoing cosmetic surgery in an outpatient surgical setting continues to increase and, because of this, the anesthesiologist is the physician most involved in the direct medical care of the patient. As much information as possible concerning the patient's medical and anesthetic history, with appropriate medical records and laboratory tests, should be obtained and reviewed in the preoperative period for a better and safer patient anesthetic experience.

REFERENCES

1. Klafka JM, Rozien MF: Current understanding of patient's attitudes toward and preparation for anesthesia: A review. *Anesth Analg* 83:1314,1996.
2. Natof HE: Pre-existing medical problems. Ambulatory surgery. *IL Med J* 166:101,1984.
3. Dix P, Howell S: Survey of cancellation rate of hypertensive patients undergoing anesthesia and elective surgery. *Br J Anaesth* 86:7889,2001.
4. Howell SJ, Hemming AE, Allman KG, et al.: Predictors of postoperative myocardial ischaemia. The role of intercurrent arterial hypertension and other cardiovascular risk factors. *Anaesthesia* 52:107,1997.
5. Muscholl MW, Hense HW, Brockel U, et al.: Changes in left ventricular structure and function in patients with white coat hypertension: Cross sectional survey. *Br Med J* 317:565, 1998.
6. Kihara S, Brimacombe J, Yaguchi Y, et al.: Hemodynamic responses among three tracheal intubation devices in normotensive and hypertensive patients. *Anesth Analg* 96:890, 2003.
7. Cannel WB: Risk stratification in hypertension: New insights from the Framingham study. *Am J Hypertension* 13:3S,2000.
8. Auerbach AD, Goldman L: Beta-blockers and reduction of cardiac events in noncardiac surgery. Scientific review. *JAMA* 287:1435,2002.
9. Auerbach AD, Goldman L: Beta-blockers and reduction of cardiac events in non-cardiac surgery. Clinical applications. *JAMA* 287:1445,2002.
10. Howell SJ, Sear JW, Foex P: Peri-operative beta-blockade: A useful treatment that should be greeted with cautious enthusiasm. *Br J Anaesth* 86:161,2001.
11. Tarhan S, Moffitt EA, Taylor WF, et al.: Myocardial infarction after general anesthesia. *JAMA* 220:1451,1972.
12. Rao TLK, Jacobs KH, El-Etr AA: Reinfarction following anesthesia in patients with myocardial infarction. *Anesthesiol* 59:499,1983.
13. Shah KB, Kleinman BS, Sami H, et al.: Reevaluation of peri-operative myocardial infarction in patients with prior myocardial infarction undergoing non-cardiac operations. *Anesth Analg* 71:231,1990.
14. Shah KB, Kleinman BS, Rao T, et al.: Angina and other risk factors in patients with cardiac diseases undergoing non-cardiac operations. *Anesth Analg* 70:240,1990.
15. Ang-Lee MK, Moss J, Yuan C: Herbal medicine and perioperative care. *JAMA* 286:208,2001.
16. Tsen LC, Segal S, Pothier M, et al.: Complementary and alternative medicine use should be included in preoperative evaluations. *Anesthesiol* 931:148,2000.

17. Kaye AD, Clarke RC, Sabar R, et al.: Herbal medicines: Current trends in anesthesiology practice – A hospital survey. *J Clin Anesth* 12:468,2000.

18. Bovil JG: Adverse drug interactions in anesthesia. *J Clin Anesth* 9 (Suppl 6):3S,1997.

19. Ernest E: The risk-benefit profile of commonly used herbal therapies: Ginko, St. John's Wort, Ginseng, Echinacea, Saw Palmetto, and Kava. *Ann Int Med* 136:42,2002.

20. Petry JJ: Surgically significant nutritional supplements. *Plast Reconstr Surg* 97:233,1996.

21. Boiven JF: Risk of spontaneous abortion in women occupationally exposed to anesthetic gases: A meta-analysis. *Occup Environ Med* 54:541,1997.

22. Mazze RI: Halothane prevents nitrous oxide teratogenicity in Sprague-Dawley rats; folic acid does not. *Teratology* 38:121,1988.

23. Shiono PH, Mills JL: Oral clefts and diazepam use during pregnancy. *N Engl J Med* 311:919,1984.

24. Mallampati SR, Gatt SP, Gugino LD, et al.: A clinical sign to predict difficult tracheal intubation: A prospective study. *Can Anaesth Soc J* 32:429,1985.

25. Khan ZH, Kashfi A, Ebrahimkhani E: A comparison of the upper lip bite test (a simple new technique) with modified Mallampati classification in predicting difficulty in endotracheal intubation: A prospective blinded study. *Anesth Analg* 96:595,2003.

27. Practice advisory for preanesthesia evaluation: A report by the American Society of Anesthesiologists task force on preanesthesia evaluation. *Anesthesiol* 96:490,2002.

28. McLeanne GJ, Cooper R: The nature of peri-operative anxiety. *Anesthesia* 45:153,1990.

29. Egbert LD, Battit GE, Turndorf H, et al.: The value of preoperative visit by the anesthetist. *JAMA* 185:553,1963.

29a. Oxorn DC, Ferris LE, Harrington E, Orser BA: The effects of midazolam on propofol-induced anesthesia: Propofol dose requirements, mood profiles, and perioperative dreams. *Anesth Analg* 85:553,1997.

30. Johnson M: Anxiety in surgical patients. *Psychol Med* 10:145,1980.

31. Gold BS, Kitz DS, Lecky JH, et al.: Unanticipated admission to the hospital following ambulatory surgery. *JAMA* 262:3008,1989.

32. Fortier J, Chung F, Su J: Unanticipated admission after ambulatory surgery: A prospective study. *Can J Anaesth* 45:612,1998.

33. Macario A, Weinger M, Carney S, et al.: Which clinical anesthesia outcomes are important to avoid? *Anesth Analg* 89:652,1999.

34. Apfel CC, Laara E, Koivuranta M, et al.: A simplified risk score for predicting postoperative nausea and vomiting. *Anesthesiol* 91:693,1999.

35. Sinclair DR, Chung F, Mezei G: Can post-operative nausea and vomiting be predicted? *Anesthesiol* 91:109,1999.

36. Visser K, Hassink EA, Bonsel GJ, et al.: Randomized controlled trial of total intravenous anesthesia with propofol versus inhalation anesthesia with isoflurane-nitrous oxide: Post-operative nausea with vomiting and economic analysis. *Anesthesiol* 95:616,2001.

37. Goll V, Ozan A, Greif R, et al.: Ondansetron is no more effective than supplemental intraoperative oxygen for prevention of postoperative nausea and vomiting. *Anesth Analg* 92:112,2001.

38. Yogendran S, Asokumar B, Cheng DC, et al.: A prospective randomized double-blinded study of the effect of intravenous fluid therapy on adverse outcomes on outpatient surgery. *Anesth Analg* 80:682–6,1995.

39. Apfel CC, Kranke P, Eberhart LH, et al.: Comparison of predictive models for postoperative nausea and vomiting. *Br J Anaesth* 88:234,2002.

40. Tram M, Moore A, McQuay H: Meta-analytic comparison of prophylactic anti-emetic efficacy for postoperative nausea and vomiting: Propofol anaesthesia vs. omitting nitrous oxide vs. total i.v. anaesthesia with propofol. *Br J Anaesth* 78:256,1997.

41. Apfel CC, Katz MH, Kranke P, et al.: Volatile anaesthetics may be the main cause of early but not delayed postoperative vomiting: A randomized controlled trial of factorial design. *Br J Anaesth* 88:659,2002.

42. Sukhani R, Vazquez J, Pappas AL, et al.: Recovery after propofol with and without intra-operative fentanyl in patients undergoing ambulatory gynecologic laparoscopy. *Anesth Analg* 83:975,1996.

43. Mniche S, Rsing J, Dahl JB, et al.: Non-steroidal anti-inflammatory drugs and the risk of operative site bleeding after tonsillectomy: A quantitative systematic review. *Anesth Analg* 96:68,2003.

44. Polati E, Verlato G, Finco G, et al.: Ondansetron versus metoclopramide in the treatment of postoperative nausea and vomiting. *Anesth Analg* 85:395,1997.

45. Scuderi PE, James RL, Harris L, et al.: Multi-modal anti-emetic management prevents early postoperative vomiting after outpatient laparoscopy. *Anesth Analg* 91:1408, 2000.

46. Zarate E, White P, Klein KW, et al.: A comparison of the costs and efficacy of ondansetron versus dolasetron for antiemetic prophylaxis. *Anesth Analg* 90:1352,2000.

47. Riley TJ, McKenzie R, Tantisira BR, et al.: Droperidol-ondansetron combination versus droperidol alone for postoperative control of emesis after total abdominal hysterectomy. *J Clin Anesth* 10:6,1998.

48. Sanchez-Ledesma MJ, Lopez-Olaondo L, Pueyo FJ, et al.: A comparison of three anti-emetic combinations for the prevention of post-operative nausea and vomiting. *Anesth Analg* 95:1590,2002.

49. Wang JJ, Ho ST, Lee SC, et al.: The use of dexamethasone for preventing postoperative nausea and vomiting in females undergoing thyroidectomy: A dose-ranging study. *Anesth Analg* 91:1404,2000.

50. Wang JJ, Ho ST, Tzeng JI, et al.: The effect of timing of dexamethasone administration on its efficacy as a prophylactic anti-emetic for post-operative nausea and vomiting. *Anesth Analg* 91:136–9,2000.

51. Domino KB, Anderson EA, Polissar NL, et al.: Comparative efficacy and safety of ondansetron, droperidol, and metoclopramide for preventing post-operative nausea and vomiting: A meta-analysis. *Anesth Analg* 88:1370,1999.

52. Sun R, Klein KW, White PF: The effect of timing of ondansetron administration in outpatients undergoing otolaryngologic surgery. *Anesth Analg* 84:331,1997.

53. Graczyk SG, McKenzie R, Kallar S, et al.: Intravenous dolasetron for the prevention of post-operative nausea and vomiting after outpatient laparoscopic gynecologic surgery. *Anesth Analg* 84:325,1997.

54. Fortney JT, Gan TJ, Graczy KS, et al.: A comparison of the efficacy, safety, and patient satisfaction of ondansetron versus droperidol as anti-emetics for elective outpatient surgical procedures. S3A-409 and S3A-410 Study Groups. *Anesth Analg* 86:731,1998.

55. ASA practice guidelines for preoperative fasting and the use of pharmacologic agents to reduce the risk of pulmonary aspiration: Application to healthy patients undergoing elective procedures. *Anesthesiol* 90:896,1999.

56. Manchikanti L, Colliver JA, Roush JR, et al.: Evaluation of ranitidine as an oral antacid in outpatient anesthesia. *South Med J* 78:818,1985.

57. Hey VMF, Ostrick DG, Mazumder JK, et al.: Pethidine, metoclopramide and gastro-oesophageal sphincter. *Anaesthesia* 36:173,1981.

58. Manchikanti L, Grow JB, Colliver JA, et al.: Bicitra® (sodium citrate) and metoclopramide in outpatient anesthesia for prophylaxis against aspiration pneumonitis. *Anesthesiol* 63:378,1985.

15 | Psychological Aspects of Cosmetic Surgery

David B. Sarwer, Ph.D., Canice E. Crerand, Ph.D., and Lauren M. Gibbons, B.A.

INTRODUCTION

According to the American Society of Plastic Surgeons (ASPS), over fifteen million Americans underwent a plastic surgical procedure in 2003.[1] The majority of plastic surgical procedures consisted of relatively new, minimally invasive, nonsurgical procedures. These numbers, while familiar to many plastic surgeons, are often staggering to other medical professionals and lay persons who have little idea of the number of Americans who turn to medicine to enhance their physical appearance. Nevertheless, these numbers likely underestimate the number of procedures performed annually, as they do not account for nonplastic surgeon physicians who offer these treatments. In particular, the preceding numbers do not reflect the surgical activity of either the American Academy of Cosmetic Surgeons (AACS) or the American Society of Dermatologic Surgeons (ASDS).

The growth in popularity of cosmetic surgery and related treatments can be attributed to several factors.[2–4] Changes in the medical and surgical communities, including improvements in safety and direct-to-consumer marketing, have likely contributed to the growth. The mass media and entertainment industries have long championed cosmetic surgery, perhaps no more so than during the current era of "reality-based" television programs such as "Extreme Makeover" and "The Swan." The virtually inescapable bombardment of mass-media ideals of beauty, coupled with the discontent that many people, particularly women, experience with regard to their physical appearance, have likely contributed as well.[5,6] Finally, society's acceptance of the use of medicine to enhance appearance, perhaps paired with a greater awareness of the importance of physical appearance in daily life, has potentially fueled cosmetic surgery's increase in popularity. Plastic surgeons and mental health professionals have long been interested in the psychological aspects of cosmetic surgery. Understanding the psychological characteristics of patients who desire and undergo cosmetic procedures is important for practical reasons. Cosmetic procedures are often considered analogous to psychological interventions; many patients report increased satisfaction with their appearance, as well as psychological improvements, postoperatively.[7] Nevertheless, these procedures are likely not appropriate for all individuals, particularly those with certain characteristics or psychiatric disorders.

Thus, an understanding of the psychological functioning of cosmetic surgery patients is an important part of maximizing treatment outcomes. This chapter reviews studies of the pre- and postoperative psychosocial functioning of persons who seek and undergo cosmetic surgery. A review of the psychological studies of individuals who have undergone the most common facial procedures begins the chapter. The second major section discusses studies of persons who have undergone cosmetic procedures of the body. The chapter concludes with a discussion of the psychiatric disorders that may be most relevant to this population—**body dysmorphic disorder** and **eating disorders**.

COSMETIC PROCEDURES OF THE FACE

Rhinoplasty

Rhinoplasty is traditionally one of the most popular cosmetic surgical procedures, with over 350,000 performed in 2003.[1] The psychological characteristics of rhinoplasty patients have received as much research attention as those of persons who have undergone any cosmetic procedure. The first reports date back to the 1940s and 1950s. These investigations, as well as studies conducted into the 1960s, relied heavily on clinical interviews and suggested that patients were highly psychopathological.[8,9] Early investigators typically conceptualized the desire for rhinoplasty from a psychodynamic perspective, the prevailing theoretical orientation in psychiatry at the time. The nose was often thought to symbolize the penis, and the desire for rhinoplasty was believed to represent the patient's unconscious displacement of sexual conflicts onto the nose.[10] For the adolescent female patient, the desire for rhinoplasty was interpreted as an attempt to remove elements of her father's personality from her own.[11]

During the 1970s and 1980s, a "second generation" of research in cosmetic surgery began to include valid and reliable measures to assess patients' psychological characteristics.[2,3] Studies of this era found less preoperative psychopathology and several noted postoperative benefits.[12–17] For example, investigations that used the Minnesota Multiphasic Personality Inventory (MMPI), likely the most widely used measure of personality, reported that the personality profiles of rhinoplasty patients were essentially normal preoperatively, and no changes were observed postoperatively.[14,15] Unfortunately, many of these studies suffered from methodological problems, such as small sample sizes and the lack of appropriate control groups, which call into question the validity of the findings. Studies through the present have used improved methodologies, including reliable and valid self-report measures and clinical interviews with established diagnostic criteria.[18–25] Most studies also have included pre- and postoperative assessments with appropriate control groups. These studies have suggested that most rhinoplasty patients are psychologically healthy individuals. As noted by at least one study,[25] the desire for rhinoplasty may be understood as an increased dissatisfaction with the size and/or shape of the nose, rather than a symptom of psychopathology. These findings are consistent with the experiences of most present-day cosmetic surgeons.

Anti-Aging Procedures

Rhytidectomy and blepharoplasty are two of the most popular surgical procedures for those interested in restoring a more youthful appearance. In 2003, 128,667 facelifts and 246,633 blepharoplasty procedures were performed in the United States.[1] (As these procedures are often performed concurrently, studies of these patient populations are reviewed together.)

Early reports suggested that facelift patients were quite psychopathological. Patients were often characterized as dependent and depressed; approximately 70% of patients received a preoperative psychiatric diagnosis.[26] However, the majority reported postoperative improvements in well-being and did not experience postoperative "emotional disturbances."[26] Studies that used standardized self-report measures noted similar improvements in psychological symptoms postoperatively.[24,27]

Other studies have examined the body-image concerns of these patients. In one of the first empirical studies investigating the body-image concerns of cosmetic surgery patients, nearly half of the patients studied sought facelift or blepharoplasty procedures.[28] They reported higher levels of dissatisfaction with the feature for which they sought surgery, but they did not report increased dissatisfaction with their overall body image.[28] Rhytidectomy and/or blepharoplasty patients have reported greater investment in their appearance as well as greater satisfaction with their overall body image as compared to women who sought rhinoplasty.[25] Postoperatively, patients reported decreases in body-image dissatisfaction for the feature that was treated but no changes in overall body image.[29]

Minimally Invasive Anti-Aging Procedures

Minimally invasive anti-aging procedures have surpassed the popularity of the more traditional anti-aging surgical procedures. For example, nearly 2.9 million botulinum toxin (Botox®) injections were performed in 2003, making it the most popular of all cosmetic treatments.[1] The toxin is typically injected into areas of the face (i.e., forehead creases, "crow's feet") in order to reduce the appearance of wrinkling. It is also effective at treating excessive sweating. Other popular minimally invasive procedures include fat injections, collagen injections, chemical peels, dermabrasion, and laser resurfacing. Like Botox® injections, these procedures can improve the appearance of wrinkled, scarred, or sun-damaged skin. In 2004, the Food and Drug Administration (FDA) approved a product specifically designed to improve lipo-atrophy in persons with HIV disease. New generations of customized facial implants also are being used to treat this condition.[30] It is quite possible that these products will also be used for cosmetic purposes in persons without HIV disease in the near future.

Despite their popularity, little is known about the psychological characteristics or body-image concerns of the patients who seek these procedures. A German study of thirty patients who received Botox® injections for facial lines examined post-treatment social outcomes and attitudes toward appearance.[31] Over half of those studied reported improvements in their appearance and nearly 50% reported greater confidence in their appearance.[31] A recent study of 178 patients seeking laser skin resurfacing reported that 18% received prior treatment for depression.[32] A third study evaluated the psychosocial benefits associated with alpha-hydroxy acid, a topical treatment that is used to reduce roughness and fine wrinkling. Patients noted significant improvements in appearance and relationship satisfaction following treatment.[33]

Other Facial Procedures
Facial skeletal procedures

Some patients request more "atypical" procedures that involve bone contouring and/or grafting as well as the insertion of cheek, chin, or other facial implants. One study described fifteen patients who sought extensive symmetrical facial skeletal recontouring procedures in order to address discontent with facial width.[34] These "facial width deformity" patients reported concerns with minor, largely *unnoticeable* anatomic deviations.

Preoperative psychiatric interviews revealed that the majority experienced significant impairment in psychosocial functioning, though only three (of fifteen) received a formal psychiatric diagnosis. The clinical descriptions of these patients, however, suggest that some may have been suffering from body dysmorphic disorder, discussed in detail herein. Postoperatively, patients reported improvements in body image and psychosocial functioning, although psychometric measures were not used to assess these changes.[34]

Although requests for some of these facial-widening procedures are rare, more patients are requesting procedures such as cheek and chin implants in order to change the structural appearance of their faces. In 2003, over 28,000 chin or cheek implantation procedures were performed.[1] The popularity of these procedures underscores the need for more research regarding the psychological characteristics and body-image concerns of these patients.

Acne treatment

Many patients present to plastic surgeons, dermatologists, or other professionals complaining of acne or acne-related scarring. This is not surprising, considering that acne affects at least 80% of adolescents.[35] The occurrence of acne typically decreases with age; however, it may persist through adulthood for a minority of persons.[36]

Historically, the psychosocial effects of acne have been dismissed, largely as it was considered a non–life-threatening, age-related cosmetic condition.[37] More health professionals now recognize the impact acne may have on psychological and social well-being. Up to 50% of adolescents experience psychological difficulties associated with acne, including body-image concerns, poor self-esteem, social isolation, and depression.[38] Studies of patients who seek acne treatment have found similar results.[37,39–41]

For some, the distress may become so severe that it contributes to suicidal ideation or suicide attempts.[40,42] Facial acne patients, compared to those with truncal acne, appear to be particularly vulnerable to the psychological effects of the disease, experiencing lower self-esteem and greater body-image dissatisfaction.[41] The distress appears to be related to the self-perceived rather than objective severity

of the acne.[43] Acne patients report impairments in quality of life on par with those of other chronic medical conditions, such as epilepsy and diabetes.[44]

Acne treatment appears to result in improvements in psychosocial functioning.[45,46] Kellett and Gawkrodger reported significant reductions in anxiety and depression, but not general emotional distress, following treatment with isotretinoin.[39] The authors concluded that some of the psychological effects of acne may remain despite successful treatment. This finding makes intuitive sense, given that acne can result in permanent scarring. Extended duration of acne and acne excoriee (skin picking) are associated with greater likelihood of scarring.[47] Even in the absence of residual cutaneous scars, emotional scars may remain. Cash and Santos found that former adolescent acne sufferers, especially women and those recalling more subjectively severe acne, reported less current facial satisfaction and more body-image dysphoria than peers who did not have facial acne as teenagers.[48] The psychosocial distress associated with acne has implications for medical professionals who treat acne-related scars. These providers may be able to assess the psychological effects of this disorder and provide appropriate mental health treatment referrals when warranted.[49]

Vitiligo

Vitiligo is a progressive condition characterized by loss of skin pigmentation, resulting in irregular hypopigmented patches.[50] Generalized vitiligo, the most common form, is characterized by bilateral, symmetric depigmentation of the face (particularly periorificial area), neck, torso, wrists, and legs.[51] The prevalence of vitiligo is estimated to be about 1–2% of the world population.[52] Age of onset is typically childhood or young adulthood.[51] Although there is no cure, medical treatments include topical cosmetics, use of psoralens and UVA light to stimulate repigmentation (PUVA), corticosteroids, and surgical skin grafting.[51,52]

Similar to acne, the psychological distress associated with vitiligo is often underestimated.[50] The condition appears to have a negative impact on the social and emotional well-being of its sufferers.[53] Patients often report difficulties with body image, self-esteem, and quality of life.[50] Similar psychological sequelae have been reported among patients with other chronic skin conditions, including eczema and psoriasis.[40,54,55]

A more extensive review of the psychological characteristics of patients who seek dermatological treatment is beyond the scope of this chapter; interested readers are directed to these reviews and books.[56–58]

Encouragingly, cognitive-behavioral psychotherapy appears to be a successful treatment for the psychological distress associated with these conditions.[50]

Hair Loss and Hair Transplantation

Head hair possesses considerable cultural, social, and personal significance.[59,60] As a result, hair loss can be a psychologically difficult experience for some. There are a number of hair-loss conditions; the most prevalent is *androgenetic alopecia* (AGA), or common genetically predisposed hair loss. AGA is a progressive condition mediated by androgenic metabolism (especially dihydrotestosterone). The receding frontal hairline and vertex balding is visibly evident in the majority of men. AGA also occurs in a significant minority of women, although the pattern of alopecia is one of diffuse thinning.

AGA can be a very distressing condition for both genders, albeit more troubling for women.[61,62] Among men, increased distress is associated with earlier onset of hair loss. It is also experienced by men who are more psychologically invested in their appearance and by younger men not involved in an intimate relationship.[63,64] The effects of AGA on women may be more extensive, including lower self-esteem.[64] As with many other conditions, the subjective severity of AGA is more related to its psychosocial impact than are objective or clinical indices of severity.[61]

Most outcome data for AGA treatment comes from large, controlled clinical trials of minoxidil and finasteride.[61,65,66] The psychological outcome measures in these studies have focused largely on patients' perceptions of, and satisfaction with, resultant hair growth and generally support the efficacy of the treatments. There is a dearth of outcomes research using more psychologically sophisticated measures. One uncontrolled study of 144 men treated with topical minoxidil confirmed moderate hair growth and improvements on hair-specific quality-of-life measures (e.g., hair-loss distress and perceived social noticeability of the hair loss) but not on more global measures of anxiety, depression, or self-esteem.[67]

In recent years, there have been major advances in surgical methods of hair replacement, including micrografting and flap techniques, especially for men with AGA.

Hair transplantation is a more certain and permanent method of hair replacement in less time. The popularity of hair transplantation has decreased in the past several years, likely due to the availability of prescription and over-the-counter medical treatments for AGA. Surprisingly, no formal studies have investigated the psychological characteristics of persons who seek hair transplantation or the psychological changes that may occur after treatment. Given the prevalence of AGA, studies are clearly warranted.

COSMETIC PROCEDURES OF THE BODY

Cosmetic Breast Augmentation

Despite the controversy surrounding silicone-gel–filled breast implants, the number of American women who have undergone cosmetic breast augmentation (primarily with saline-filled implants) has increased by no less than 600% in the past decade.[1] The dramatic increase is remarkable considering that in 1992 the FDA issued a moratorium on the use of silicone-gel–filled implants because of concerns related to the physical safety of the implants. Several studies and literature reviews since have suggested that silicone breast implants are *not* associated with specific diseases, including cancer and connective tissue disease.[68–72] These findings, along with others, motivated two breast-implant manufacturers to reapply for FDA approval for silicone-gel–filled implants in early 2005.

Many studies have examined the psychological characteristics of women who undergo cosmetic breast augmentation. Some have provided important information on the characteristics of women interested in the procedure. Others have investigated the psychological changes typically experienced postoperatively.

Descriptive characteristics and motivational factors

The average breast augmentation patient appears to be quite different than the stereotypical one. The typical woman is European-American, in her late twenties or early thirties, and is married with children.[73–83] Many of these women pursue augmentation with the goal of returning their breasts of their former, pre-childbirth size and shape. In contrast, the stereotypical patient is thought to be younger, single, and interested in breast augmentation as a way to facilitate the development of a romantic relationship. Nevertheless, women from their late teens to mid forties of varying ethnic backgrounds and relationship status present for breast augmentation. Given the increasing popularity of the procedure, there likely is no "typical" patient.

Several factors likely motivate women to undergo breast augmentation.[84] Intrapsychic factors describe the internal motivations for surgery and the resulting effects on psychological status. Interpersonal factors concern the importance of the appearance of the breasts in marital, sexual, and social relationships. Women anticipate an improved quality of life, body image, and self-esteem, as well as increased marital and sexual satisfaction following breast enlargement.[77,82,83,85–88] Informational and medical factors also are thought to play a role in the decision to seek augmentation. Women who undergo breast augmentation obtain a great deal of information about breast implants from the mass media[85,89,90] and appear to be aware of many of the risks associated with the procedure.[85,87,91]

Nevertheless, women who receive breast implants differ from their peers in several ways. Women with breast implants are more likely to have had more sexual partners, report a greater use of oral contraceptives, be younger at their first pregnancy, and have a history of terminated pregnancies as compared to other women.[92–95] They have been found to be more frequent users of alcohol and tobacco.[93–95] They also have a higher divorce rate.[82,83] Finally, they have been reported to have a below-average body weight,[85,92–96] leading to concern that some may be experiencing eating disorders (*vide infra*).

Studies of pre- and postoperative psychological status

Numerous studies have investigated the preoperative psychological status of women interested in breast augmentation. As with the studies of persons interested in facial procedures, the early generations of research in this area relied primarily on clinical interviews to assess psychological functioning.[84] More often than not, these studies described breast-augmentation patients as experiencing increased symptoms of depression, anxiety, guilt, and low self-esteem.[81–83,97,98] Fewer studies have examined the effects of breast augmentation on psychological functioning. Most of these studies have reported improvements, or at least no change, in self-esteem and depressive symptoms postoperatively.[74,81,97] Subsequent studies were more likely to use valid and reliable psychometric measures to assess relevant characteristics. They typically

have found significantly less psychopathology than the interview-based investigations. For example, two studies of breast-augmentation patients who used psychometric measures, including the MMPI, found little evidence of psychopathology.[76,79] Few investigators have used psychometric measures to assess changes following surgery. One study found a decrease in depressive symptoms after surgery; another reported increased symptoms in 30% of patients in the immediate postoperative period.[99,100] Although generally considered more valid and reliable than the clinical interview studies, these studies have also suffered from methodological problems.

Nevertheless, two tentative conclusions can be drawn from this research.[2,101,102] First, breast-augmentation candidates likely present for surgery with a variety of psychological symptoms and conditions. Whether some of these conditions serve as contraindications for surgery has yet to be established. Second, given the limited number of studies that have specifically investigated the psychosocial benefits of breast augmentation, it is premature to definitively conclude that the procedure confers more general psychological benefits.

Body-image dissatisfaction

The most profound psychological effects of breast augmentation may occur in the realm of body image. An increasing amount of attention has been paid to the relationship between body image and cosmetic surgery over the past decade.[2,7,102–104] Empirical studies have suggested that cosmetic-surgery patients report increased body-image dissatisfaction prior to surgery.[25,85,96,103,105,106] Others have found postoperative improvements in body image.[29,87,107–110]

The body-image concerns of breast-augmentation patients have been described in several reports.[76,77,79] For example, more than 50% of breast-augmentation patients reported significant behavioral avoidance (e.g., avoidance of being seen undressed) in response to negative feelings about their breasts.[111] Compared to women similar in breast size not pursuing breast augmentation, surgery candidates reported greater dissatisfaction with their breasts, greater investment in their overall appearance, and greater concern with their appearance in social situations.[85,96] Augmentation candidates also rated their ideal breast size, as well as the breast size preferred by women, as significantly larger than did controls.[96] Finally, prospective patients reported more frequent teasing about their physical appearance and more frequent use of psychotherapy than controls, suggesting that some breast-augmentation candidates may be experiencing negative emotional consequences as a result of their breast dissatisfaction.[96]

Women who undergo breast augmentation experience improvements in their body image postoperatively, as suggested by clinical reports and empirical studies.[29,76,78,81,87,108] In one of the largest studies of psychosocial outcomes following breast augmentation, greater than 90% of patients reported an improved body image two years postoperatively.[87]

Psychosocial outcomes and postoperative complications

Clinical reports and empirical studies suggest that the vast majority of women are satisfied with the outcome of breast augmentation.[78,87,99,112,113] Patient satisfaction and body-image improvements, however, may be tempered by the occurrence of a postoperative complication. Up to 25% of women experience a surgical or implant-related complication.[114–116] The most common complications are implant rupture/deflation, capsular contracture, pain, breast asymmetry, scarring, loss of nipple sensation, and breast-feeding difficulties.[68,–72,114–118]

Approximately 10% of women who receive breast implants for cosmetic purposes experience a complication within five years of implantation.[114,115]

In a study of 749 women who received breast implants in the United States before 1991 (prior to the FDA ban on silicone-gel–filled implants), 23.8% experienced complications severe enough to require additional surgery.[115] The most common complication was capsular contracture (73.6% of complications, 17.5% of women), followed by implant rupture (24.2% of complications, 5.7% of women), hematoma (24.2% of complications, 5.7% of women), and wound infection (10.7% of complications, 2.5% of women). Large-scale studies in Europe have corroborated these findings.[69,70,116–118]

At least three studies have suggested that the experience of a complication is negatively related to postoperative satisfaction.[87,91,119] In a large prospective study, Cash and colleagues[87] found that although women typically report improvements in self-image and body image after breast augmentation, those who experienced postoperative complications reported less favorable improvements. At six

months after surgery, women who experienced a "socially detectable" complication, such as significant capsular contracture, expressed less surgical and body-image satisfaction compared to women with nonsocially detectable or no complications. By twenty-four months after surgery, the groups did not differ in satisfaction. However, women with "socially detectable" complications viewed the risk-benefit ratio of surgery less favorably compared to those with less visible or no complications.

Breast implants and suicide

In the past few years, four large epidemiological studies in the United States and Europe designed to investigate the relationship between breast implants and mortality found an unexpected relationship between breast implants and suicide.[120–123] The suicide rate (as obtained from patients' death records) was two to three times greater among patients with breast implants as compared to either patients who underwent other cosmetic surgical procedures or population estimates.

The exact nature of the relationship between breast implants and suicide is unclear. Some psychological variable(s), yet to be specified, may explain this relationship. Some women may enter into surgery with unrealistic expectations about the effect that breast augmentation will have on their lives. When these expectations are not met, they may become despondent, depressed, and potentially suicidal. Alternatively, women who experience postoperative complications, particularly those that they believe are a consequence of their implants but that have not been found to be statistically associated with breast implants (e.g., autoimmune and connective tissue diseases), may become depressed as a result of a lack of perceived or real attention from the medical community. Although speculative, both of these hypotheses have some intuitive appeal.

As described earlier, women seeking breast augmentation may present for surgery with certain unique preoperative personality characteristics that may predispose them to commit suicide. Several are, in and of themselves, associated with an increased risk of suicide. Joiner has argued that these personality characteristics could actually account for an even higher suicide rate than found in the epidemiological investigations.[124] He further suggests that postoperative improvements in body image may produce a protective effect from the otherwise increased risk. Jacobsen and colleagues found an increased prevalence of preoperative psychiatric hospitalizations in women who received breast implants as compared to women who underwent other forms of cosmetic surgery or breast reduction.[121] These results suggest that the increased suicide rate among women who have breast implants likely reflects some underlying psychopathology rather than a direct relationship with the implants.[125–126] Obviously, additional prospective epidemiological and empirical studies of the relationship between breast implants and suicide are needed.

Lipoplasty and Abdominoplasty

The United States is in the midst of an obesity epidemic. Approximately two thirds of American adults are now considered to be overweight or obese, as defined by a body mass index (BMI) >25 kg $\cdot$ m^{-2}.[127] Obesity is associated with increased body-image dissatisfaction as well as several significant comorbidities, including coronary heart disease, hypertension, type II diabetes, osteoarthritis, and sleep apnea.[128] Although Americans spend billions of dollars annually in efforts to lose weight, successful long-term weight control proves elusive for most. Although designed for body-contouring purposes, many individuals erroneously believe that lipoplasty (liposuction) and adominoplasty are permanent solutions to weight problems.

Lipoplasty

Over 320,000 men and women underwent lipoplasty in 2003, making it the most popular surgical procedure.[1] Unlike the sizable literature on the psychological characteristics of breast-augmentation patients, few, if any, studies have specifically investigated the pre- and postoperative psychological status of liposuction patients. As with all cosmetic procedures, patients' expectations of the postoperative result are critical to a successful outcome. Many patients mistakenly believe that liposuction leads to significant weight loss. The typical weight loss associated with liposuction has not been well documented. One pilot study of fourteen overweight women reported a mean weight loss of 5.1 kg by six weeks postoperatively, with an additional 1.3 kg weight loss by four months.[129] Studies investigating changes in lipids and insulin sensitivity following liposuction have been equivocal.[130–132]

Many patients erroneously believe that fat deposits will *never* return to the treated areas. Although liposuction

reduces the number of fat cells in a local area of the body, the remaining fat cells may still expand if weight increases. The "average" person has about two million fat cells.

Similarly, some patients may believe that liposuction will result in "washboard abs" and smooth thighs. Unfortunately, if fat cells are not removed in a consistent fashion, residual pockets of fat may remain. Most patients, however, report satisfaction with their results and maintain a more proportional shape, even if they do gain some weight postoperatively.[133,134] Between 40% and 50% reported weight gain after surgery and up to 29% claimed that their fat returned to the site of the surgery.[133,134]

Persons with excessive weight or shape concerns require particular attention prior to lipoplasty. Women and men with formal eating disorders, as discussed in detail herein, may seek lipoplasty as an inappropriate compensatory behavior to control their weight. In a case report of two women with bulimia nervosa who underwent lipoplasty, the request for surgery was accompanied with an unrealistic expectation that surgery would result in an improvement of eating-disorder symptoms.[135] Postoperatively, both women reported a worsening of their bulimic and depressive symptoms, and one woman reported a weight gain of twenty-five pounds in three months.[135] Unfortunately, little else is known about the relationship between eating disorders and lipoplasty.

Abdominoplasty

The number of men and women who seek abdominoplasty has increased steadily over the past decade. The popularity may be a result of the increasing numbers of individuals with extreme obesity who are now undergoing bariatric surgery ("stomach stapling") for weight loss. Bariatric procedures typically result in a weight loss of approximately one third of operative body weight. In addition, the procedure often results in significant improvements in obesity-related comorbidities and psychosocial status.[136] Unfortunately, many patients are left with excess folds of skin and fat on the abdomen, arms, and thighs following the massive weight loss. This redundant skin may contribute to increased body-image dissatisfaction[128] and, as a result, may lead patients to seek abdominoplasty and related procedures. In 2003, approximately 52,000 individuals underwent abdominoplasty and other body-contouring procedures following weight loss associated with bariatric surgery.[1] Although no formal studies exist, case reports suggest that these individuals experience psychosocial improvements and a decrease in the physical discomfort associated with the excess skin.[137]

Only one study has documented the psychosocial changes associated with abdominoplasty. Eight weeks after the surgery, women reported significant improvements in overall body-image dissatisfaction, abdominal dissatisfaction, and self-conscious avoidance of body exposure during sexual activity.[107] Patients did not report significant improvements in self-concept or general life satisfaction. These results are consistent with other postoperative studies, suggesting that the impact of cosmetic surgery procedures may be limited to specific improvements of body-image discontent but not necessarily more general psychosocial functioning.[29]

Other Body Enhancement Procedures

There are an almost limitless number of procedures that can be performed to enhance the body. The following discussion will focus on body-contouring implants, genital enhancement, and tattoos and body piercing.

Body-contouring implants

An increasing number of individuals are using pectoral, calf, gluteal, and other body-contouring implants to improve their appearance. Very little is known about the psychological motivations and characteristics of persons who seek these implants or the psychological changes that may occur postoperatively.[138] Many of the features shaped by these implants are typically covered by clothing. As a result, the changes in appearance are not readily visible to others. Thus, it is quite possible that some individuals who undergo these procedures may be suffering from body dysmorphic disorder or its associated condition, muscle dysmorphia, which are discussed later. Some of these patients, may also be HIV positive and have had loss of muscle mass secondary to their disease process.

Genital enhancement

An unknown number of men and women who are dissatisfied with the appearance of their genitalia pursue what has been called "genital enhancement" or "genital beautification" procedures. Men may undergo procedures to lengthen or widen their genitals. Women may seek surgery to reduce the size of the labia minora. Although these "defects" are sometimes thought to be functional (impeding urination or adversely affecting sexual functioning), there is a significant aesthetic component. Patients typically report that they are motivated for surgery out of embarrassment, either when undressed or wearing tight clothing.[139–140] Little else, however, is known about the psychological characteristics of these patients.[138] Considering the nature of these procedures, it is possible that a significant percentage of these patients are suffering from body dysmorphic disorder or other psychiatric disorders with a delusional or psychotic component. The plastic-surgery literature includes several case reports of individuals who have performed "do-it-yourself" surgeries, such as injecting their genitals with various oils and substances.[141–143]

Tattoos and body piercing

Up to twenty million Americans are estimated to have tattoos.[144] Tattoos are found on 3–8% of the general population and 10–13% of adolescents (ages twelve to eighteen).[145] More than half are found on women.[146] Interestingly, requests for tattoo removal appear to be on the rise as well, perhaps because of the development of more effective laser removal tools.[146] In a study of 105 individuals seeking tattoo removal, 61% reported embarrassment as a consequence of their tattoo(s), and 26% reported a less positive body image.[146]

Accurate estimates of the number of Americans who have undergone body piercing are lacking. Body piercing, particularly when ear piercing is considered, may be even more prevalent than tattoos, as piercings are less expensive, less difficult to obtain, and may be considered less permanent. However, they can result in lifelong complications such as scarring and blood-borne infectious diseases, as well as more temporary complications such as abscesses.[147,148] In a study of 454 college students, 51% had at least one body piercing (including ears), with 17% experiencing a medical complication (e.g., bleeding, local trauma, and bacterial infections).[149] Tongue piercings can be prone to infection and can result in swelling, chipped teeth, speech impediment, and nerve damage.[150]

The presence of tattoos or body piercings in adolescents may be a marker for other risk-taking behavior.[145]

Adolescents with tattoos and/or body piercings were more likely to have engaged in risky behaviors such as drug use and sexual activity and were at increased risk for disordered eating and suicide.[145] Crawford and Cash found that pierced and/or tattooed college students scored higher on a measure of excitement seeking and were more likely to smoke cigarettes and engage in binge drinking relative to their "unmarked" peers.[151] Pierced/tattooed students also reported more body-image dissatisfaction, despite being very pleased with their "body art." Perhaps body dissatisfaction is an impetus to obtain body art to "improve" one's appearance.

PSYCHIATRIC DISORDERS AMONG COSMETIC SURGERY PATIENTS

All of the major psychiatric diagnoses can likely be found within the large population of cosmetic-surgery patients. There is some evidence that body dysmorphic disorder may occur with greater frequency among cosmetic-surgery populations as compared to the general population. Given the relationship of body-image dissatisfaction and cosmetic surgery, eating disorders such as anorexia and bulimia also warrant consideration.

Body Dysmorphic Disorder

Body dysmorphic disorder (BDD) is defined as a preoccupation with an imagined defect in appearance (or if a slight physical defect is present, the person's concern is exaggerated) that results in significant emotional distress or impairment in functioning.[152] Although not recognized as a formal psychiatric disorder in the United States until 1987,[152] descriptions of persons with the distinctive symptoms first appeared in the American dermatology and plastic-surgery literatures much earlier. Reports in the dermatology literature described patients presenting with "dermatological nondisease,"[154] whereas those in the plastic-surgery literature detailed "minimal deformity" and "insatiable" patients.[155,156] These patients typically reported dissatisfaction with their postoperative results.

BDD is estimated to occur in 0.5% to 2% of the general population.[157,158] Rates of 2.5% to 5% have been reported in university samples.[159,162] The condition, however, appears to be far more common among patients presenting for cosmetic surgery. The first study in the

United States suggested that 7% of female cosmetic-surgery patients met criteria for BDD.[28] A recent study of patients seeking only facial cosmetic procedures found that 8% met diagnostic criteria.[163] Among international samples, rates of BDD among cosmetic-surgery patients range from 9% to 53%.[164–167] Rates of 9–15% have been reported in patients seeking dermatological treatment, most commonly for acne.[168–170] Methodological differences in the assessment of symptoms are likely responsible for the wide range of rates reported. Though prevalence rates are unknown, patients with BDD also request treatment from orthodontists, maxillofacial surgeons, and paraprofessionals.[171–174]

Clinical features

Age of onset for BDD is typically late adolescence. The disorder occurs with *equal* frequency among men and women. Most clinical and demographic features appear to be similar between genders.[175,176] Although any body part can be a source of preoccupation, patients typically report concerns with the skin, face, nose, and hair.[171,175,176] Preoccupation with more than one feature is common.[171] Although the course of BDD tends to be chronic, symptom severity, areas of concern, and insight may vary over time.[175,177]

Patients often experience intrusive thoughts about their "defects." Some may recognize the exaggerated nature of these concerns, whereas others may hold more delusional beliefs about their appearance.[178,179] Patients with BDD often engage in compulsive behaviors, such as skin picking, mirror checking, camouflaging, and reassurance seeking often as a means of decreasing their distress.[177,180–184] The condition frequently results in significant emotional distress, impairment in social and occupational functioning, and decreased quality of life.[184–187] Self-harm and suicidality are relatively common.[175,177,181,186,187]

Nonpsychiatric and psychiatric treatments

Individuals with BDD often seek cosmetic and dermatological treatments as a means of decreasing their appearance concerns.[171,173,175,186,187] In the largest study to date of the use of aesthetic treatments by BDD patients (n = 250), 76% sought and 66% received treatment, with dermatological procedures and cosmetic surgery being the most popular.[171] Similarly, in a sample of 200 persons with BDD, nonpsychiatric treatment was sought by 71% and received by 64%.[173] The most commonly received treatments were topical acne agents, rhinoplasty, collagen injections, electrolysis, and tooth whitening.[173]

Studies suggest that nonpsychiatric treatments often are ineffective at reducing the preoccupation with appearance. Greater than 80% have been found to be dissatisfied with the results of cosmetic treatments.[187] Two studies have indicated that the majority of nonpsychiatric treatments received by patients with BDD result in either no change or a worsening in symptoms.[171,173] Following treatment, some patients develop new appearance preoccupations. Others may threaten or enact legal action and/or violence against their surgeons.[188-190] Because of these issues, the presence of BDD is often considered a contraindication for cosmetic procedures.[104,191,192] Selective-serotonin-reuptake-inhibitor antidepressant medications and cognitive-behavioral therapy appear to be more effective strategies for treating BDD.[193-205]

Variants of BDD

Muscle dysmorphia, referring to a preoccupation with being insufficiently large and muscular, is considered a form of BDD.[206] Patients with muscle dysmorphia tend to weight lift and diet in a compulsive manner; they also engage in other checking and camouflaging behaviors (i.e., layering clothing to appear larger). Some use anabolic steroids in order to compensate for their perceived lack of muscularity. Individuals with muscle dysmorphia typically experience significant social and occupational impairment, often because their exercise and eating regimens are so time-consuming. The prevalence of muscle dysmorphia is unknown. Estimates suggest that 5% of nonprofessional weightlifters and 9% of individuals with BDD have the condition.[207]

Another possible variant of BDD, "botulinophilia," was recently described. The condition is characterized by persistent demands for Botox® injections to treat excessive sweating (hyperhidrosis), despite any clinical evidence of a physical problem.[208]

In summary, a significant minority of cosmetic-surgery patients appear to have BDD. Cosmetic treatments, however, appear to be an ineffective treatment for the condition. Treatment providers need to be aware of the potential for BDD in their patients and to provide appropriate mental health referrals when necessary.[191,192,209]

Eating Disorders

Given the disproportionate amount of concern that individuals with anorexia and bulimia nervosa place on their appearance, these disorders may occur with increased frequency among those who seek cosmetic surgery.[138] The distinguishing feature of anorexia nervosa is a fanatical pursuit of thinness related to an overwhelming fear of becoming fat.[152] Patients with bulimia nervosa are generally distinguished from those with anorexia on the basis of relatively normal weight and the presence of binge eating and purging.[152] The normal weight of bulimic patients frequently makes them more difficult to identify than anorexic patients. Persons with both conditions may erroneously believe that cosmetic surgery will improve their immense dissatisfaction with their bodies and self-esteem.

Presently, there is no information on the rate of anorexia or bulimia among cosmetic-surgery patients; investigation has been limited to case reports. Women with both disorders have experienced an exacerbation of their eating-disorder symptoms following breast augmentation, lipoplasty, rhinoplasty, and chin augmentation.[135,210,211] Interestingly, a case report of five breast-reduction patients with bulimia suggested that four of the five women experienced an improvement in their eating-disorder symptoms and psychological distress postoperatively.[212] Impressively, the improvement in eating-disorder symptoms was maintained ten years postoperatively.[213]

SUMMARY

Studies suggest that persons who seek cosmetic procedures experience a wide variety of psychological symptoms. Although early studies conceptualized the desire for cosmetic treatments as being indicative of psychopathology, *recent investigations utilizing improved methodologies suggest that most cosmetic-surgery patients are psychologically "normal."* This finding is consistent with the experiences of most cosmetic-treatment providers today. Body-image dissatisfaction, rather than psychopathology, appears to provide a more reasonable explanation as to why individuals seek to change their appearance.

Future studies are needed to address the motivations of patients who seek cosmetic procedures (particularly body-contouring procedures) and the relationship of body image and preoperative psychopathology to treatment outcome. Although more men now seek cosmetic enhancements, particularly for hair loss, empirical evaluations of gender differences in body image and other psychological characteristics among those who seek cosmetic procedures are lacking. Future studies should incorporate appropriate control groups and standardized pre- and postoperative assessments (including structured clinical interviews and psychometrically sound self-report measures). Although several studies have suggested that patients experience psychosocial improvements after surgery, studies investigating the endurance of these changes beyond the first or second postoperative year are needed.

The studies reviewed in this chapter have implications for clinical practice. Clearly, it is not uncommon for patients requesting cosmetic procedures to experience psychosocial distress, particularly those seeking treatments for chronic skin conditions. Furthermore, a minority of patients likely present with serious psychiatric disorders, such as BDD and eating disorders. Patients complaining of minimal appearance flaws or excessive emotional distress should be evaluated for BDD. Additionally, patients presenting for body procedures, such as lipoplasty, abdominoplasty, and breast augmentation, should be assessed for symptoms of eating disorders. Because persons with these disorders may be more likely to present for surgical rather than psychiatric treatment, cosmetic-treatment providers are in a unique position to identify such patients and to provide appropriate referrals to mental health professionals.

REFERENCES

1. American Society of Plastic Surgeons. *National clearinghouse of plastic surgery statistics.* Arlington Heights, IL: ASPS;2004.
2. Sarwer DB, Crerand CE: Body image and cosmetic medical treatments. *Body Image: Internat J Res* 1:99,2004.
3. Sarwer DB, Magee L, Crerand CE: Cosmetic surgery and cosmetic medical treatments, in JK Thompson (ed.), *Handbook of Eating Disorders and Obesity.* Hoboken, John Wiley & Sons, Inc., 2004;p718.
4. Cash TF: Body image and cosmetic surgery, in Sarwer DB, Pruzinsky T, Cash TF, Goldwyn RM, Persing LA, Whitaker LA (eds.), *Psychological Aspects of Reconstructive and Cosmetic Surgery: Empirical, Clinical, and Ethical Issues.* Philadelphia, Lippincott, Williams & Wilkens, in press.
5. Sarwer DB, Magee L, Crerand CE: Cosmetic surgery and cosmetic medical treatments, in Thompson JK (ed.), *Handbook of eating disorders and obesity.* Hoboken, John Wiley & Sons, Inc. 2004;p718.
6. Sarwer DB, Magee L: Physical appearance and society, in Sarwer DB, Pruzinsky T, Cash TF, Goldwyn RM, Persing LA, Whitaker LA (eds.), *Psychological Aspects of Reconstructive and Cosmetic Surgery: Empirical, Clinical, and Ethical Issues.* Philadelphia, Lippincott, Williams & Wilkens, in press.
7. Sarwer DB, Wadden TA, Pertschuk MJ, et al.: The psychology of cosmetic surgery: A review and re-conceptualization. *Clin Psychol Rev* 18:1,1998.
8. Linn L, Goldman IB: Psychiatric observations concerning rhinoplasty. *Psychosom Med* 11:307,1949.
9. Hill G, Silver AG: Psychodynamic and esthetic motivations for plastic surgery. *Psychosom Med* 12:345,1950.
10. Book HE: Sexual implications of the nose. *Compr Psychiatry* 12:450,1971.
11. Gifford S: Cosmetic surgery and personality change: A review and some clinical observations, in Goldwyn RM (ed.), *The Unfavorable Result in Plastic Surgery: Avoidance and Treatment,* 1st ed., New York, Little, Brown, 1973; p 1.
12. Hay GG: Psychiatric aspects of cosmetic nasal operations. *Br J Psychiatry* 116:85,1970.
13. Robin AA, Copas JB, Jack AB, et al.: Reshaping the psyche: The concurrent improvement in appearance and mental state after rhinoplasty. *Br J Psychiatry* 152:539,1988.
14. Wright MR, Wright WK: A psychological study of patients undergoing cosmetic surgery. *Arch Otolaryngol* 101:145, 1975.
15. Micheli-Pellegrini V, Manfrida GM: Rhinoplasty and its psychological implications: Applied psychology observations in aesthetic surgery. *Aesth Plast Surg* 3:299,1979.
16. Hay GG, Heather BB: Changes in psychometric test results following cosmetic nasal operations. *Br J Psychiatry* 122: 89,1973.
17. Marcus P: Psychological aspects of cosmetic rhinoplasty. *Br J Plast Surg* 37:313,1984.
18. Ercolani M, Baldaro B, Rossi N, et al.: Short-term outcome of rhinoplasty for medical or cosmetic indication. *J Psychosom Res* 47:277,1999.
19. Ercolani M, Baldaro B, Rossi N, et al.: Five-year follow-up of cosmetic rhinoplasty. *J Psychosom Res* 47:283,1999.
20. Goin MK, Rees TD: A prospective study of patients' psychological reactions to rhinoplasty. *Ann Plast Surg* 27:210,1991.
21. Hern J, Hamann J, Tostevin, P, et al.: Assessing psychological morbidity in patients with nasal deformity using the CORE questionnaire. *Clin Otolaryngol* 27:359,2002.
22. Hern J, Rowe-Jones J, Hinton A: Nasal deformity and interpersonal problems. *Clin Otolaryngol* 28:121,2003.
23. Borges-Dinis P, Dinis M, Gomes A: Psychosocial consequences of nasal aesthetic and functional surgery: A controlled prospective study in an ENT setting. *Rhinology* 36:32, 1998.
24. Rankin M, Borah GL, Perry AW, et al.: Quality-of-life outcomes after cosmetic surgery. *Plast Reconstr Surg* 102:2139, 1998.
25. Sarwer DB, Whitaker LA, Wadden TA, et al.: Body image dissatisfaction in women seeking rhytidectomy or blepharoplasty. *Aesth Surg J* 17:230,1997.

26. Webb WL, Slaughter R, Meyer E, et al.: Mechanisms of psychosocial adjustment in patients seeking 'face-lift' operation. *Psychosom Med* 27:183,1965.
27. Goin MK, Burgoyne RW, Goin JM, et al.: A prospective psychological study of 50 female facelift patients. *Plast Reconstr Surg* 65:436,1980.
28. Sarwer DB, Wadden TA, Pertschuk MJ, et al.: Body image dissatisfaction and body dysmorphic disorder in 100 cosmetic surgery patients. *Plast Reconstr Surg* 101:1644, 1998.
29. Sarwer DB, Wadden TA, Whitaker LA: An investigation of changes in body image following cosmetic surgery. *Plast Reconstr Surg* 109:363,2002.
30. Binder WJ, Bloom DC: The use of custom-designed midfacial and sub-malar implants in the treatment of facial wasting syndrome. *Arch Facial Plast Surg* 6:394,2004.
31. Sommer B, Zschocke I, Bergfeld D, et al.: Satisfaction of patients after treatment with botulinum toxin for dynamic facial lines. *Dermatol Surg* 29:456,2003.
32. Koch RJ, Newman JP, Safer DL: Psychological predictors of patient satisfaction with laser skin resurfacing. *Arch Facial Plast Surg* 5:445,2003.
33. Fried RG, Cash TF: Cutaneous and psychosocial benefits of alpha hydroxyl acid use. *Percept Mot Skills* 86:137,1998.
34. Edgerton MT, Langmann MW, Pruzinsky, T: Patients seeking symmetrical recontouring for 'perceived' deformities in the width of the face and skull. *Aesth Plast Surg* 14:59, 1990.
35. Krowchuk DP: Managing acne in adolescents. *Ped Clin N Am* 47:841,2000.
36. White GM: Recent findings in the epidemiologic evidence, classification, and subtypes of acne vulgaris. *J Am Acad Dermatol* 39:S34,1998.
37. Koo J: The psychosocial impact of acne: Patients' perceptions. *J Am Acad Dermatol* 32:S26,1995.
38. Baldwin HE: The interaction between acne vulgaris and the psyche. *Cutis* 70:133,2002.
39. Kellett SC, Gawkrodger DJ: The psychological and emotional impact of acne and the effect of treatment with isotretinoin. *Br J Dermatol* 140:273,1999.
40. Gupta MA, Gupta AK: Depression and suicidal ideation in dermatology patients with acne, alopecia areata, atopic dermatitis, and psoriasis. *Br J Dermatol* 139:846,1998.
41. Papadopoulos L, Walker C, Aitken D, et al.: The relationship between body location and psychological morbidity in individuals with acne vulgaris. *Psychology, Health, and Medicine* 5:431,2000.
42. Cotterill JA, Cunliffe WJ: Suicide in dermatological patients. *Br J Dermatol* 137:246,1997.
43. Krowchuk DP, Stancin T, Keskinen R, et al.: The psychosocial effects of acne in adolescents. *Pediatric Dermatol* 8:332,1991.
44. Mallon E, Newton JN, Klassen A, et al.: The quality of life in acne: A comparison with general medical conditions using generic questionnaires. *Br J Dermatol* 140:672,1999.
45. Rubinow DR, Peck GL, Squillace KM, et al.: Anxiety and depression in cystic acne patients after successful treatment with isotretinoin. *J Am Acad Dermatol* 17:25,1987.
46. MacDonald Hull S, Cunliffe WJ, et al.: Treatment of the depressed and dysmorphic acne patient. *Clin Exp Dermatol* 16:210,1991.
47. Layton AM: Optimal management of acne to prevent scarring and psychological sequelae. *Am J Clin Dermatol* 2:135,2001.
48. Cash TF, Santos M: *Remembrance of things past: The vestigial psychological effects of adolescent acne in early adulthood.* Unpublished manuscript, Old Dominion University, Norfolk, VA;2004.
49. Crerand CE, Cash TF, Whitaker LA: Cosmetic surgery of the face, in Thompson JK (ed.), *Handbook of eating disorders and obesity.* Hoboken, John Wiley & Sons, Inc., 2004;p718.
50. Papadopoulos L, Bor R, Legg C: A preliminary investigation into the effects of cognitive-behavioural therapy. *Br J Med Psychol* 72:385,1999.
51. Kovacs SO: Vitiligo. *J Am Acad Dermatol* 38:647,1998.
52. Hartmann A, Brocker EB, Becker JC: Hypopigmentary skin disorders: Current treatment options and future directions. *Drugs* 64:89,2004.
53. Kent G, Al'Abadie M: Psychologic effects of vitiligo: A critical incident analysis. *J Am Acad Dermatol* 35:895,1996.
54. Rapp SR, Feldman SR, Exum ML, et al.: Psoriasis causes as much disability as other major medical diseases. *J Am Acad Dermatol* 41:401,1999.
55. Novartis. Eczema patients face a lifetime of isolation, bullying, discrimination, and under-performance at school and work (2004). www.novartis.com. International Study of Life with Atopic Eczema. Results presented at the European Academy of Dermatology and Venereology, Florence, Italy.
56. Koo J, Lebwohl A: Psychodermatology: The mind and skin connection. *Am Fam Physician* 64:1873,2001.
57. Gupta MA, Gupta AK: Psychiatric and psychological co-morbidity in patients with dermatological disorders: Epidemiology and management. *Am J Clin Dermatol* 4:833,2003.
59. Kligman AM, Freeman B: History of baldness: From magic to medicine. *Clin Dermatol* 6:83,1988.
60. Morris D: Bodywatching: *A field guide to the human species.* New York, Crown, 1985.
61. Cash TF: The psychosocial consequences of androgenetic alopecia: A review of the research literature. *Br J Dermatol* 141:398,1999.
62. Cash TF: The psychology of hair loss and its implications for patient care. *Clin Dermatol* 19:161,2001.
63. Cash TF: Psychological effects of androgenetic alopecia among men. *J Am Acad Dermatol* 26:926,1992.
64. Cash TF, Price V, Savin R: The psychosocial effects of androgenetic alopecia on women: Comparisons with balding men and female control subjects. *J Am Acad Dermatol* 29:568,1993.
65. Kaufman KD, Olsen EA, Whiting D, et al.: Finasteride in the treatment of men with androgenetic alopecia. *J Am Acad Dermatol* 39:578,1998.
66. Pharmacia & Upjohn Co. Rogaine® Extra Strength for Men (5% Minoxidil Topical Solution) for non-prescription use. Data presented at FDA Non-prescription Drug Advisory

Committee Meeting. July 16, 1997. Pharmacia & Upjohn, Kalamazoo, MI.

67. McNulty P, Buesching DP, Patrick DL, et al.: Change in quality of life in a study of male minoxidil users. *Drug Info J* 27:871,1993.

68. Bondurant S, Ernester VR, Herdman R: Committee on the Safety of Silicone Breast Implants, Division of Health Promotion and Disease Prevention. Safety of Silicone Breast Implants. Washington, DC: National Academy Press; 2000.

69. Holmich LR, Kjoller K, Fryzek JP, et al.: Self-reported diseases and symptoms by rupture status among unselected Danish women with cosmetic silicone breast implants. *Plast Reconstr Surg* 111:723,2003.

70. Jensen B, Wittrup IH, Friss S, et al.: Self-reported symptoms among Danish women following cosmetic breast implant surgery. *Clin Rheumatol* 21:35,2002.

71. Sanchez-Guerrero J, Colditz GA, Karlson EW, et al.: Silicone breast implants and the risk of connective-tissue diseases and symptoms. *N Engl J Med* 332:1666,1995.

72. Silverman BG, Brown SL, Bright RA, et al.: Reported complications of silicone gel breast implants: An epidemiologic review. *Ann Intern Med* 124:744,1996.

73. Edgerton MT, McClary AR: Augmentation mammaplasty: Psychiatric implications and surgical indications. *Plast Reconstr Surg* 21:279,1958.

74. Edgerton MT, Meyer E, Jacobson WE: Augmentation mammaplasty II: Further surgical and psychiatric evaluation. *Plast Reconstr Surg* 27:279,1961.

75. Druss RG: Changes in body image following augmentation breast surgery. *Int J Psychoanal Psychother* 2:248,1973.

76. Baker JL, Kolin IS, Bartlett ES: Psychosexual dynamics of patients undergoing mammary augmentation. *Plast Reconstr Surg* 53:652,1974.

77. Schlebusch L: Negative bodily experience and prevalence of depression in patients who request augmentation mammaplasty. *S Afr Med J* 75:323,1989.

78. Young VL, Nemecek JR, Nemecek DA: The efficacy of breast augmentation: Breast size increase, patient satisfaction, and psychological effects. *Plast Reconstr Surg* 94:958,1994.

79. Shipley RH, O'Donnell JM, Bader KF: Personality characteristics of women seeking breast augmentation. *Plast Reconstr Surg* 60:369,1977.

80. Goin JM, Goin MK: *Changing the body: Psychological effects of plastic surgery*. Baltimore, Lippincott, Williams & Wilkens, 1981.

81. Sihm F, Jagd M, Pers M: Psychological assessment before and after augmentation mammaplasty. *Scan J Plast Surg* 12:295,1978.

82. Beale S, Lisper H, Palm B: A psychological study of patients seeking augmentation mammaplasty. *Br J Psychiatry* 136:133,1980.

83. Schlebusch L, Levin A: A psychological profile of women selected for augmentation mammaplasty. *S Afr Med J* 64:481,1983.

84. Sarwer DB, Nordmann JE, Herbert JD: Cosmetic breast augmentation surgery: A critical overview. *J Womens Health* 9:843,2000.

85. Didie ER, Sarwer DB: Factors that influence the decision to undergo cosmetic breast augmentation surgery. *J Womens Health* 12:241,2003.

86. Birtchnell S, Whitfield P, Lacey JH: Motivational factors in women requesting augmentation and reduction mammaplasty. *J Psychosom Res* 34:509,1990.

87. Cash TF, Duel LA, Perkins LL: Women's psychosocial outcomes of breast augmentation with silicone gel-filled implants: A 2-year prospective study. *Plast Reconstr Surg* 109:2112,2002.

88. Meyer L, Ringberg A: Augmentation mammaplasty-psychiatric and psychosocial characteristics and outcome in a group of Swedish women. *Scand J Plast Reconstr Surg* 21:199,1987.

89. Larson DL, Anderson RC, Maksud D, et al.: What influences public perceptions of silicone breast implants? *Plast Reconstr Surg* 94:318,1994.

90. Palcheff-Wiemer M, Concannon MJ, Cohn VS, et al.: The impact of the media on women with breast implants. *Plast Reconstr Surg*, 92:779,1993.

91. Handel N, Wellisch D, Silverstein MJ, et al.: Knowledge, concern and satisfaction among augmentation mammaplasty patients. *Ann Plast Surg* 30:13,1993.

92. Brinton LA, Brown SL, Colton T, et al.: Characteristics of a population of women with breast implants compared with women seeking other types of plastic surgery. *Plast Reconstr Surg* 105:919,2000.

93. Cook LS, Daling JR, Voigt LF, et al.: Characteristics of women with and without breast augmentation. *JAMA* 277:1612,1997.

94. Fryzek JP, Weiderpass E, Signorello LB, et al.: Characteristics of women with cosmetic breast augmentation surgery compared with breast reduction surgery patients and women in the general population of Sweden. *Ann Plast Surg* 45:349,2000.

95. Kjoller K, Holmich LR, Fryzek JP, et al.: Characteristics of women with cosmetic breast implants compared with women with other types of cosmetic surgery and population-based controls in Denmark. *Ann Plast Surg* 50:6,2003.

96. Sarwer DB, LaRossa D, Bartlett S, et al.: Body image concerns of breast augmentation patients. *Plast Reconstr Surg* 112:83,2003.

97. Ohlsen L, Ponten B, Hambert G: Augmentation mammaplasty: A surgical and psychiatric evaluation of the results. *Ann Plast Surg* 2:42,1978.

98. Napoleleon A: The presentation of personalities in plastic surgery. *Ann Plast Surg* 31:193,1993.

99. Schlebusch L, Marht I: Long-term psychological sequelae of augmentation mammaplasty. *S Afr Med J* 83:267, 1993.

100. Meyer L, Ringberg A: Augmentation mammaplasty—Psychiatric and psychosocial characteristics and outcome in a group of Swedish women. *Scand J Plast Reconstr Surg* 21:199,1987.

101. Honigman R, Phillips KA, Castle DJ: A review of psychosocial outcomes for patients seeking cosmetic surgery. *Plast Reconstr Surg* 113,1229,2004.

102. Sarwer DB, Gibbons LM, Crerand CE: Body dysmorphic disorder and aesthetic surgery, in Nahai F (ed.), *The art of aesthetic surgery: Principles and techniques.* Quality Medical Publishing (in press).

103. Sarwer DB, Pertschuk, MJ, Wadden TA, et al.: Psychological investigations in cosmetic surgery: A look back and a look ahead. *Plast Reconstr Surg* 101:1136,1998.

104. Sarwer DB, Didie ER: Body image in cosmetic surgical and dermatological practice, in Castle DJ, Phillips KA (eds.), *Disorders of Body Image.* Petersfield, UK, Wrightson Biomedical Publishing Ltd.,2002; p 37.

105. Pertschuk MJ, Sarwer DB, Wadden TA, et al.: Body image dissatisfaction in male cosmetic surgery patients. *Aesth Plast Surg* 22:20,1998.

106. Simis KJ, Verhulst FC, Koot HM: Body image, psychosocial functioning, and personality: How different are adolescents and young adults applying for plastic surgery? *J Child Psychol Psychiatry* 42:669,2001.

107. Bolton MA, Pruzinsky T, Cash TF, et al.: Measuring outcomes in plastic surgery: Body image and quality of life in abdominoplasty patients. *Plast Reconstr Surg.* 112:619, 2003.

108. Banbury J, Yetman R, Lucas A, et al.: Prospective analysis of the outcome of subpectoral breast augmentation: Sensory changes, muscle function, and body image. *Plast Reconstr Surg* 113:701,2004.

109. Dunofsky M: Psychological characteristics of women who undergo single and multiple cosmetic surgeries. *Ann Plast Surg* 39:223,1997.

110. Kilman PR, Sattler JI, Taylor J: The impact of augmentation mammaplasty: A follow-up study. *Plast Reconstr Surg* 80:374,1987.

111. Sarwer DB, Bartlett SP, Bucky LP, et al.: Bigger is not always better: Body image dissatisfaction in breast reduction and breast augmentation patients. *Plast Reconstr Surg* 101:1956,1998.

112. Park AJ, Chetty U, Watson ACH: Patient satisfaction following insertion of silicone breast implants. *Brit J Plast Surg* 49:515,1996.

113. Wells KE, Cruse CW, Baker JL, et al.: The health status of women following cosmetic surgery. *Plast Reconstr Surg* 93:907,1994.

114. Cunningham BL, Lokeh A, Gutowski KA: Saline-filled breast implant safety and efficacy: A multicenter retrospective review. *Plast Reconstr Surg* 105:2143,2000.

115. Gabriel SE, Woods JE, O'Fallon WM, et al.: Complications leading to surgery after breast implantation. *N Engl J Med* 336:677,1997.

116. Kjoller K, Holmich LR, Jacobsen PH, et al.: Epidemiological investigation of local complications after cosmetic breast implant surgery in Denmark. *Ann Plast Surg* 48:229,2002.

117. Fryzek JP, Signorello LB, Hakelius L, et al.: Self-reported symptoms among cosmetic breast implant and breast reduction surgery. *Plast Reconstr Surg* 107:206,2001.

118. Fryzek JP, Signorello LB, Hakelius L, et al.: Local complications and subsequent symptom reporting among women with cosmetic breast implants. *Plast Reconstr Surg* 107:214,2001.

119. Fiala TG, Lee WPA, May JW: Augmentation mammoplasty: Results of a patient survey. *Ann Plast Surg* 30:503,1993.

120. Brinton LA, Lubin JH, Burich MC, et al.: Mortality among augmentation mammoplasty patients. *Epidemiology* 12:321,2001.

121. Jacobsen PH, Holmich LR, McLaughlin JK, et al.: Mortality and suicide among Danish women with cosmetic breast implants. *Arch Intern Med* 164:2450,2004.

122. Koot VC, Peeters PH, Granath F, et al.: Total and cause specific mortality among Swedish women with cosmetic breast implants: A prospective study. *Br Med J* 326:527,2003.

123. Pukkala E, Kulmala I, Hovi SL, et al.: Causes of death among Finnish women with cosmetic breast implants, 1971–2001. *Ann Plast Surg* 51:339,2003.

124. Joiner TE: Does breast augmentation confer risk of or protection from suicide? *Aesth Surg J* 23:370,2003.

125. McLaughlin JK, Lipworth L, Tarone RE: Suicide among women with cosmetic breast implants: A review of the epidemiologic evidence. *J Long Term Eff Med Implants* 13:445,2003.

126. Sarwer DB: Discussion of causes of death among Finnish women with cosmetic breast implants, 1971–2001. By Pukkala E, et al. *Ann Plast Surg* 51:343,2003.

127. Hedley AA, Ogden CL, Johnson CL, et al.: Prevalence of overweight and obesity among US children, adolescents and adults, 1999–2002. *JAMA* 291:2847,2004.

128. Sarwer DB, Thompson JK, Cash TF: Obesity and body image in adulthood. *Psych Clin NA* 28:69,2005.

129. Giese SY, Bulan EJ, Commons GW, et al.: Improvements in cardiovascular risk profile with large-volume liposuction: A pilot study. *Plast Reconstr Surg* 108:510,2001.

130. Baxter RA: Serum lipid changes following large-volume suction lipectomy. *Aesth Surg J* 17:213,1997.

131. Klein S, Fontana L, Young VL, et al.: Absence of an effect of liposuction on insulin action and risk factors for coronary heart disease. *N Engl J Med* 350:2549,2004.

132. Samdal F, Birkeland KI, Ose L, et al.: Effect of large-volume liposuction on sex hormones and glucose and lipid metabolism in females. *Aesth Plast Surg* 19:131,1995.

133. Dillerud E, Haheim LL: Long term results of blunt suction lipectomy assessed by a patient questionnaire survey. *Plast Reconstr Surg* 92:35,1993.

134. Rohrich RJ, Broughton G, Horton B, et al.: The key to long-term success in liposuction: A guide for plastic surgeons and patients. *Plast Reconst Surg* 114:1945,2004.

135. Willard SG, McDermott BE, Woodhouse L, et al.: Lipoplasty in the bulimic patient. *Plast Reconstr Surg* 98:276,1996.

136. Sarwer DB, Wadden TA, Fabricatore AN: Psychosocial and behavioral aspects of bariatric surgery. *Obesity Res*, in press.

137. Rhomberg M, Pulzi P, Piza-Katzer H: Single-stage abdominoplasty and mastopexy after weight loss following gastric banding. *Obesity Surg* 13:418,2003.

138. Sarwer DB, Didie ER, Gibbons LM: Cosmetic surgery of the body, in Thompson JK (ed.), *Handbook of eating disorders and obesity.* Hoboken, John Wiley & Sons, Inc., 2004; p 718.

139. Choi HY, Kim KT: A new method for aesthetic reduction of labia minora (the de-epithelialized reduction labioplasty). *Plast Reconstr Surg* 105:419,2000.

140. Perovic SV, Radojicic ZI, Djordjevic ML, et al.: Enlargement and sculpturing of a small and deformed glans. *J Urol* 170:1686,2003.

141. Behar TA, Anderson EE, Barwick WJ, et al.: Sclerosing lipogranulomatosis: A case report of scrotal injection of automobile transmission fluid and literature review of subcutatneous injection of oils. *Plast Reconstr Surg* 91:352,1991.

142. Bhagat R, Holmes IH, Andrzjej K, et al.: Self-injection with olive oil: A cause of lipoid pneumonia. *Chest* 107:875,1995.

143. Cohen JL, Kreoleian CM, Krull EA: Penile paraffinoma: Self-injection with mineral oil. *J Am Acad Dermatol* 45:S222,2001.

144. Greif J, Hewitt W, Armstrong ML: Tattooing and body piercing: Body art practices among college students. *Clin Nurs Res* 8:368,1999.

145. Carroll ST, Riffenburgh RH, Roberts TA, et al.: Tattoos and body piercings as indicators of adolescent risk-taking behaviors. *Pediatrics* 109:1021,2002.

146. Armstrong ML, Stuppy DJ, Gabriel DC, et al.: Motivation for tattoo removal. *Arch Dermatol* 132:412,1996.

147. Wright J: Modifying the body: Piercing and tattoos. *Nurs Stand*10:27,1995.

148. Tweeten SS, Rickman LS: Infectious complications of body piercing. *Clin Infect Dis* 26:735,1998.

149. Mayers LB, Judelson DA, Moriarty BW, et al.: Prevalence of body art (body piercing and tattooing) in university undergraduates and incidence of medical complications. *Mayo Clin Proc* 77:29,2002.

150. Farah CS, Harmon DM: Tongue piercing: Case report and review of current practice. *Aust Dent J* 43:387,1998.

153. Crawford Y, Cash TF: Tattooing and body piercing among college students: Relationships with personality and body image. Unpublished manuscript, Old Dominion University, Norfolk, VA.

154. American Psychiatric Association. *Diagnostic and statistical manual of mental disorders.* 4th ed., text rev. Washington, D. C., APA Press, 2000.

155. American Psychiatric Association. *Diagnostic and statistical manual of mental Disorders.* 3rd ed., rev. Washington, D. C., APA Press,1987.

156. Cotterill JA: Dermatological non-disease: A common and potentially fatal disturbance of cutaneous body image. *Br J Dermatol* 104:611,1981.

157. Edgerton MT, Jacobson WE, Meyer E: Surgical-psychiatric study of patients seeking plastic (cosmetic) surgery: Ninety-eight consecutive patients with minimal deformity. *Br J Plast Surg*13:136,1960.

158. Knorr NJ, Edgerton MT, Hoopes JE: The 'insatiable' cosmetic surgery patient. *Plast Reconstr Surg* 40:285,1967.

159. Otto MW, Wilhelm S, Cohen LS, et al.: Prevalence of body dysmorphic disorder in a community sample of women. *Am J Psychiatry* 158:2061,2001.

160. Faravelli C, Salvatori S, Galassi F, et al.: Epidemiology of somatoform disorders: A community survey in Florence. *Soc Psychiatry Psychiatr Epidemiol* 32:24,1997.

161. Bohne A, Keuthen NJ, Wilhelm S, et al.: Prevalence of symptoms of body dysmorphic disorder and its correlates: A cross-cultural comparison. *Psychosomatics* 43:486,2002.

162. Bohne A, Wilhelm S, Keuthen NJ, et al.: Prevalence of body dysmorphic disorder in a German college student sample. *Psychiatry Res* 109:101,2002.

163. Cansever A, Uzun O, Donmez E, et al.: The prevalence and clinical features of body dysmorphic disorder in college students: A study in a Turkish sample. *Compr Psychiatry* 44:60,2003.

164. Sarwer, DB, Cash, TF, Magee, L et al.: Female college students and cosmetic surgery: An investigation of experiences, attitudes, and body image. *Plast Reconstr Surg* 115:931,2005.

165. Crerand CE, Sarwer DB, Magee L, et al.: Rate of body dysmorphic disorder among patients seeking facial plastic surgery. *Psychiatric Annals* 34:958,2004.

166. Aouizerate B, Pujol H, Grabot D, et al.: Body dysmorphic disorder in a sample of cosmetic surgery applicants. *Eur Psychiatry.* 18:365,2003.

167. Vindigni V, Pavan C, Semenzin M, et al.: The importance of recognizing body dysmorphic disorder in cosmetic surgery patients: Do our patients need a preoperative psychiatric evaluation? *Eur J Plast Surg* 25:305,2002.

168. Ishigooka J, Iwao M, Suzuki M, et al.: Demographic features of patients seeking cosmetic surgery. *Psychiatry Clin Neurosci* 52:283,1998.

169. Vargel S, Ulusahin A: Psychopathology and body image in cosmetic surgery patients. *Aesth Plast Surg* 25:474,2001.

170. Phillips KA, Dufresne RG, Wilkel C, et al.: Rate of body dysmorphic disorder in dermatology patients. *J Am Acad Dermatol* 42:436,2000.

171. Dufresne RG, Phillips KA, Vittorio CC, et al.: A screening questionnaire for body dysmorphic disorder in a cosmetic dermatologic surgery practice. *Dermatol Surg* 27:457, 2001.

172. Uzun O, Basoglu C, Akar A, et al.: Body dysmorphic disorder in patients with acne. *Compr Psychiatry* 44;415,2003.

173. Phillips KA, Grant JE, Siniscalchi J, et al.: Surgical and nonpsychiatric medical treatment of patients with body dysmorphic disorder. *Psychosomatics* 42:504,2001.

174. Cunningham SJ, Feinmann C: Psychological assessment of patients requesting orthognathic surgery and the relevance of body dysmorphic disorder. *Br J Orthod* 25:293,1998.

175. Crerand CE, Phillips KA, Menard W, et al.: Non-psychiatric medical treatment of Body Dysmorphic Disorder. *Psychosomatics* (in press).

176. Cunningham SJ, Bryant CJ, Manisali M., et al.: Dysmorphophobia: Recent developments of interest to the maxillofacial surgeon. *Br J Oral Maxillofac Surg.* 34:368,1996.

177. Phillips KA, Diaz S: Gender differences in body dysmorphic disorder. *J Nerv Ment Dis* 185:570,1997.

178. Perugi G, Akiskal HS, Giannotti D, et al.: Gender-related differences in body dysmorphic disorder (dysmorphophobia). *J Nerv Ment Dis* 185:578,1997.

179. Phillips KA, McElroy SL, Keck PE, et al.: Body dysmorphic disorder: 30 cases of imagined ugliness. *Am J Psychiatry* 150:302,1993.

180. Phillips KA, McElroy SL: Insight, overvalued ideation, and delusional thinking in body dysmorphic disorder: Theoretical and treatment implications. *J Nerv Ment Dis* 181:699,1993.

181. Phillips KA, McElroy SL, Keck PE, et al.: A comparison of delusional and non-delusional body dysmorphic disorder in 100 cases. *Psychopharmacol Bull* 30:179,1994.

182. Phillips KA, Castle DJ: Body dysmorphic disorder, in Castle DJ, Phillips KA (eds.), *Disorders of body image*. Hampshire, England, Wrighton Biomedical Publishing, 2002; p 101.

183. Phillips KA, Taub SL: Skin picking as a symptom of body dysmorphic disorder. *Psychopharmacol Bull* 31:279,1995.

184. Koblenzer CS: Psychodermatology of women. *Clin Dermatol* 15:127,1997.

185. Rosen JC, Reiter J, Orosan P: Cognitive-behavioral body image therapy for body dysmorphic disorder. *J Consult Clin Psychol* 63:263,1995.

186. Phillips KA: The broken mirror. New York, Oxford University Press, 1996.

187. Phillips KA: Quality of life for patients with body dysmorphic disorder. *J Nerv Ment Dis* 188:170,2000.

188. Veale D: Outcome of cosmetic surgery and 'DIY' surgery in patients with body dysmorphic disorder. *Psychiatr Bull R Coll Psychiatr* 24:218,2000.

189. Veale D, Boocock A, Gournay K, et al.: Body dysmorphic disorder: A survey of fifty cases. *Br J Psychiatry* 169:196,1996.

190. Sarwer DB: Awareness and identification of body dysmorphic disorder by aesthetic surgeons: Results of a survey of American Society for Aesthetic Plastic Surgery members. *Aesth Surg J* 22:531,2002.

191. Leonardo J: New York's highest court dismisses BDD case. *Plastic Surgery News* 2001 July:1–9.

192. Yazel L: The serial-surgery murder. *Glamour* 1999 May:108–114.

193. Sarwer DB, Pertschuk MJ: Cosmetic Surgery, in Kornstein SG, Clayton AH (eds.): *Textbook of Women's Mental Health*. New York, NY, Guilford, 2002; p 481.

194. Sarwer DB: Psychological considerations in cosmetic surgery, in Goldwyn, Cohen (eds.), *The Unfavorable Result in Plastic Surgery*. Philadelphia, Lippincott, Williams, & Wilkens, 2001; p 14.

195. Hollander E, Allen A, Kwon J, et al.: Clomipramine vs. Desipramine crossover trial in body dysmorphic disorder. *Arch Gen Psychiatry* 56:1033,1999.

196. Hollander E, Liebowitz M, Winchel R, et al.: Treatment of body-dysmorphic disorder with serotonin reuptake blockers. *Am J Psychiatry* 146:768,1989.

197. Perugi G, Giannotti D, Di Vaio S, et al.: Fluvoxamine in the treatment of the body dysmorphic disorder (dysmorphophobia). *Int Clin Psychopharmacol* 11:247,1996.

198. Phillips KA. Body dysmorphic disorder: Clinical aspects and treatment strategies. *Bull Menninger Clin* 62:A33,1998.

199. Phillips KA, Dwight MM, McElroy SL: Efficacy and safety of fluvoxamine in body dysmorphic disorder. *J Clin Psychiatry* 59:165,1998.

200. Phillips KA, Albertini RS, Siniscalchi JM, et al.: Effectiveness of pharmacotherapy for body dysmorphic disorder: A chart review study. *J Clin Psychiatry* 62:721,2001.

201. Phillips KA, Albertini RS, Rasmussen SA: A randomized placebo-controlled trial of fluoxetine in body dysmorphic disorder. *Arch Gen Psychiatry* 59:381,2002.

202. Phillips KA, Najjar F: An open-label study of citalopram in body dysmorphic disorder. *J Clin Psychiatry* 64:715,2003.

203. Looper KJ, Kirmayer LJ: Behavioral medicine approaches to somatoform disorders. *J Consult Clin Psychol* 70:810, 2002.

204. Neziroglu FA, Yaryura-Tobias JA: Exposure, response prevention, and cognitive therapy in the treatment of body dysmorphic disorder. *Behav Ther* 24:431,1993.

205. Veale D, Gournay K, Dryden W, et al.: Body dysmorphic disorder: A cognitive behavioural model and pilot randomised controlled trial. *Behav Res Ther.* 34:717,1996.

206. Wilhelm S, Otto MW, Lohr B, et al.: Cognitive behavior group therapy for body dysmorphic disorder: A case series. *Behav Res Ther* 37:71,1999.

207. Sarwer DB, Gibbons LM, Crerand CE: Treating body dysmorphic disorder with cognitive-behavior therapy. *Psychiatric Annals* 34:934,2004.

208. Pope HG, Gruber AJ, Choi P, et al.: Muscle dysmorphia: An under-recognized form of body dysmorphic disorder. *Psychosomatics* 38:548,1997.

209. McIntosh VV, Britt E, Bulik CM: Cosmetic breast augmentation and eating disorders. *N Z Med J* 107:151,1994.

210. Olivardia, R: Mirror, mirror on the wall, who's the largest of them all? The features and phenomenology of muscle dysmorphia. *Harvard Rev Psychiatry* 9:254,2001.

211. Harth W, Linse R: Botulinophilia: Contraindication for therapy with botulinum toxin. *Int J Clin Pharmacol Ther* 39:460,2001.

212. Sarwer DB, Crerand CE, Didie ER: Body dysmorphic disorder in cosmetic surgery patients. *Facial Plast Surg* 19:113, 2003.

213. Yates A, Shisslak CM, Allender JR, et al.: Plastic surgery and the bulimic patient. *Int J Eat Disord* 7:557,1988.

214. Losee JE, Serletti JM, Kreipe RE, et al.: Reduction mammaplasty in patients with bulimia nervosa. *Ann Plast Surg* 39:443,1997.

215. Losee JE, Jiang S, Long DE, et al.: Macromastia as an etiologic factor in bulimia nervosa: 10-year follow-up after treatment with reduction mammoplasty. *Ann Plast Surg* 52:452, 2004.

16 | The Business of Office-Based Anesthesia for Cosmetic Surgery

Marc E. Koch, M.D., M.B.A.

INTRODUCTION

The practice of office-based anesthesiology (OBA) is nearly a century old.[1] However, published articles on the subject did not appear in the medical literature until 1981.[2] As with traditional applications, the goal of anesthesia in the office setting is to provide patients with a lack of awareness of surrounding events, to keep the patient still to allow the surgery to take place, to enable access for the surgeon through muscles to bones and body cavities. All cosmetic surgery avoids body cavities and is therefore, minimally curative to prevent dangerous surges in hemodynamics.

Compared to hospitals and licensed ambulatory surgery centers, office-based medical practices currently have to abide by significantly fewer regulations. Therefore, it is imperative that physicians adequately investigate areas taken for granted in the hospital or ambulatory surgical facility, such as organizational structure, governance, facility construction, and logistical equipment, as well as policies and procedures, including fire, safety, drugs, emergencies, staffing, training, and unanticipated patient transfers.[3]

In addition to the core functions of any business, OBA possesses many unique elements compared to traditional hospital-based practice. At its core, OBA more closely resembles any other community-based referral practice with a long list of business considerations. The benefits of OBA have made it one of the fastest growing sectors in anesthesiology. Patients enjoy the heightened privacy, efficiency, and familiarity of an office setting (lower costs, too). Surgeons appreciate the increased convenience and control of operating in their own offices. Many save time in travel and eliminate many of the hassles associated with hospitals and surgery centers. For an anesthesiologist, an office-based practice can usually provide a better lifestyle with unique challenges. Catching this wave of the future requires careful consideration of these unique circumstances, pressures, and challenges.

There are many business issues an anesthesiologist experiences when entering the cosmetic surgery market. This chapter covers some of the more important business issues that any physician should consider before embarking in a career that, either in whole or in part, includes cosmetic and plastic surgery.

CHOOSING AN APPROPRIATE CLIENT

Due Diligence and Surgeon's Credentials

The first thing one needs to take care of is due diligence. This means carefully researching and making sure that things are what they seem to be and that the circumstances of the opportunity have been adequately and appropriately represented. The main concern here is not to enter a situation where the economic and clinical well-being of the anesthesiologist can be held in the balance.

Cosmetic surgery is one of those specialties that are inhabited by various competitors from multiple specialties. For instance, the "gold" standard in cosmetic surgery is certainly a board-certified plastic surgeon. Plastic surgeons have generally completed a residency in general surgery, a fellowship in plastic surgery, and some additional training in special techniques. These physicians are board-certified by the ABMS specialty of plastic and reconstructive surgery. A 2006 court case in California held that board-certified cosmetic surgeons were equivalent to ABMS-certified plastic surgeons. The California Medical Board is considering an appeal. Having said that, one must note that cosmetic surgery is also peformed by dentists, oral surgeons, dermatologists, general surgeons, ENTs, obstetrician-gynecologists, and even gastroenterologists. In this regard, the specialty is unlike anesthesiology. Anesthesia may be administered by anesthesiologists, nurse anesthetists, and anesthesia assistants. The medical specialty of anesthesiology is practiced only by anesthesiologists.

Oral surgeons and dentists have become involved through extension of their related area of expertise. In other words, oral and maxillofacial surgery, which was once a profession that was limited to the teeth and the structures that support the mouth, has now expanded to the point where some oral surgeons are performing rhinoplasty, facelift, liposuction on the neck, and facial laser resurfacing. Anesthesiologists need to understand that these alternate providers are the people who are actually providing care. Some of them may or may not have completed medical school, internship, and formal residency training.

Although not a hard and fast rule, it seems as though most oral and maxillofacial surgeons tend to limit their cosmetic surgery to the head, neck, and related structures. If, in fact, the oral surgeon is providing service in an area that is already somewhat saturated by cosmetic surgeons, it may not be unusual that competition will be based on price. Anesthesiologists should be especially cautious of alternate providers, such as oral and maxillofacial surgeons, if during negotiations for anesthesia fees the contractee appears to be aggressive.

Dermatology is another example of a specialty that has been competing on the cosmetic surgery front. No deaths were reported from dermatologic cosmetic surgical offices in Florida between 2000 and 2003 in the Coldiron paper.[4] Liposuction was formerly a procedure associated with general anesthesia and a substantial amount of blood loss. One of the reasons this technique was safe and successful was that it utilized an anesthesiologist. In 1987, it was shown that by using a high volume of dilute local anesthesia with epinephrine, and by encouraging homeostasis, less tissue trauma and a safer overall technique for patients would result.[5,6] Just as there are good and bad board-certified plastic surgeons, there are dermatologists (and other cosmetic surgeons) who are aware and those who are *unaware* of the pharmaceutical limitations of high-volume local anesthetics (see Chapter 8).

Ask questions (*vide infra*) and make sure that the anesthesiologist who is embarking on a career that includes the coverage of cosmetic surgery clients obtains all the information necessary. Only then can the anesthesiologist gauge his comfort level and determine if it meshes well with the opportunity at hand.

Beyond establishing the surgeon's credentials, do not forget about real life experience. With rapidly emerging changes in technology, it is not unusual for new techniques, new drugs, and new procedures to be offered to patients. The skill of the surgeon, however, needs to be evaluated. Is this the first time a given surgeon is providing a procedure? Is this the tenth time? Is this the twentieth time? Nevertheless, it is important that each individual anesthesiologist set their own guidelines as to what they consider a necessary and indicated amount of experience prior to providing anesthesia to a given client. Another hint about the surgeon's experience is to inquire about the "redo" or reoperation rate. In most competent practices, it is 1–2%. A 5–10% redo rate should raise a red flag! A marginally competent practice may be completely unprepared to provide those statistics because a "redo" would not be considered particularly unusual.

BE PREPARED

The Stark Act, Malpractice Liability, and Compliance Issues

The Stark Act is generally known as the "self-referral" law because it basically prohibits physicians from referring Medicare patients for certain health services to entities in which they (or immediate family members) have a financial relationship. Office-based cosmetic surgery practices are not affected by the Stark Act. These health services include laboratories, physical/occupational/speech therapy, radiology and imaging, radiation therapy, DME, home health, prosthetics, outpatient prescriptions, and inpatient and out-patient hospital services, among others. Originally, there was an exception for physicians referring Medicare patients to an entity where they had an ownership interest. However, under the 2003 Medicare Modernization Act, that exception was limited to exclude specialty hospitals.

It is rare that a cosmetic procedure will be covered by insurance, especially by Medicare.

The basic issues are no different from malpractice liability for anesthesiologists providing anesthesia services during any other kind of procedure or venue (see Chapter 18). In order for malpractice liability to have occurred, two conditions must be met. First, the patient must be harmed. Second, the anesthesiologist must depart from the standard of care. Thus, theoretically at least, a patient with an undesirable outcome must still prove that the anesthesiologist's care was not within the standards of other anesthesiologists under the same circumstances. With that said, however, one cannot rule out the sympathy that a jury might feel for a patient who suffers an injury while undergoing cosmetic surgery. It is sometimes difficult to overcome the juror's prejudice regarding cosmetic surgery. The average juror often feels that the surgery is probably unnecessary in the first place and that the physicians are undertaking a purely money-making pursuit rather than helping a truly sick patient.

Another consideration is that, unlike a hospital, a company employing the anesthesiologist is vicariously liable for the anesthesiologist's negligence. It therefore behooves any such company to obtain separate and additional insurance.

Compliance issues are somewhat less significant for the anesthesiologist providing care in the office-based cosmetic surgery setting. On the assumption that the vast majority of cosmetic surgeries are not paid for by any insurance carrier, the usual Health Insurance Portability and Accountability Act (HIPAA) requirements do not apply. The federal Anti-kickback Statute is not applicable, nor is the Federal False Claims Act and its requirements regarding proper coding and billing. However, rules regarding physician conduct are enforceable.

However, in those cases in which the cosmetic surgery is, in fact, paid for by an insurance company, including the Center for Medicaid and Medicare Services (CMS), all of these statutes must be complied with.

SELF-PROMOTION

Sales, Marketing, and Business Development

One of the most important components of OBA is spreading the word about one's services and capabilities. Therefore, marketing, sales, and business development is a crucial investment for OBA providers. Developing new clients within the specialty of cosmetic surgery can be a challenge. When presenting an anesthesia solution to cosmetic surgeons, there are two questions that immediately arise:

1. Are your anesthesiologists board-certified?
2. What are your fees?

Board certification is important in part because of a large number of cosmetic surgery practices being accredited by national accrediting agencies such as AAAASF, AAAHC, and JCAHO. Although these organizations do not require that the anesthesiologist be board-certified, they do require that the anesthesia provider have the appropriate credentials to manage patients at whatever level of sedation and anesthesia is achieved. In addition, owing to the length of the cases, along with the level of invasiveness of many of them, working with a board-certified anesthesiologist may also help the surgeon with malpractice insurance and liability.

Because members of the American Society of Plastic Surgeons (ASPS) are required to obtain accreditation in order to operate in their office, accreditation is a major component in marketing to plastic and cosmetic surgery clients.

In order to market oneself as a premier anesthesia group, consider aligning oneself with the three major office-based surgery accreditation organizations (JCAHO, AAAASF, and AAAHC). This signifies to a cosmetic surgeon that the anesthesiologist is dedicated to patient safety. The necessary policies, procedures, and processes will be in place in order to administer a safe anesthetic. Sometimes, cosmetic surgeons may even advertise the fact that they utilize an accredited anesthesia group.

Anesthesia cash fees vary from town to town depending on the availability of anesthesiologists, as well as the competitive marketplace of cosmetic surgeons. In the New York metropolitan area, for example, there is a high volume of cosmetic surgeons, making it an extremely competitive marketplace. The cosmetic surgeons who have lowered their fees in an effort to attract their share of the market will frequently expect the anesthesiologist to do the same. If an anesthesiologist is working primarily at a hospital and is covering a cosmetic surgeon to *supplement* his income, he may choose to negotiate his fees downward. However, if the cosmetic surgeon is using an anesthesia group that is specializing in outpatient anesthesia, then there may be less room to negotiate because of the anesthesia group's higher overhead and overall costs.

In general, the anesthesia rates will be charged hourly, with the first hour ranging between $400 and $600 and subsequent hours ranging from $225 to $400. These hourly rates are charged on a per-case basis. Some practices will charge flat fees per case; however, this is normally done after performing the surgery a minimum of three times with the surgeon to gauge how long the procedure takes them and to price it accordingly. The offering of a flat day rate is cost effective for surgeons who can schedule two or more cases, or five or more hours of anesthesia time. Flat day rates range from $1800 to $3000 and may or may not include medications and supplies or ancillary staff.

Logistical arrangements vary and the anesthesiologist may bring their own medications and supplies at an added fee of $175–$250 per case. It behooves the surgeon to review closely what materials and personnel the anesthesiologist is supplying and to make sure that he is equipped to handle any untoward event. One possible scenario is for the anesthesia group, or solo provider, to adhere to state guidelines and/or accreditation guidelines. The surgeon then knows that a high level of patient safety issues has been addressed. Once this is realized, the surgeon may conclude that he is better off having the anesthesia medications and supplies provided by the anesthesiologist, since he may bring an added layer of protection.

Although the lowest hourly rate may win the surgeons' business initially, they may soon realize they are compromising their schedules to work with the lower fee anesthesia providers who may provide coverage only during non-hospital hours. Weighed in with the knowledge that they may be receiving the anesthesia provider post-call, after eight to twelve hours of work, the cost-savings rationale often dissipates and inquiries into additional coverage options resume.

The cosmetic surgeons who appear to be most satisfied with their anesthesia coverage arrangement and have been successful in maintaining a lengthy relationship with their group are more often than not the ones who view the anesthesia service as an extension of their own surgical practice. Therefore, the surgeons may place a high "worth" on what is brought to the table.

Marketing to cosmetic surgeons is very different than marketing to other office-based specialties. One significant difference is that, in most cases, the patient pays out-of-pocket for the anesthesia instead of billing an insurance company. In order to be successful, OBA providers must offer the most competitive daily and hourly rates. Since patients are primarily responsible for the costs, accepting all types of payments, including credit cards, makes good business sense.

Cosmetic surgeons often cater to an educated, affluent population. These are generally people who look for seals of approval, such as board certification and accreditation. For this particular clientele, it is important to build one's practice with exemplary physicians and highlight their impressive credentials in promotional materials.

It is vitally import that an anesthesiologist demonstrate respect for the patient, surgeon, and office staff. Marketing materials should stress the fact that the anesthesiologist is a guest in the plastic surgeon's office. Promise to deliver the quality of care that their patients expect or even demand.

The cosmetic surgery specialty necessitates flexibility and reliability from anesthesia providers. Promote the fact that a large group will guarantee coverage for regular clients and can often provide last-minute or back-up coverage for cosmetic surgeons utilizing other, often smaller, anesthesia groups.

WHO'S THE COMPETITION?

Competition is present in any kind of business. Medicine and cosmetic surgery is no exception. The cosmetic surgeons compete as do anesthesiologists who primarily work in the ambulatory environment. One strives to provide excellent clinical care and to keep on the forefront of the latest techniques that improve outcomes and patient satisfaction. Cosmetic surgeons and their patients want great anesthesiologists too, but unlike other specialties, the surgeons are very cost conscious. One might even say cost savvy.

There is no insurance claim. Instead, the patient writes a check or uses a credit card. This patient wants it all—a great surgery team and a cost perceived as affordable. Cosmetic surgeries are growing at an astounding rate. Patients are price shopping and are not shy about comparing prices.

Competition for the anesthesia component of cosmetic surgery comes in a variety of forms. First, there is the surgeon himself, who may opt to do a local anesthetic. Alternatively, a "conscious sedation" may be administered with the nurse (hopefully) monitoring the patient. Surgeon-administered anesthesia is becoming progressively less frequent as cases emerge that have had negative outcomes. The ASPS and other cosmetic surgery organizations have encouraged their members to conform to standards, such as becoming accredited or state licensed. This is also the case for the surgeon supervising a nurse anesthetist, without the presence of an anesthesiologist; another (potentially) risky situation for all involved.

There are also varying types of anesthesiologist-to-anesthesiologist competition for cosmetic cases. These cases can be very desirable to many doctors, as it is cash in hand and no paperwork. Additionally, the setting is often very "posh." The patients are normally younger and healthy, so complications tend to be minimal. Many hospital-based anesthesiologists vie for these cases and moonlight on their post-call day, vacation, or holiday time off. It is a great way to supplement one's income, especially for doctors recently out of residency. There is even a growing trend of full-time freelancers that transit from office to office. A doctor can work a 9 to 5 schedule and have a great deal of freedom. These two types of arrangements offer pretty much just the doctor's services. Moonlighters and freelancers often require the cosmetic surgeon to supply all the anesthesia equipment, medications, supplies, and so forth. This arrangement may not be a suitable one for all cosmetic surgery practices.

On the other hand, there are anesthesia groups that have found their way into the cosmetic surgery niche. Again, the lure of upfront payment and no insurance claims to deal with is an attraction to groups with idle full-time equivalent (FTE) time. Because cosmetic surgery is a booming market, groups are also adding to their staff to accommodate the cosmetic surgery office-based surgical facilities (OBSFs). These groups can be the type that has a large hospital contract and does cosmetic surgery at an ambulatory surgery center (ASC). Or they can be the type that provides service at a smaller community hospital and does multiple ASCs and OBSFs. And last there is the unique type of group that focuses solely on ambulatory anesthesia, devoting full time to OBSFs and ASCs.

The arrangement with these anesthesia groups does vary from providing only the anesthesiologist's service (as in the moonlighter or freelancers) to providing everything related to anesthesia. Still, other permutations may be everything in between these two extremes. Because the full-time groups are larger and have a behind-the-scenes staff, the cosmetic surgeon can negotiate the type of service arrangement that fits best with his practice. When in this competitive environment, it is important to know one's competition and make sure that proposals are "apples-to-apples" comparisons. Otherwise, another group's rates may look more attractive than one's own rates.

Competition in cosmetic surgery will probably get more intense as the type of procedures increase and the technology enhancements enable more cases to be done in the ambulatory setting. When partnering with cosmetic surgeons to provide anesthesia, concentrate on longevity. Try to become a trusted member of the team, not just another charge on the bill. Work with the surgeon. Be flexible and keep abreast of market conditions that affect rates. Volunteer to do comarketing events. Contribute to the cost of advertising. Do one's best to promote the cosmetic surgery industry and that surgeon's individual practice. Create a win-win, mutually beneficial partnership to help ensure a long-term relationship that will also be financially rewarding.

MAINTAINING ONE'S CLIENTELE

As more and more anesthesia providers dabble in the office and ambulatory arena, it's important to develop policies that distinguish one's group from the rest. Once clients are brought on board, one needs to maintain and nurture those business relationships. Having a dedicated staff person or "client advocate" to address concerns on a consistent and one-on-one basis will yield high dividends for the future.

Cosmetic surgeons oftentimes have sporadic schedules and untimely surgical procedures; therefore, scheduling is an evolving and dynamic process. One of the major aspects of scheduling is to ensure every physician is scheduled to cover the correct facility according to licensure, certifications, type of procedures, and travel time. Each facility should have a core group of three to four physicians who consistently provide that client's anesthesia according to the credentialing idiosyncrasies mentioned previously.

BILLING AND COLLECTIONS FOR COSMETIC SURGERY CASES—BILLING AND PAYMENT

Be flexible. That's the bottom line for anesthesia billing. Plastic-surgery cases can fall under two categories:

Elective cosmetic surgery—These procedures are not medically necessary. There are flat-fee agreements according to procedures and special agreements per surgeon: in 2005 dollars, for example, $600 for the first hour of anesthesia services, $300 for each additional hour, and $200 for medications and supplies used for anesthesia. ($600/$300/$200). To be accommodating, it's advisable to accommodate surgeons' individual policies of collecting payment from patients. There are surgeons who collect *both* the procedure and anesthesia fee from patients prior to the procedure. In this case, the payment is forwarded to the anesthesia provider.

Other surgeons collect a combined fee for the procedure and the anesthesia. These surgeons will then cut a check for the anesthesia portion. In a third scenario, usually for sporadic cosmetic surgeons, patients are given an estimated anesthesia fee, and a check or credit card is given to the anesthesiologist/billing staff. If at the end of the proce-

dure the estimated time is higher or lower than originally quoted, the patient is credited or charged the difference.

Charge entry is performed as usual (patient demographics, procedure, and diagnosis are entered referencing the anesthesia grid and/or surgeon's superbill). Upon charge entry, it's a good idea to reconcile the number of cases billed versus the number of cases scheduled and completed. This also ensures that payments are received according to specific fee schedules.

Medical necessity plastic surgery—These cases are usually billed through insurance carriers and are subject to individual payor contracts and negotiated reimbursement rates. In some cases, patients will be responsible for deductibles, coinsurances, and/or copays. Some insurance carriers request and require medical-necessity notes from the surgeon in order to proceed with the anesthesia payment. If payment claims are denied, patients should be billed according to the surgeon's agreement.

The following are some example cases that have constituted as medical necessity depending on the diagnosis:

1. A severed limb/digit hand or foot
2. Breast reduction due to back problems
3. Cleft lip
4. Insertion of prosthesis (mastectomy due to breast cancer)
5. Bell's palsy paralysis (corrective eye surgery)

Whether elective or medically necessary, all cosmetic/plastic cases must provide and complete the following:

1. A detailed anesthesia record
2. A signed consent form
3. Q/A form
4. Demographics
5. Insurance, when applicable

CONCLUSION

The business of OBA has a multitude of unique attributes compared to the hospital and surgery center environments. Comfortable working hours and a more intimate relationship with patients and physicians can provide the forum for a considerable amount of professional resonance. In addition, the limited resources, the itinerant nature of the practice, and the need to innovate on the spur of the moment can make for both variety and excitement. The gamut of anesthesia techniques, patient comorbidities, and surgeon expectations is generally no more homogeneous than that found in traditional locations. But, then again, no specific area of anesthesia practice or venue is devoid of challenges. Although OBSFs are very different from other settings, this distinction does not necessarily make it superior or inferior. There is little doubt that some of the growing pains experienced by trailblazing ambulatory surgery centers have been and will continue to be felt by nascent OBSF practices as the industry evolves and develops. For the anesthesiologist, a meld between business person and clinician is becoming more a rule than an exception, and efforts to maintain and promote professional sovereignty will help forge continued growth of this unique practice setting.

REFERENCES

1. Waters RM: The downtown anesthesia clinic. *Am J Surg* 33:71, 1919.
2. Vinnik CA: An intravenous dissociation technique for outpatient plastic surgery: tranquility in the office surgical facility. *Plast Reconstr Surg* 67:199,1981.
3. Mihalcik JA: The anesthesiologist and office-based anesthesia practice. *ASA Newsletter*. Park Ridge, IL, American Society of Anesthesiologists. 60:20,1996.
4. Koch ME, Giannuzzi R, Goldstein RC: Office anesthesiology. *North Am Clin* 17:395,1999.
5. Coldiron B, Shreve BA, Balkrishnan R, et al.: Patient injuries from surgical procedures performed in medical offices: Three years of Florida data. *Dermatol Surg*, 30:1435,2004.
6. Klein JA: The tumescent technique for liposuction surgery. *J Am Acad Cosmetic Surg* 4:263,1987.
7. Klein JA: Tumescent Liposuction. *Saint Louis*, MO, Mosby, 2000.

17 | The Politics of Office-Based Anesthesia

David Barinholtz, M.D.

INTRODUCTION

Whereas Parts I and II of this book is dedicated to discussing clinical issues regarding anesthesia for cosmetic surgery, this chapter delves into the broad-based issues surrounding the locale where much of cosmetic surgery is being done, the physician's office.

Over the past twenty years, the number of cosmetic as well as other invasive procedures performed in the office-based setting has skyrocketed. Unfortunately, along with this increase have come **a few**, *highly publicized*, bad outcomes resulting in patient's deaths. Along with these deaths comes the question, why? Why are these things occurring in office-based surgical (OBS) facilities at a higher rate than hospitals or ambulatory surgery centers (ASCs) (or are they)? The answer to this highly charged, complex issue is itself highly charged and complex, and playing out all over the country at the state legislative level, state regulatory level, between professional societies, among the accrediting bodies, and, of course, the payers. At the moment, however, the patient's lives are at stake.

In this chapter, the salient issues are elucidated regarding office-based surgery (OBS) and office-based anesthesia (OBA). However, the reader is cautioned. This chapter can discuss and present only what specifically is going on as of the time of its writing. There is constantly evolving activity at many levels. Anyone who is pondering becoming involved in this practice should exercise due diligence regarding the regulatory/legislative climate in the state in which one is contemplating an office-based anesthesia practice.

WHAT IS OBS/OBA?

OBS/OBA refers to procedures being performed within the confines of a physician's office suite, not licensed by the state as a hospital or ASC. (However, some states do require OBS settings to be licensed.) Other defining features include (1) the idea that the *majority* of activity in the office suite is office visits, **not** ambulatory surgery, and (2) the procedure room/OR is open only to physicians who are members of that medical practice.

OBA Trends

According to SMG Marketing Group, in 1984 fewer than 500,000 surgical procedures nationwide were being performed in a physician's office-based setting (POBS).

SMG was a marketing research company based in Chicago that had been following ambulatory surgery trends since the late 1970s. SMG was acquired by Verispan and, in 2004, the surgical-trends project was terminated. By 2005, the

Table 17-1. 2004 top 5 female[a] cosmetic surgical procedures

1. Liposuction	292,402
2. Breast implants	264,041
3. Eyelid surgery	200,667
4. Nose reshaping	195,504
5. Facelift	103,994

[a]According to the ASAPS, women accounted for 87% of the nine million cosmetic surgery patients.*
*Editor's note: *These figures do not include the same procedures performed by members of the AACS or ASDS and likely significantly underestimate the true numbers.* —BLF

number of OBS was estimated to be approximately ten million (Table 17-1). In 2004, according to ASAPS, nine million cosmetic procedures were performed. This figure does not include cosmetic procedures performed by members of the American Academy of Cosmetic Surgeons (AACS) or members of the American Society of Sermatologic Surgeons (ASDS). Both AACS and ASDS members perform cosmetic surgery. Therefore, the figure ten million is likely a *substantial* underestimation.

To put this in perspective, the total number of outpatient surgeries in the United States in 2005 was projected to be approximately forty million. Of these, approximately half, or twenty million, would be performed in hospital outpatient departments (HOPD). The other twenty million are virtually equally divided between ASCs and POBS[1] (Fig. 17-1). Why has this trend developed?

The main force behind this trend is clearly *economic*. During the 1980s and 1990s, third-party payers paid fees for procedures done in freestanding ASCs that were substantially lower than the identical procedures done in the HOPD. In the 1990s and beyond, these same payers paid fees that were even lower in OBS. Over the past fifteen years, payers have been nudging and, more recently, forcing procedures into the office. This is evidenced most recently by CMS's elimination of ASC codes.[2] Elimination of these codes mean ASCs can no longer be reimbursed for these procedures. CMS (formerly Medicare) has simultaneously created significant site-of-services differentials, reimbursing physicians more to perform these procedures in the office. One of the main reasons surgeons started taking their cosmetic procedures to the office is to have control over the costs that were spiraling out of control in the hospitals and ASCs. Added to the cost considerations are the

facts that many physicians have been seeing their professional reimbursements cut and malpractice costs rising. Facility fees generated by procedures done in-office can augment one's net income or "bottom line."

Other benefits of OBS include control over the OR, from the scheduling of cases to the drugs, supplies, equipment, and personnel. Convenience for the surgeon, efficiency of an office-based surgical practice, as well as patient preference, comfort, and privacy round out the reasons why OBS has grown in popularity. Recent technologic advances have also moved procedures from the traditional OR to the POBS.[3] Procedures for liposuction, benign prostatic hypertrophy (BPH), sterilization, and endometrial bleeding are but a few examples.

Problems/Issues That Have Emerged

On the surface, these trends all *appear* positive. The payers are paying out less. Physicians are experiencing increased remuneration *and* more control over their practices. Patients are delighted to be cared for in the doctor's office and to not have go to a hospital or ASC. However, under the surface, dark clouds are gathering. In most states, physicians are licensed to "practice medicine in all of its branches." Additionally, most states do not or have not (until very recently) regulated surgery in POBS. There have emerged physicians who are performing procedures in their offices beyond the scope of their education, training, and experience.

What follows generally in these office-based situations are inadequate environments that were improperly staffed and equipped. This is a recipe for disaster, and disaster is just what has happened.

A few highly publicized tragedies occurred. A woman dies having liposuction in her plastic surgeon's office in California.[4] A woman dies having laser surgery in her ophthalmologist's office in Atlanta.[5] Some people die in offices in Florida having liposuction.[6] A plastic surgeon performs a breast augmentation on a healthy woman in his office in Florida, is unable to resuscitate her, and she dies.[7]

If one looks into the details surrounding these deaths and many others that have occurred in POBS over the past several years, the same theme emerges. Virtually every one of the cases involved an anesthesia mishap: overdose of local anesthetic; overdose of sedatives and analgesics; prolonged surgery without DVT prophylaxis; inadequate monitoring; inadequate or nonexistent emergency

Table 17-2. Procedure-related office-based deaths (13) in Florida, March 2000 and March 2003[10]

Procedure	Surgeon	Facility	Boards	Hospital priv
1. Abdominoplasty Liposuction	Plastic	AAAASF	yes	yes
2. Breast reduction	Plastic	None	yes	yes
3. Abdominoplasty	Plastic	None	yes	yes
4. Rhinoplasty	Facial plastic	None	yes	yes
5. Liposuction laser resurf	Plastic	AAAASF	yes	yes
6. Abdominoplasty, hernia	Plastic	AAAHC	yes	yes
7. Facelift	Plastic	AAAASF	yes	yes
8. TAB	OB/GYN	None	yes	yes
9. Hemodialysis cath insert	Radiol	AAAHC	yes	yes
10. Dialysis cath repl	Radiol	None	yes	yes
11. Colonoscopy	GI	None	yes	yes
12. Colonoscopy	GI	None	yes	yes
13. Liver biopsy	Radiol	None	yes	yes

Editor's note: Seven of thirteen deaths were in cosmetic surgery offices! —BLF

resuscitation, drugs, and equipment; inadequate personnel properly trained in anesthesia, resuscitation and airway management. Combinations of one or more of these were involved in these cases. What is going on? (See Table 17-2.)

Morbidity and mortality

Obviously, patient safety must remain at the heart of OBS concerns. Are people having more complications requiring hospitalization and/or dying more frequently in POBS than in HOPD and ASCs? The answer is presently unknown!

DEFINING THE PROBLEM. In 2005, there wasn't comprehensive, definitive data quantifying the exact numbers of procedures done in each of these settings, nor was there data on the relative morbidity and mortality rates. All of the accrediting bodies had the data from each individual organization they accredit, including numbers of procedures, hospitalizations, deaths, types of anesthesia, and so forth. Unfortunately, the data had not been pooled. With pooled data, at least the morbidity and mortality rates in HOPD, ASCs, and the approximately 2,000 accredited POBS practices would be known. Differences, *if* they exist, could be dissected out. Until then, there are smaller databases from sources such as Medicare and The National Ambulatory Medical Care Survey, from which data was extrapolated. More recently, there is the data from the state of Florida.

Unfortunately, small differences of opinion in which pieces of data are to be considered, and differences in data collection methods among settings, can result in distinctly different conclusions (*vide infra*).

INTERPRETING THE DATA. One of the first studies to alert the medical community that a serious problem *may* exist with POBS was published in 2000 by Grazer and deJong.[8] Based on results of voluntary *surveys* sent out to board-certified plastic surgeons, a study was published that claimed that the mortality rate for in-office lipoplasty is approximately 1 in 5,000. The major cause of death in this study was pulmonary embolism, followed by anesthesia-related mishaps. This study has been widely criticized for its methods and data interpretation. The statistical shortcomings of this article precluded its publication in the anesthesia literature. It is highly improbable that these figures would stand if extrapolated to the number of liposuction cases performed nationally. Grazer and deJong's[8] figure is widely at variance with the mortality rate of approximately 1 in 250,000 usually cited by the anesthesia community.

In 1999, the state of Florida passed a moratorium on OBS requiring *general anesthesia* after approximately eighteen people died over a period of *two years* between 1997 and 1999 in POBS. Following those deaths and that moratorium, Florida has since enacted some of the strictest regulations governing OBS. Within those regulations is a requirement for mandatory reporting of all deaths and/or hospital transfers from POBS.

The Florida data has been analyzed, but opinions differ on the *interpretation* of the data. In 2003, Vila et al. published a study in *Archives of Surgery* utilizing the Florida data that had been collected from April 1, 2000, to April 1, 2002.[9] Based on the analysis and interpretation of the data, Vila et al. concluded that the relative risk of adverse incidents and death was twelve times greater in POBS than ASCs.[9]

In December 2004, Coldiron and Venkat published two studies in *Dermatologic Surgery*.[10,11] These studies used three years of Florida data collected from March 2000 to March 2003. The conclusions these studies made were in stark contrast to Vila's conclusions. In Venkat's study, it was concluded that surgery in a POBS was approximately 50% to 90% *safer* than surgery performed in an ASC.[11] Coldiron's evaluation of the data was even more interesting. Coldiron[10] criticized the Vila et al.[9] interpretation of and inclusion of some data. Based on two IV sedation deaths compared with five general anesthesia deaths, Coldiron concluded that this increased risk was mostly due to cosmetic surgeries performed under general anesthesia.[10]

Coldiron suggests a ban on general anesthesia in POBS as the way to solve the problem.[10] Requirements such as board certification, accreditation, and hospital privileges would do little to alter the situation.[10]

So, is there a problem or not? Are there more deaths and/or adverse occurrences in POBS than in ASCs or HOPD? Or do different mandatory reporting requirements in POBS versus ASCs or HOPD make it appear so? Are anesthesiologists and board-certified plastic surgeons responsible for most of the problem? Is accreditation a good idea or not?

These are discussed here in, along with other issues that have been considered and/or implemented in the name of patient safety in POBS (*vide infra*).

PROPOSED SOLUTIONS TO PERCEIVED PROBLEMS

Banning General Anesthesia

As Coldiron pointed out in his evaluation of the Florida data, 52% of the cases of death or hospital transfer involved cosmetic surgery performed under general anesthesia.[10] In a discussion of his findings in the March 2005 issue of *Cosmetic Surgery Times*, Guttman suggests a ban on general anesthesia in the office setting.[12]

Further supporting Coldiron's argument is the fact that during the ninety-day moratorium on general anesthesia in POBS, there were *no* deaths related to general anesthesia. Most anesthetic-related mishaps in hospitals and ASCs are also related to general anesthesia. Most surgical patients in hospitals and ASC are there for medically indicated surgery.

Banning general anesthesia in these hospitals and ASCs would also save many lives. Two very highly publicized cosmetic surgery deaths in 2004 occurred as complications of general anesthesia at Manhattan Eye and Ear Hospital, not an office.

General anesthesia is inherently risky, and the anesthesia community is to be credited with making great strides in patient safety. In the regulated, accredited world of hospitals and ASCs, one thing is certain: the only practitioners credentialed and privileged to administer and/or supervise deep sedation or general anesthesia are persons who demonstrate adequate training, education, and experience as determined by very specific criteria outlined in the process. Hence, only fully qualified anesthesiologists and nurse anesthetists will obtain these privileges. Furthermore, people with a history of significant problems—serious malpractice issues, medical board issues, and so forth—will not be granted these privileges.

In contrast, in the office-based environment this process frequently is in the hands of the surgeon/owner.

Without the benefit of a peer-review process, no detailed and agreed-on specifics exist among the accrediting bodies as to what defines "adequate training, education, and experience." With surgeons motivated to have cost-effective anesthesia in their office, one can see how an unsafe provider might fall through the cracks. However, if one adopts mechanisms for credentialing and privileging in POBS similar to those in hospitals and ASCs for anesthesia providers, one may achieve similar success. **However, general anesthesia is never risk free.**

One point Coldiron also brought up in his discussion is that "restrictions on office procedures could potentially limit patients' access to necessary medical care."[10] In that spirit, let's not throw out the baby with the bathwater. Banning of general anesthesia would seriously limit access to necessary care for hundreds of thousands of patients per year. Hospitals and ASCs could not absorb the ten million procedures per year, most of which are performed under deep sedation/general anesthesia, and most of which are medically necessary. Oral surgery, pediatric dentistry, gastroenterology, orthopedic surgery, podiatric surgery, urology, gynecology, and otolaryngology are but a handful of specialties where patients would be significantly impacted by this restriction, and it is not necessary.

In practices where these processes of credentialing and privileging are followed, the safety record is indeed impressive. Data compiled by two AAAHC-accredited office-based anesthesia practices over the past ten years demonstrate almost 200,000 anesthetics (virtually every one deep sedation or general anesthesia) in POBS settings without a single death or other negative outcome.[14] A series of over 23,000 patients in eighteen years was recently published in *Plastic and Reconstructive Surgery* without a death or negative outcome.[15]

In 2003, the *Journal of Oral and Maxillofacial Surgery* published the results of a prospective study involving seventy-nine oral surgeons at fifty-eight study sites and data from 34,578 patients cared for between January and December of 2001.[16] In this study, 71.9% of patients received deep sedation/general anesthesia (24,737 patients) without a death.

Two patients required hospitalization—one for an allergic reaction to cefazolin and one who aspirated. Both patients recovered fully. Based on data collected by the Oral Maxillofacial Surgery National Insurance Corporation (OMSNIC), between 1988 and 2001 the incidence of death or serious brain injury was 1.28 per 1 million anesthetics administered. Clearly, when practiced correctly by qualified practitioners in appropriate environments, general anesthesia in the office-based setting *can* be as safe as or safer than in hospitals and ASCs.

Requiring Accreditation in the Office-Based Setting

At the core of every state's hospital treatment act, ambulatory surgery center treatment act, and office-based legislative and regulatory initiatives is accreditation by one of the major accrediting bodies. The Joint Commission on Accreditation of Healthcare Organizations (JCAHO) accredits virtually every hospital. The Accreditation Association for Ambulatory Health Care (AAAHC) accredits

most ASCs, with the balance being JCAHO accredited. In the office arena, the majority of facilities that have achieved accreditation have done so through the American Accreditation Association for Ambulatory Surgical Facilities (AAAASF), formerly the American Accreditation Association for Plastic Surgical Facilities (AAAPSF), an organization founded by plastic surgeons in 1980 to address the accreditation needs of the office-based plastic surgical facilities. Most of the remaining offices are accredited by AAAHC through their office-based accreditation program.

Even JCAHO and, more recently, the American Osteopathic Association (AOA) have developed office-based accreditation programs.

What is accreditation?

With subtle yet sometimes significant differences, the essential elements of accreditation are the same. When an accrediting body with the help of its surveyor(s) examines an organization, they all address the same core issues (Table 17-3). The differences between the accrediting bodies as they relate to office-based anesthesia and surgery are outlined in Table 17-4. Coldiron and many others argue that accreditation in POBS would have *no impact* on patient safety and hence is an unnecessary intrusion.[10] Coldiron states, in the paper's abstract, "requiring office accreditation, board certification and hospital privileges, would have *little effect* on overall safety of surgical procedures."[10]

Certainly, compelling arguments are made especially in the situation where local anesthetics are used alone or in combination with minimal sedation. In these situations of Level or Class A facilities, little is to be gained by requiring the accreditation process. In fact, states that do regulate OBS recognize this and don't require accreditation for these facilities (Table 17-5).

Table 17-3. Core issues of accrediting bodies

1. Facilities and environment
2. Governance and administration
3. Quality of care
4. Medical records
5. Peer review and quality improvement
6. Credentialing and privileging
7. Emergency preparedness

Table 17-4. AAAASF level of surgery and facility definition

Level of Surgery	Facility Class	Definition
I	A	Provides for minor surgical procedures performed under topical and local Infiltration blocks with or without oral or intramuscular preoperative sedation. **Excluded** are spinal, epidural, axillary, stellate ganglion blocks, regional blocks (e.g., interscalene), supraclavicular, infraclavicular, and intravenous regional anesthesia. These methods are appropriate for Class B and C facilities.
II	B	Provides for minor and major surgical procedures performed in conjunction with oral, parenteral, or intravenous sedation or under analgesic or **dissociative** drugs.
III	C	Provides for major surgical procedures that require general[a] or regional block anesthesia and support of vital bodily functions.

[a]Editor's note: The MIA™ technique is not "general anesthesia." See Chapter 1, Appendix 1-1. —BLF

However, Surgery Level II or III (B or C Class Facilities) are another matter. In these facilities, more invasive surgeries with deeper levels of anesthesia are being performed, and it is in those facilities where the majority of problems arise. It is also these facilities that account for the bulk of the increased caseload in POBS as procedures shifted from HOPD and ASCs. Is it possible the perceived increase in complications is an uncovering of a "hidden epidemic" of similar occurrences in hospitals and ASCs as they shift to POBS? The only way to know for sure is to adopt the same reporting mechanisms in all settings. However mandatory reporting does not necessitate mandatory accreditation. In the meantime, be conservative.

For over fifty years in hospitals and twenty-five years in ASCs, the medical community and the public have accepted accreditation as the minimum acceptable standards of care. The same minimum standards could be applied to offices that offer identical services. Coldiron points out in the Florida data that four (57%) of the seven cosmetic surgery deaths were in accredited offices.[10] Particularly in light of the small numbers, accreditation to guarantee patient safety is not an especially compelling argument.

Barinholtz will be the first to admit accreditation is no panacea. Bad things do happen in accredited facilities (as illustrated by the two aforementioned deaths at the prestigious Manhattan Eye and Ear Hospital).

Table 17-5. Similarities and differences between various accreditation organizations

Accreditation body	AAAASF	AAAHC	JCAHO
Medicare Deemed Status	Yes	Yes	Yes
Board Certification of Surgeon	Yes	No	No
Physician Supervision of Anesthesia[a]	Yes	Yes	Yes
Additional Education Requirements for Nonanesthesiologists Supervising	Yes	No	No
Accreditation Cycle	3 yrs	6 mos, 1 yr, or 3 yrs	3 yrs
Approximate Base Cost[b]	$675–$1,000	$2,990	$3,975
Corporate Website	aaaasf.org	aaahc.org	jcaho.org

[a]This requirement may not apply in the event a state's governor has opted out of the physician supervision of nonanesthesiologist anesthesia-providers requirement.
[b]Cost for an accreditation survey may be influenced by the number of offices to be accredited, the number of surgeons and surgical specialties, and whether or not a facility is asking for Medicare "deemed" status.

Accrediting bodies are constantly evaluating the standards and how to improve on them. The Office of the Inspector General of the Department of Health and Human Services issued a report in 2002 stating that the accrediting bodies and state agencies have to do a better job with quality oversight.[17]

No one, however, is suggesting abandoning the accreditation process. Identify the problems and fix them. Patients and practitioners in Surgery Level II or III (B or C Class Facilities) may benefit. The best way to benefit is to live the standards every day.

In hospitals and ASCs, many practitioners from many disciplines as well as nurses and administrators provide a check-and-balance system to assure standards are being complied with on a daily basis, not just every two or three years. Offices, on the other hand, are isolated, and it is usually up to one surgeon, one anesthesia provider, and one nurse (the latter two often being employed by the surgeon) to make sure the standards are being followed. The advantages of accreditation are lost without a commitment by all involved.

Requiring Hospital Privileges/Board Certification

As significant numbers of procedures have moved from hospitals and ASCs to POBS, another concern has arisen. Are practitioners performing procedures in their offices because they could not obtain privileges in a peer-reviewed institution owing to inadequate training, education, and experience?

Are physicians with "inadequate training, education, and experience" responsible for a disproportionate share of adverse outcomes? Alternatively, are some very qualified, very capable practitioners being kept off staff of hospitals and ASCs for political and/or economic reasons? The answers to both questions are yes. This is the crux of the controversy surrounding the issue of whether only board-certified physicians with hospital privileges should be allowed to perform the same procedures in the office-based setting.

Hospital privileges and board-certification requirements are very touchy subjects. However, the solutions are not as complicated and cumbersome as one might think. The overwhelming majority of physicians would agree that although licensed to practice medicine in all of its branches, not all physicians are qualified to practice every specialty. Hospitals and ASCs have created credentialing committees to evaluate whether practitioners have the qualifications to perform the procedures they request. By and large, the process works well, but sometimes the reasons for denial of privileges has nothing to do with qualifications and everything to do with politics.

One example may be when plastic surgeons influence committees to deny cosmetic privileges to ENT surgeons, dermatologists, and maxillofacial surgeons despite adequate training. Another example may be when orthopedic surgeons keep podiatrists off staff. These are just a couple of examples of political/economic credentialing. So how does one discern between these situations and those where privileges are denied because of lack of qualifications? It is not currently possible. The answer may lie in an alternative credentialing mechanism.

As states regulate OBS and attempt to assure the public that practitioners are safe, several have adopted multiple ways to accomplish this. One is to require accreditation. Accrediting bodies address standards qualifications for practitioners. The problem is that accrediting bodies don't specifically describe what constitutes adequate education, training, and experience. The only one that goes into detail is the AAAASF, which requires proof of board certification and hospital privileges. AAAHC and JCAHO are much more vague. In order for accreditation to adequately address this, those organizations must define specifically what constitutes proper education, training, and experience. Another way is for the state to require hospital privileges, but this has significant limitations (*vide supra*). Yet one other solution is for the state medical board to develop alternative credentialing mechanisms for people that don't have hospital privileges. There *are* ways to assure the public practitioners performing procedures in every setting have proper qualifications without unfairly restricting one's ability to practice. However, *specific* ways to assure the public would have been more constructive than the preceding generalization.

What about board certification? Is that necessary?

According to the American Board of Medical Specialties (ABMS) website, approximately 90% of physicians practicing in the United States are board certified.

So this question is germane to only 10% of physicians. Should these people be allowed to perform surgery in-office (or anywhere)?

Most hospitals and ASCs won't grant privileges to non–board-certified/eligible physicians. Many third-party payers won't enter into contracts with non–board-certified/eligible physicians.

Most medical malpractice carriers won't write policies for non–board-certified/eligible physicians. (Coverage may not be available for activities outside these physicians' primary field.) So the reality is that few of these people are out there. Unfortunately, in the case of office-based cosmetic surgery, there are some people who don't disclose to their carrier what procedures they perform, are subject to no regulations in the office, and are licensed to practice medicine in all of its branches. Thus, they can and do perform all manner of procedures for which they *may not* be qualified.

Are these people responsible for more complications? According to the American Society of Aesthetic Plastic Surgeons (ASAPS), an analysis of the Florida data shows an approximately threefold increase in the risk of an in-office death in the hands of a non–board-certified cosmetic surgeon compared to a board-certified plastic surgeon. A fact not supported by the Coldiron study.[10]

The plastic surgeons [ASAPS] didn't dissect out the data on board-certified dermatologists performing tumescent liposuction under local anesthesia. *Significantly, there were no deaths in this group.* It would appear that board certification *per se* has little merit. In its recent publication of "Core Principles for Office-Based Surgery," The American College of Surgeons advocates board certification for physicians.[18] This document was unanimously approved by all three major accrediting bodies—American Society of Aesthetic Plastic Surgeons (ASAPS), American Society of Cosmetic Surgery (ASCS), and the Dermatologic Surgical Society (DSS)—as well as a host of other surgical and anesthesia societies.

Placing Limits on Procedures

Another tactic that has been employed in the name of patient safety has been to limit what procedures can be performed in the office and on whom. States have enacted limits on the length of surgery, liposuction volumes, and combinations of certain procedures. The concern here is that this has been done by legislation. That is not to say these measures don't have merit; it is, however, very disconcerting when lay legislators decide to legislate medical judgment. These issues could be dealt with at the accred-

itation and medical-board level. The limits are discussed herein.

Limits on patients

Widely supported is that not all patients are appropriate candidates for outpatient surgery, let alone in an office-based setting. Furthermore, *not all settings are equal.*

Compared to an office-based setting, the hospital has an ICU, a code team, respiratory therapy, and other services that make this setting most appropriate for any patient at perceived increased risk to require these services.

No matter how prepared a freestanding outpatient facility is (ASC or POBS), it does not possess the personnel and resources for emergencies that a hospital does. This is why patients have to be chosen with care in POBS. Only ASA physical status I and II patients should be routinely cared for in this setting. ASA physical status III and IV patients are *generally* not appropriate candidates. **In the final analysis, it is more prudent to avoid emergencies than to be prepared to handle them when they arise.**

Limits on procedures

Most states that regulate OBS, as well as the ASA, surgical societies, and accrediting bodies, have statements to the effect that procedures should be of such duration and complexity as to expect them to be completed in a reasonable period of time, and the patient should be able to be discharged in a reasonable amount of time. However, specifics are notoriously absent. Some states have legislated limits. Unless this slippery slope is to continue and every individual procedure is to be legislated, the medical boards and accrediting bodies must take a stand.

Limiting time

Some states have adopted regulations limiting the time a surgical procedure can be done safely in the office-based setting. Typically, these limits range from four to six hours. Although common sense may dictate this, there are no data to support this. It is, however, reasonable to assume that the longer the procedure, the more potential for anesthetic morbidity, hypothermia, hypovolemia, and thromboembolic phenomena.

It would behoove the medical community to extract and look at the data of adverse incidents as related to length of procedure. In the meantime, some commonsense limits would be appropriate. Most hospitals, ASCs, and offices that have limits do not allow elective outpatient procedures anticipated to take more than six hours. This would appear to be appropriate.

Limiting combination of procedures

Because Florida had a cluster of deaths after liposuction combined with abdominoplasty, a ninety-day moratorium was placed on liposuction performed within fourteen days of an abdominoplasty in 2004. Upon further review, the office surgery rules in January of 2005 were amended, limiting the amount of liposuction performed in conjunction with any procedure. The incidences were more likely due to combinations of procedures resulting in a prolonged (greater-than-six-hour) anesthetic than to a specific combination of procedures. Establishing reasonable time limits should adequately address this situation.

Limits on liposuction

Because a seemingly disproportionate number of patients having liposuction in the office-based setting experience complications, some states have put specific limits on liposuction volumes. Others are considering this. Again, this is more an issue in the *duration of surgery* than a specific problem with liposuction. Liposuctions beyond 5,000–6,000 cc generally take more than six hours. It may be difficult to justify going beyond that in one session for the stated reason.

On average, 1 liter of tumescent solution contains 50 cc of 1% lidocaine or 500 mg. Five liters amounts to 2,500 mg or 35 mg · kg^{-1} for a 70-kg person. Current "industry standards" recommend no more than 35–50 mg · kg^{-1} of lidocaine when administered in the dilute concentration for liposuction (see Chapter 8). These limits seem reasonable and certainly should not impact patients' access to care.

Mandatory Reporting of Adverse Events

As stated earlier, one of the problems in discussing patient safety in OBS is that there are no comprehensive and accurate data. Florida made the reporting of adverse events mandatory in all settings, a requirement other states should follow.

This way each entity would be able to track adverse incidences and spot trends, if they exist (i.e., in differences between settings, providers, procedures). Rational deter-

minations could then be made based on undisputed facts as to which measures make sense and which don't.

What the states are doing/have done?

CONs. Historically, in order to assure proper allocation of healthcare resources and avoid duplicative, wasteful services to exist in any given area, many states adopted Certificate of Need (CON) laws. Under these programs, the governor of the state appoints a board whose job is to review applications for licensure of new healthcare facilities. The board is supposed to evaluate the proposed new healthcare facility and—based on issues such as location, existence of similar facilities that offer similar services, population trends, sources of funding, and overall soundness of the plan—make a determination as to whether the facility is needed in the community. If the determination is positive, then a CON is issued, clearing the way for state licensure. If the determination is negative, no CON is issued, and the project does not go forward. Currently, thirty-seven states have laws requiring CONs for state licensure of hospitals, twenty-seven states require CONs for ASCs, and thirteen states have no CON law. A few states—Connecticut, Pennsylvania, and Rhode Island—have recently established laws requiring a CON and licensure of single-specialty, office-based surgical facilities (Table 17-6). Other states are considering expanding or resurrecting CON laws to include OBS facilities as well. Is this a good idea?

If one asks the federal government, the answer to this question appears to be "no." In July of 2004, the Federal Trade Commission and Department of Justice in Washington, D.C., issued the results of a five-year study evaluating CON programs in states that still have them. The main conclusion of this report is that CON boards and the CON process is a *corrupt system* fraught with undue influence of special-interest groups such as local hospitals and the hospital lobby. The CON boards create an anticompetitive environment that restricts consumer access to care and keeps health-care costs artificially high. Based on the results of this study, those departments recommended that states that still have CON laws abolish them.[19] Why then, in the light of this study's results, are some states expanding and resurrecting CON laws?

CON laws are, undoubtedly, influenced by the hospital lobbies. They argue a doomsday scenario in which there is a hospital and/or ASC on every corner, diluting and duplicating health-care resources to such an extent

Table 17-6. States with CON laws, summary prepared 02/05/2002

Certificate of need (CON)	CON laws exempting ASCs	No CON
1. Alabama	1. Arkansas	1. Arizona
2. Alaska	2. Florida	2. California
3. Connecticut	3. Louisiana	3. Colorado
4. Delaware	4. Missouri[b]	4. Idaho
5. District of Columbia	5. Nebraska	5. Indiana
6. Georgia	6. New Jersey	6. Kansas
7. Hawaii	7. Ohio	7. Minnesota
8. Illinois	8. Oklahoma	8. New Mexico
9. Iowa	9. Oregon	9. North Dakota
10. Kentucky	10. Wisconsin	10. Pennsylvania
11. Maine	11. South Dakota	
12. Maryland	12. Texas	
13. Massachusetts	13. Utah	
14. Michigan	14. Wyoming	
15. Mississippi		
16. Montana		
17. Nevada[a]		
19. New Jersey		
20. New York		
21. North Carolina		
22. Rhode Island		
23. Tennessee		
24. Vermont		
25. Virginia		
26. Washington		
27. West Virginia		

[a]Las Vegas, Reno, and all ASC includes major medical are exempt from CON equipment over $1 million.
[b]CON may be required in other counties over 100K.

as to make it impossible for any health-care institution to survive. One need only look at states without CON laws to see how ludicrous this contention is. In fact, in these states, market forces have not only worked to assure adequate distribution of healthcare resources but have also kept costs under control by healthy free-market competition. Clearly, CONs are not the answer. What about state licensure?

STATE LICENSES. CONs aside, state licensure is simply the process by which one applies for and receives a license to operate a health-care facility. Typically, the sequence is as follows: Once a completed application is received, the state will require the organization to undergo an accreditation survey by one of the major accrediting organizations, a state inspection, and a Medicare inspection. Upon successful completion, a time-limited license is granted. At the time of renewal, the process is repeated. Virtually every hospital in the United States is licensed by the state using this process. Forty-three states require licensure of ASCs. To date, three states, Connecticut, Pennsylvania, and Rhode Island, require state licensure of OBS facilities. Arizona requires licensure of such organizations that provide general anesthesia. But is licensure necessary in OBS/OBA? Is it realistic to expect states to inspect and license all 50,000 OBS facilities? *Both answers are "no."*

As stated earlier, at the core of state licensure is the requirement for accreditation. The accrediting bodies JCAHO, AAAHC, and AAAASF have done an admirable (though, admittedly, not perfect) job of assuring patient safety and quality of care in hospitals, ASCs, and OBS facilities.

If Medicare reimbursement is expected by the facility, it must also undergo a Medicare survey. All of the accrediting bodies have been given "deemed status" by Medicare to perform these surveys. The state inspection is probably the most redundant and superfluous part of the process. Rarely do state inspections uncover a problem missed by the accrediting bodies. Also, it is unrealistic to expect state medical boards and/or regulatory bodies to have the manpower with the appropriate expertise to inspect every OBS facility.

The accrediting bodies, on the other hand, already inspect and accredit more than 5,000 hospitals, almost 4,000 ASCs, and approximately 2,000 OBS facilities, and counting.

All the major accrediting bodies have developed accreditation programs for OBS facilities and are currently increasing their surveyor ranks to accommodate the rapidly increasing demand for surveys. Other accrediting organizations, such as the American Osteopathic Association (AOA) program, have been developed. In assuring safety and quality of care in hospitals and ASCs, who better to turn to to assure a similar standard of care in OBS than the experts?

SCOPE-OF-PRACTICE ISSUES

As states grapple with all of these concerns, there are other issues heating up at the state level. These battles generally involve scope-of-practice issues (*vide infra*).

Anesthesiologists vs. nurse anesthetists

There are few issues in medicine that garner more debate than the scope-of-practice battle between anesthesiologists and nurse anesthetists. This battle played out nationally in the late 1990s as the American Association of Nurse Anesthetists (AANA) lobbied the U.S. Congress to have the Medicare rule requiring physician supervision of nurse anesthetists abolished. In the end, the rule was maintained but with the ability of individual state governors to opt out (see Table 17-7).

At the heart of this matter is a discussion of patient safety. The anesthesiologists' argument was that when an anesthesiologist is involved in a patient's care, the risk of adverse outcomes is lower and quality of care is better. A University of Pennsylvania (U of P) study demon-

---

Table 17-7. States that have opted out of the nurse anesthetist physician supervision rule

1. Alaska
2. Idaho
3. Iowa
4. Kansas
5. Minnesota
6. Montana
7. Nebraska
8. New Hampshire
9. New Mexico
10. North Dakota
11. Oregon
12. Washington
13. South Carolina
14. Tennessee (considering an opt-out)

---

strated a substantially higher failure-to-rescue rate when a patient under the care of a nurse anesthetist *not* supervised by an anesthesiologist suffers an adverse event compared to the rate when an anesthesiologist is involved.[20] The nurse anesthetists responded that the U of P study was flawed, that unsupervised nurse anesthesia care is every bit as safe as supervised nurse anesthesia care, and that the motivations of the anesthesiologists were economic and political.

Aside from the thirteen opt-out states, in the remaining thirty-seven states an anesthesiologist or the operating practitioner (i.e., the surgeon) by law must supervise nurse anesthetists. It is the rare hospital or ASC that doesn't have staff anesthesiologists directly administering or supervising the administration of every anesthetic. Over 95% of anesthetics in the United States in hospitals and ASCs are either directly administered or supervised by anesthesiologists. Even in the small number of institutions that don't have an anesthesiologist on staff, there are other clinical and ancillary resources to respond in case of an adverse event (e.g., code team, ER staff, ICU staff).

In the office-based setting, approximately ten million patients per year are being treated. The rate of adverse outcomes in this setting is unknown. There is no breakdown on the percentage of these ten million patients having cosmetic surgery as opposed to medically indicated procedures. The relative percentages of anesthesiologist and nurse anesthetist administered anesthetics are also unknown. Last, it is also unknown how many anesthetics are administered (or directed) by the operating practitioner without the involvement of an anesthesia professional. What is known is that 2,000 of the 50,000 OBS facilities are accredited. It is unknown how many of the remaining 48,000 OBS facilities may be inadequately staffed and equipped. It may be that the staff in these 48,000 facilities is inadequately trained in many or all aspects of care. This may even include the surgeon. Some surgeons are not only performing procedures in-office for which they do not have ABMS training (*vide supra*), but they are also choosing to perform or supervise anesthetics that go beyond their scope of training and expertise. However the same argument could be made for an ABMS plastic surgeon, trained before the advent of liposuction, who took a weekend post-graduate course or learned from the liposuction supply salesman.

POBS are facilities with one operating room, one surgeon, one anesthesia provider, and no code team. It is not unreasonable to expect the same minimum standard of care that exists in hospitals and ASCs. However, without a dedicated code team this standard may be difficult to achieve.

The accrediting bodies all address administration of and supervision of anesthesia. Although the specifics of the standards may vary, all accrediting bodies attempt to assure that persons administering and/or supervising anesthesia have the proper education, training, and experience. So, why then do the AANA and its state component societies oppose making accreditation mandatory in the office-based setting? The main argument made by the nurse anesthetists against mandatory accreditation, and the basis of several lawsuits brought by state nurse anesthesia societies, is that it will restrict their ability to practice. However, nurse anesthetists currently practice in hospitals and ASCs, all of which are accredited. The accrediting bodies would have no reason to deny accreditation in a facility where nurse anesthetists are being properly supervised as required by law in thirty-seven states. The argument makes no sense.

Operator/anesthetist

If there is one thing that anesthesiologists and nurse anesthetists can agree on, it's that few other healthcare professionals possess the skills and abilities to perform anesthetics safely. With that being said, by state law, there are several other categories of practitioners that *can* provide anesthetics. In every state physicians (MDs and DOs) are licensed to practice medicine in all of its branches. Oral surgeons are trained and licensed in deep sedation/general anesthesia. Podiatrists are licensed in most states to provide and/or supervise all levels of sedation *but not* general anesthesia.

There is now a movement afoot, fueled by the leadership of the gastroenterology societies, to allow RNs (not nurse anesthetists) to administer propofol for endoscopies. Although these practitioners can and do safely provide sedation and analgesia in hospitals and ASCs, these settings are regulated and accredited. These practitioners must demonstrate proficiency and adequate training prior to receiving privileges. JCAHO, AAAHC, and AAAASF all have standards addressing this.

The specific standards may differ between accrediting bodies

Many professional organizations, including the ASA, American College of Surgeons, AANA, and AMA, have comprehensive guidelines regarding surgery and anesthesia in the office-based setting. ASAPS mandates to its membership that their facilities be accredited or they risk losing membership.[21]

In February of 2005, the Board of Regents of the American College of Surgeons voted unanimously to adopt a similar policy. Virtually every one of these organizations frowns on the operating practitioner providing (either directly or by having staff, usually an RN, provide) anesthetics beyond local anesthesia and "conscious sedation."

If accreditation was adopted as the standard of care in the office-based setting, then the same minimum standards that exist in hospitals and ASCs *could* be applied to the office-based setting.

Practitioners would have to demonstrate adequate education, training, and experience as well as assure environments are adequately staffed and equipped. The states would merely have to police whether the facility is accredited.

Plastic vs. cosmetic surgeons

If the largest scope-of-practice issue in OBS is between anesthesiologists and nurse anesthetists, then the second largest one is between plastic and cosmetic surgeons.

For the purpose of this discussion, "plastic" surgeons refers to ABMS board-certified/eligible plastic surgeons who perform cosmetic procedures. "Cosmetic" surgeons are physicians in other specialties who also perform cosmetic procedures.

In the 1980s, as cosmetic surgeons began operating in their offices, Grazer and other plastic surgeons raised the "hospital privileges" issue to "warn" the public that they should not have office surgery with a physician who did not have hospital or ASC privileges. Anesthesiologists practicing in the office-based setting need to be aware of differences in training as well as proficiency in performing surgery. A crude guideline to proficiency can be procedural times. Two hours in surgery for a "virgin" breast augmentation is reasonable; six hours is not. Four hours in surgery for a standard open rhytidectomy (facelift) with no added procedures is about average; eight hours in surgery is bordering on the unreasonable. Another index of competency may be the reoperation or "redo" rate. In most practices, 1–2% would be reasonable to expect, 10% would be unreasonable.

A (potentially) good rule of thumb to assure one is working with an ABMS certified/eligible surgeon is to require proof of hospital privileges for surgeons requesting to perform in-office surgery. The gray area occurs when practitioners claim to have adequate training but are being kept off hospital staffs for political and/or economic reasons, as discussed previously.

Some states have developed alternative credentialing programs for these practitioners. Also the accrediting bodies are generally blind to board certification as long as the surgeon can demonstrate appropriate education, training, and experience. The issue here is not to enter into the turf battle between plastic surgeons, facial plastic ENT surgeons, or dermatologic surgeons on *who* should be performing rhinoplasties, facelifts, and liposuction. The issue is to know when one is working with the family practitioner (FP) performing liposuction or the oral surgeon doing breast augmentation.

The accreditation process *may* help assure that only *properly qualified* practitioners are performing procedures in the office-based setting.

Dentists

As previously stated, dentists are also licensed by the states to administer anesthetics. Basically, dentists fall into three categories: general dentists, oral surgeons, and dentist anesthesiologists.

GENERAL AND PEDIATRIC DENTISTS. In virtually every state, if general or pediatric dentists wish to perform anesthesia in their office (aside from local anesthesia and nitrous oxide), they must apply for a special permit. There are basically two types of special permits, one that covers conscious to moderate sedation, and one that provides for deep sedation to general anesthesia. Both permits require the dentist to go through extra training. Generally, the lesser permit (frequently referred to as Special Permit A) requires a training course of 50 to 100 hours and has clinical requirements. The permit for deep sedation/general anesthesia requires training in the 1,000- to 2,000-hour range (frequently referred to as Special Permit B). Most general or pediatric dentists who want to provide sedation obtain the lesser permit. In most states (except for the opt-out states), dentists can supervise nurse anesthetists only to the extent they are licensed. So a dentist with a Special Permit A cannot supervise a nurse anesthetist providing general anesthesia (requiring a Special Permit B).

When a pediatric dentist has an uncooperative child requiring dental work, the dentist needs a way to be able to safely control the child. Many of these dentists try to take these children to a hospital or ASC for general anesthesia. Unfortunately, the reimbursement climate is such that the dental insurance carriers say general anesthesia is a "medical service" and refuse payment. On the other side, the medical insurance carriers claim this is a dental and not a medical problem and refuse payment. Even if the dental carrier will cover general anesthesia, dental plans have annual maximums in the $1,000 to $3,000 range. After the dental work is paid for, there is little left to cover anesthesia and facility expenses. This has forced many pediatric dentists into treating children in their office with various combinations of physical and pharmacological restraints without a qualified anesthesia provider present, with predictably disastrous outcomes (see Chapter 5).

After some highly publicized cases and segments on television shows like "60 Minutes," "Dateline," and "20/20," states are starting to respond. Since 1995, twenty-eight states have passed laws requiring third-party medical insurance carriers to pay for general anesthesia for these patients.[22] Although a good start, these laws still have many loopholes that render them ineffective.

ORAL SURGEONS. Aside from anesthesiologists and nurse anesthetists, the largest group of providers with significant anesthesia training is oral/maxillofacial surgeons. Oral surgery residency training programs provide six months to one year of training exclusively in anesthesia. In these programs the oral surgery residents are being taught side-by-side with anesthesia residents. States recognize this and grant oral surgeons licensure to provide deep sedation/general anesthesia. By and large, the oral surgery community has done an admirable job with patient safety (see Chapter 5). The American Association of Oral and Maxillofacial Surgeons (AAOMS) has an accreditation program whose anesthesia standards mirror the other accrediting bodies. By the rules imposed on them by their own professional society, all oral surgeons performing surgery and anesthesia in their offices must go through accreditation by this program in all fifty states.

Oral surgeons perform cosmetic surgery. At first thought one might say, "These people are dentists, of course they can't perform cosmetic surgery!" However, oral surgeons perform all manner of reconstructive surgery on the face, maxilla, mandible, and skull. Why can't an oral surgeon do a chin implant or blepharoplasty? Frequently, this comes down to hospital and local politics. It has more to do with "turf" battles and medical elitism than common sense. Oral surgeons who have the training and experience and frequently do orthognathic procedures are qualified to perform all manner of facial cosmetic procedures. On the other hand, there is no amount of oral surgical training that will qualify one to perform breast augmentation or abdominoplasties. Many states are currently addressing this issue. For example, the California Medical Board quashed a move by the oral surgeons to include facial cosmetic surgery under the "mouth and related structures" portion of the dental regulations. However, recent efforts by these surgeons have succeeded. Botox®, Restylane®, and rhytidectomy can now be had at the dental office. Caveat emptor.

DENTIST ANESTHESIOLOGISTS. There is a small group of dental professionals—called dentist anesthesiologists—who complete an anesthesia residency training program after dental school. There are only a few anesthesia residencies that will accept dental-school graduates. There is no separate, recognized subspecialty board certification for these individuals. Hence, in the United States there are only approximately 200 of these individuals. Although most of these professionals practice exclusively in the den-

tal community, some do work with physicians. In Pennsylvania, there are dental anesthesiologists who work with cosmetic surgeons. At the University of Illinois, dentist anesthesiologists ran the anesthesia division at the Eye and Ear Infirmary for many years, training medical anesthesia residents and oral surgery residents performing anesthetics for ophthalmic and ENT surgery. Other than granting permits or licenses for general anesthesia, there is no separate licensure or certification for dentist anesthesiologists. In Japan, where there is separate licensure and certification, dentist anesthesiologists make up a significant portion of the anesthesia professionals in that community. It might behoove the American Dental Association to consider creating a separate certification program for this subspecialty in order to encourage more professionals to take this path. This could help alleviate the anesthesia-provider shortage in the United States (see Chapter 5).

Podiatrists

No discussion on state regulations and legislative issues regarding anesthesia would be complete without discussing podiatrists. Podiatrists are individuals who attend a four-year podiatric medical school. Upon completion (and sometimes doing a residency, although this is not mandatory), podiatrists can perform surgery on the foot and ankle.

Podiatrists are allowed by state laws to provide and/or supervise local anesthesia, regional anesthesia, and/or intravenous sedation for podiatric procedures, with the specific exclusion of general anesthesia. Currently, many podiatrists have their own freestanding facilities and perform all manner of surgeries such as procedures on bunions, hammertoes, and ankle arthroscopies requiring anesthesia.

In many of these centers, podiatrists are supervising nurse anesthetists. When states amend laws addressing OBA/OBS, it is imperative that they include the podiatrists. Mandatory accreditation for OBA/OBS would assure these settings are proper and safe.

Anesthesiologist "extenders"

The increasing demand for anesthesia services in North America has led to two different types of anesthesiologist "extenders." In Canada, respiratory technicians have been pressed into service under anesthesiologist supervision in the hospital-based socialized system. Once patients are induced, intubated, placed on a ventilator, and have their vital signs stabilized, maintenance of the anesthetic is turned over to a respiratory technician. By contrast, in the United States, the services of a new class of helper, called the anesthesia assistant (AA), has evolved to serve a similar function. Currently, only a few states recognize this type of provider. The nurse anesthetist community is not enamored with this development.

Propofol and RNs

As any anesthesia provider who practices ambulatory anesthesia knows, propofol is a godsend. This short-acting, quick-recovery drug has revolutionized outpatient anesthesia.

The anesthesia community has a commendable safety record with regard to propofol. However, the anesthesia community appears to be the victim of its own success. There is such a good safety record with propofol that a false sense of security has emerged. Other non–anesthesia-trained practitioners are now attempting to administer propofol. In March of 2004, all three major gastroenterology societies came out with a joint statement advocating nurse-administered propofol sedation (NAPS).[23] In this statement, they erroneously classify propofol administration as "conscious sedation." The reality of NAPS is that when propofol is administered for endoscopy, it is a level of hypnosis compatible with general anesthesia (i.e., BIS 45–60). (See Chapter 1, Appendix 1.1.)

Licensed and/or accredited hospitals and ASCs, through their own credentialing and privileging process, by and large do not allow non–anesthesia providers to administer propofol. However, as freestanding endoscopy centers are popping up all over the country, this is quickly becoming a large patient-safety issue. Most of these centers are not subject to state CON and licensing laws, and few jurisdictions require accreditation. As the population is aging and more of these procedures are done outside hospitals and ASCs and in centers without institutional support such as code teams, something needs to be done. Already thirteen states, by nursing statute, specifically *prohibit* RNs (except nurse anesthetists) from administering propofol in any setting.[24] Six states, however, do allow this, and the issue is not specifically addressed by standards requiring an anesthesia professional to administer propofol in any of its accredited facilities. AAAHC and JCAHO are also addressing this issue.

Current Status of Office-Based Activities at the State Level

Now that myriad office-based issues involved have been elucidated, what has been done thus far to assure patient safety and quality of care in the office-based setting?

Table 17-7 summarizes the current status of legislative regulatory and medical board activities in the states that address them. Currently, approximately twenty-four states have addressed OBS/OBA. There are seven additional states with activities in development. This still leaves nineteen states with **no** regulatory legislative activities. The ways this has been approached varies from state to state, with some states requiring accreditation, some having recreated the accreditation process at the state regulatory level, others having addressed only specific elements of patient safety (e.g., requiring ACLS certification of providers of OBS/OBA) while ignoring other critical elements, and still others having issued only guidelines and recommendations. To help decipher and understand the table, one may find the following definitions of terms helpful.

LEGISLATION. Legislation means that a law was passed by the state mandating these changes. Persons not in compliance are in direct violation of the law. If apprehended, violators can face significant penalties.

REGULATIONS. Regulations are rules adopted by the state medical board or its equivalent. These rules have as much enforceability as laws, the only difference being that the regulatory agency already has statutory authority, obviating the need for additional legislation. There is some disagreement over what statutory authority the regulatory body has, and many of these regulations have been challenged in court.

GUIDELINES. Guidelines are more like suggestions. Although many organizations have adopted guidelines for the safe practice of OBS/OBA, at the end of the day, they are unenforceable. These guidelines can supply a wonderful template for states looking for guidance in developing standards, but without it becoming a law or a regulation, it has no enforceability or "teeth."

Professional Society Activities

In 1995, in response to the lack of attention the organized anesthesia community was giving to anesthesia and surgery in the office-based setting, Barry L. Friedberg, M.D., formed the Society for OFfice Anesthesiologists (**SOFA**). The purpose of this society was to bring together anesthesiologists who practice in this setting to share ideas in the name of elevating patient safety and quality of care. In 1996, a small group of anesthesiologists, including this author, at the University of Illinois in Chicago started the Society for Office-Based Anesthesia (**SOBA**), an organization with similar goals. Soon, SOFA and SOBA merged. Over the next few years, membership expanded to over 500, and several educational meetings were held. Word of these activities reached the ASA and SAMBA, and these organizations began addressing the unique issues in the office-based environment. In 1999, the ASA convened a task force, and in October of that year issued "Guidelines for Office-Based Anesthesia."[25]

Also in 1994, the American College of Surgeons issued "Guidelines for Optimal Office Based Surgery," a manual that addresses all the salient issues to assure safe surgical practices in the office-based setting. Interestingly, this manual virtually recreates the accreditation process (a second edition was published in 2000).[26]

In 2000, ASAPS issued a statement to its membership. This statement mandated to the membership that if Level I or II surgery was being performed in their office facility, the facility be accredited. Failure to comply could result in loss of membership in the society.[21]

In 2002, the Federation of State Medical Boards (FSMB) in its "Report of the Special Committee on Outpatient Surgery" published guidelines for the safe practice of anesthesia and surgery in POBS.[27] Within these guidelines is a recommendation that all states require accreditation or create their own standards (using FSMB model guidelines).

Then, in 2003, the American Medical Association (AMA) and the American College of Surgeons (ACS) both issued public policy statements on improving patient safety in office-based surgery.[18] These statements both contain the same ten core principles. The principles are well thought out and address all the issues that have been discussed in this chapter. Furthermore, these core principles have been endorsed by all of the accrediting bodies, all of the major surgical societies and organizations (including the ASAPS, AACS, and ASDS), the ASA, Federation of State Medical Boards, and many state medical societies. Clearly, virtually all of organized medicine is now speaking with one voice when it comes to office-based surgery. There probably isn't a reader of this chapter who doesn't belong to or isn't affiliated with one of these organizations. From a patient-safety and/or regulatory perspective, and certainly from a medico-legal perspective, one should strive to become familiar with these core principles and insure compliance. Ignore them at one's (and one's patient's) peril.

Federal Government Issues

Traditionally, when it comes to regulating the practice of medicine, the federal government has deferred to the states. However, there are exceptions. Federal law requires physicians and nurse anesthetists who receive Medicare reimbursement to follow the physician supervision rule. The federal law did provide a mechanism for states to opt out. Recently, there have been other federal actions that may impact OBS/OBA.

Stark Law amendments

Last year, on the heels of the Stark Law amendments that ban physician ownership of surgical hospitals, initiatives were introduced to extend this to ASCs. If passed it would make it illegal for physicians to own any part of an ASC at which they operate. Some versions of this amendment are attempting to include single-specialty OBS facilities. This would mean that if physicians want to do surgery in their own offices, they are not allowed to own their office. This is clearly a Catch-22.

Effect of government issues on reimbursement

Whereas reimbursement for elective cosmetic surgery and anesthesia is primarily done on a cash basis, many anesthesia providers also work in settings where third-party payers largely control reimbursement. The third-party payers do recognize the cost savings in the OBS setting. However, various political and bureaucratic issues present several obstacles to reimbursement.

REASONS FOR DENIAL OF PAYMENT IN POBS

State Licensure. The reasons for denial of reimbursement abound, but at the top of the list is state licensure. It is the policy of Blue Cross (BC) /Blue Shield (BS) and Medicare that a facility not licensed by the state as a hospital or ASC will not be reimbursed for facility-related expenses.

However, this is not entirely true (vide infra). Because BC/BS and Medicare are the two largest payers in the country, their policies have a significant impact on the ability of physicians to run a successful office-based surgical practice. Many states have CON requirements for licensure, which makes it very difficult if not impossible for a physician to obtain a license for an OBS center.

Accreditation. Many other third-party payers, such as Aetna, Cigna, and United Healthcare, will reimburse OBS facilities for their facility-related expenses as long as they are accredited by one of the major accrediting bodies. It is the attitude of these carriers that accredited facilities provide care that is just as safe as licensed hospitals and ASCs. And because they can simultaneously assure their subscribers safe care and save money, to them it's a "no-brainer."

OTHER REIMBURSEMENT ISSUES

Site-of-Service Differentials. Medicare and BC/BS will not *directly* reimburse nonlicensed facilities for facility-related expenses (*vide supra*). Instead, they have created the "site-of-service differential." Recognizing the cost savings on a whole host of procedures (urologic, gynecologic, orthopedic, podiatric, and gastroenterologic, to name a few), third-party payers are reimbursing physicians performing these procedures in their office a *higher* professional fee than they would if the same procedures were done in the hospital or ASC. The differential can range from a few hundred to over a thousand dollars a case. Physicians don't have to have their facility licensed or accredited to get the increased fee. These carriers appear to be talking out of both sides of their mouths. Indeed, Medicare, in 2005, published over 100 CPT codes for which they will no longer reimburse hospitals or ASCs. The reason given for the elimination of many of these codes is that they are being performed in OBSs more than 50% of the time. Clearly, the intent is to force procedures into the more cost-effective office-based environment. But they are picking and choosing with the potential for compromising patient safety by not requiring accreditation or licensure.

Taxes. As market forces have shifted 50% of outpatient surgery outside the hospital, the better payers tend to make up a higher proportion of these cases, as discussed previ-

ously. The hospitals are left with higher proportions of the poorer paying Medicare, Medicaid, and BC/BS. Hospitals are feeling this financial loss and turning to state legislatures for relief. Some of the initiatives have focused on expanding CON and licensure requirements, others have focused on banning physician ownership of ASCs, and yet others are imposing new taxes.

In 2004, the state of New Jersey enacted two laws impacting outpatient surgery. One law imposes a 6% tax on cosmetic surgeons on gross revenues received for all cosmetic procedures (including Botox® injections). The other law imposes a 3.5% tax on gross revenues of for-profit ASCs.

Illinois is considering a similar cosmetic surgery tax. The monies from these taxes are *supposed* to go to support charity care at hospitals (in Illinois the money is earmarked for stem-cell research). Hopefully, these laws will be successfully challenged on constitutional and commonsense grounds. These laws make no sense.

What *does* make sense is creating a level playing field for outpatient surgery by requiring accreditation of all such facilities, HOPD, ASC, and POBS, and making BC/BS and Medicare reimburse all accredited facilities (thereby saving taxpayers and subscribers potentially billions of dollars). *Allow the free-market economy to do what it does best.* Balance quality with cost. Hospitals need to step up to the plate, cut their bureaucratic bloat and other waste, and compete instead of lobbying state legislatures to continue to buoy up their inefficient, obsolete model.

THE FUTURE

The future of office-based surgery and anesthesia appears to be on the right track. The states are addressing it, and the professional societies appear to have a clear consensus and have created a reasonable set of standards to guide the states. The accrediting bodies are specifically addressing POBS with reasonable, unobtrusive, inexpensive, one-day surveys to help to assure patients receive safe care in this setting. Although some fine-tuning of scope-of-practice issues, accreditation standards, alternative credentialing mechanisms, and a few other issues needs to occur, patient-care issues appear to be on the right track. Mandatory reporting and the ability to track trends will be beneficial—not only in POBS but also in all arenas where procedures are being performed—in making reasonable, rational decisions on what needs to be done in the efforts to continuously improve patient safety and quality of care.

REFERENCES

1. SMG Marketing Group: Forecast of surgical volume in hospital/ambulatory setting: 1981–2006. 1999; p27.
2. Federal Register, Part III, Department of Health and Human Services, Centers for Medicare and Medicaid Services, 42 CFR Part 416, Medicare Program: Update of Ambulatory Surgical Center List of Covered Procedures; Proposed Rule, November 26, 2004, p69182.
3. Klein JA: The tumescent technique for liposuction surgery. *J Am Acad Cosmetic Surg* 4:263,1987.
4. Allen JE: Boom in liposuction treatment carries risk. Associated Press, August 24, 1997.
5. Hayden T, Sieder JJ: Death by Nip and Tuck. *Newsweek* August 9, 1999, p58.
6. Associated Press: Report: 18 died after basic cosmetic surgery. *The Palm Beach Post,* March 7, 1999, p28A.
7. Associated Press: Expert: Sarasota doctor used too much anesthesia in fatal surgery. *HeraldToday.com* January 6, 2005.
8. Grazer FM, deJong, RH: Fatal outcome from liposuction: census survey of cosmetic surgeons. *Plast Reconstr Surg* 105:436,2000.
9. Vila H, Soto R, Cantor A, et al.: Comparative outcomes analysis of procedures performed in physician offices and ambulatory surgery centers. *Arch Surg* 138:991,2002.
10. Coldiron B, Shreve E, Balkrishnan R: Patient injuries from surgical procedures performed in medical offices: Three years of Florida data. *Dermatol Surg* 30:1435, 2004.
11. Venkat AP, Coldiron B, Balkrishnan R, et al.: Lower adverse event and mortality rates in physician offices compared with ambulatory surgery centers: A reappraisal of adverse event data. *Dermatol Surg* 30:1444,2004.
12. Guttman C: Office-Based Surgery Deaths: Who is Most at Fault? *Cosmetic Surgery Times* March 2005; p4.
13. Laurito CE: Anesthesia provided at alternative sites, in Barasch PG, Cullen BF, Stoelting RK (eds.), *Clincal Anesthesia,* 4th ed., Philadelphia, Lippincott, Williams & Wilkins, 2001; p1343.
14. Koch M, Barinholtz D: Combined data from two AAAHC accredited office-based anesthesia practices over a ten year period. Personal Communication, March 2005.
15. Hoeffin SM, Bornstein JB, Martin G, et al.: General anesthesia in an office-based plastic surgical facility: A report on more than 23,000 consecutive office-based procedures under general anesthesia with no significant anesthetic complications. *Plast Reconstr Surg* 107:243,2001.
16. Perrot DH, Yuen J, Andreson RV, et al.: Office-based ambulatory anesthesia: Outcomes of clinical practice of oral and maxillofacial surgeons. *J Oral Maxillofacial Surg* 61:983,2003.
17. Rehnquist J: Quality Oversight of Ambulatory Surgical Centers: A System in Neglect. Department of Health and Human Services, Office of Inspector General, February 2002, OEI-01–00–00450.
18. American College of Surgeons: Statement on Patient Safety Principles for Office-Based Surgery Utilizing Moderate Sedaton/Analgesia, Deep Sedation/Analgesia, or General Anesthesia. Bulletin of the American College of Surgeons 2004; p89.
19. Department of Justice/Federal Trade Commission: Improving Health Care: A Dose of Competition. July 2004, Chapter 8.
20. Silber, Williams SV, Krakauer H, et al.: Hospital and patient characteristics associated with death after surgery. A study of adverse occurrence and failing to rescue. *Medical Care* 30:65A,1992.
21. ASAPS Communications Department, American Society of Plastic Surgeons, American Society for Aesthetic Plastic Surgery, Inc., Policy Statement on Accreditation of Office Facilities, Society Statement issued February 2000.
22. American Dental Association, Department of State Government Affairs, #47 Associated Medical Costs, July 25, 2003.
23. AGA News Release: Three Gastroenterology Specialty Groups Issue Joint Statement on Sedation in Endoscopy. American Gastroenterological Association, March 8, 2004.
24. Meltzer, B: RNs Pushing Propofol. *Outpatient Surgery Magazine,* Paoli, PA, Herrin Publishing Partners LP, 7:28,2003.
25. ASA Statement: Guidelines for Office-Based Anesthesia. Approved by ASA House of Delegates, October 13, 1999.
26. American College of Surgeons: Guidelines for Optimal Office-Based Surgery, 2nd Ed., 2000.
27. Federation of State Medical Boards, "Report of the special committee on outpatient surgery (BD Rpt 02–3)," 2002.

18 | Staying Out of Trouble: The Medicolegal Perspective

Ann Lofsky, M.D.

INTRODUCTION

From a pricing standpoint, malpractice carriers do not routinely rate anesthesiologists who work in plastic surgery offices any differently from those who work in hospital operating rooms, but the claims they generate often do have issues that are unique to the plastic surgery population or to an office environment. An anesthesiologist working in an office is often the only one there who is skilled in airway and fluid management, and any additional help required, in terms of personnel or equipment, may be located some distance away. Office operating rooms are regulated by state requirements that vary widely, and anesthesia equipment typically runs the gamut from state of the art to frankly antique.

Despite all these considerations, from a legal standpoint, the standard of care—which is defined as what a similarly trained, competent physician might have chosen to do given the same circumstances—does not vary between office and hospital operating rooms. An anesthesiologist working in a small plastic surgery suite OR is held to the same standard of care as if the case were done in the operating room of a large metropolitan hospital a few miles away. This practice also includes the handling of any and all unforeseen complications that might occur.

Complications resulting in malpractice litigation against anesthesiologists can stem from problems in any stage of the process, from the patient preoperative evaluation through discharge. The following is a review of the most common categories of these claims with an emphasis on the factors that make claims resulting from cosmetic surgeries unique.

PATIENT SELECTION

Cosmetic surgery cases are, by definition, elective. When complications occur related to the preoperative condition of the patient, the argument that "This patient needed to have the surgery regardless" never applies. This places an extra burden on anesthesiologists to ensure that each patient is optimized for surgery preoperatively and that pertinent medical conditions have been sufficiently evaluated. (N.B. All claims described in this chapter in italics are composites, incorporating details from numerous closed malpractice cases.)

A twenty-year-old woman, 95 lbs. and 5′ 2″, presented to an office surgery center for breast augmentation under general anesthesia. She gave no pertinent medical history and had no prior surgeries. She tolerated the surgery and anesthesia without incident, but in the recovery room, she became obtunded and began seizing, which did not stop with intravenous benzodiazepines. She developed wide-complex bradycardia, progressing to a full cardiac arrest. The paramedics were called and she was resuscitated and transferred to a hospital, where she was ultimately declared brain dead.

One of the issues in this case was that well known to the patient's family and primary care practitioner, she had struggled with anorexia and had lost more than 30 pounds in the three months prior to her surgery. Laboratory work after the arrest demonstrated severe electrolyte abnormalities thought to have contributed to the intractable seizures and arrhythmia. The anesthesiologist and surgeon were both criticized for failing to question the patient about recent weight changes (see BDD in Ch. 15) and for requiring neither a history and physical nor clearance from the patient's primary care physician. The office preoperative questionnaire contained no inquiries about illicit drug or diuretic use.

This case is somewhat unusual in that a patient may have intentionally failed to disclose pertinent medical information, possibly owing to fears that the surgery might not have gone forward. It is not a secret, however, that sometimes patients do seek cosmetic surgery for largely psychological reasons, and the anesthesiologist should at least be alert for "red flags" that might indicate patients are not entirely forthcoming regarding their medical condition or habits. If still unsure, a physician can ask that a patient be sent for a complete preoperative evaluation and clearance.

A sixty-five-year-old woman was scheduled for a facelift. She gave a history of smoking, high blood pressure, and elevated cholesterol. Her preoperative evaluation consisted of a CBC and EKG , both felt by the anesthesiologist to be within normal limits. The surgery was performed under local sedation. Two hours into the procedure, she developed ST segment changes and nitroglycerin paste was applied with some improvement. Her blood pressure then fell but responded to ephedrine and fluids. The procedure was completed in four hours, but in recovery, the patient remained hypotensive and the EKG monitor showed multifocal PVCs. She was transferred to a university hospital, where she ruled-in for acute myocardial infarction. The cardiologist there read her preoperative EKG as showing left ventricular strain and possible lateral ischemia. In deposition, he stated that, had he seen that EKG preoperatively, he would have ordered a treadmill exam or stress echocardiogram before clearing this patient for surgery.

An allegation in this case was the fact that the anesthesiologist had failed to seek cardiology evaluation or clearance for this patient prior to surgery. Consider the possibility of undiagnosed underlying disease. From a medical-legal standpoint, if physicians fail to obtain indicated consultations, they can be held to the standard of care of physicians in the specialty they *could have* referred to, which in this case would be cardiology. If a reasonable and prudent cardiologist would have cancelled the case based on the preoperative EKG, an anesthesiologist might also be found negligent for failing to do so.

In the real world of anesthesia practice, comfortable working relationships develop between surgeons and anesthesiologists. An anesthesiologist who works solely in one physician's office may feel that he or she is in essence an employee and therefore required to do whatever the surgeon needs. The standard of care for any anesthesia provider, however, requires independent judgment. No one is better able to assess a patient's ability to withstand a given anesthetic than someone trained in that specialty. An anesthesiologist should always be prepared to defend the choice of the anesthetic for any patient and for the decision to proceed with the surgery.

From the medical-legal perspective, the anesthesiologist is the final gatekeeper. Regardless of what the surgeon has planned or what the specialists have cleared the patient for, the ultimate decision of whether or not to proceed with the case is always in the hands of the person who pushes the induction dose. If something doesn't feel right—perhaps a patient with an active upper respiratory infection, or someone who appears pale or lethargic—it is always within the anesthesiologist's rights and responsibilities to either reschedule the case or obtain additional information.

Again, because there is *never* an urgent threat to life or limb in cosmetic surgery cases, they can always be safely delayed for medical reasons or to obtain additional studies. Although perhaps a genuine fact of life and something anesthesiologists do take into consideration, concerns such as "The surgeon never would have used me again if I had cancelled another case" or "additional testing would have been too expensive for this patient" will not likely be viewed sympathetically by jury members in court.

FACILITY SELECTION

Cosmetic surgery cases may be performed in hospital operating rooms, surgery centers, or office-based ORs. The explanation for why any given case was done at a certain facility should, hopefully, be something more substantial than "that was just where it was scheduled." Many factors are obviously taken into account, including the surgeons' and anesthesiologists' schedules, patients' preferences, their insurance statuses, and patients' medical conditions. Medicolegally, the patient's medical concerns take precedence over all others. One never wants to be sheepishly forced to admit that you made a decision primarily based on financial issues.

One surgeon, doing a facelift on a high-profile patient, opened his office OR on a Saturday, when it was normally closed, and had only one nurse present in addition to the anesthesiologist. As everyone was anxious to leave the office, the patient was discharged home thirty minutes after the procedure finished. The patient subse-

quently developed intractable vomiting with rupture of a suture line. Her caretaker was forced to call the paramedics, who transported her to a large metropolitan emergency room for treatment, as the office had then closed. Although this patient suffered no complications (other than severe embarrassment), it was argued this was simply a surgical case done in the wrong place at the wrong time with the wrong staffing.

Another issue is whether, for any given patient, the facility is appropriate for the surgery anticipated. Some surgery centers and offices have rules as to whether they will accept ASA 3 and 4 patients. Higher risk patients such as the morbidly obese, insulin-dependent diabetics, and sleep apnea patients might not be appropriate for every setting. Should a patient with moderately severe asthma have surgery at a facility without access to respiratory therapy and breathing treatments?

Should a procedure with a possible large blood loss be done at a site without access to a blood bank? Should a patient with an extensive cardiac history be done only in a facility with the ability to urgently admit and monitor overnight, if needed?

These are questions that need to be addressed on a case-by-case basis, but it is always better if the surgeon, anesthesiologist, and medical director (if one exists) have previously agreed on policies in place as to which patients are and are not appropriate for the outpatient office setting.

A thirty-two-year-old female, 5′ 3″ and 335 lbs., had bilateral breast reduction performed in an office surgery facility under general anesthesia. Postoperatively, she developed respiratory difficulty and had rales consistent with pulmonary edema. She was reintubated, and the paramedics were called for transfer to the local hospital. This was technically difficult because the gurney did not fit into the building's elevator and they had to carry her down six flights of stairs, delaying her arrival at the emergency room. She alleged cognitive difficulties secondary to prolonged hypoxia.

For procedures that may be excessively long or complicated, facilities with the ability to admit and monitor patients overnight might be more appropriate. According to Dr. Mark Gorney, a past president of the American Society of Plastic Surgeons and former medical director of The Doctors Company, a medical malpractice insurance carrier, reviews of malpractice claims indicate that plastic surgery procedures longer than six hours do seem to have a higher complication rate overall. "That doesn't mean you shouldn't do them, but you should take that into account in your decision making process."[1] Surgeries expected to last exceedingly long might be better scheduled in more acute care environments, or consideration could be given to staging them into two or more smaller and shorter procedures.

When problems develop, a common question posed by plaintiffs' attorneys is "Why did you decide to operate on the patient there?" Even though it is often the surgeon's decision where to book a case, the final decision over whether or not a patient can be safely anesthetized in any given situation is still considered to be the anesthesiologist's.

No one can force you to start a case wherein you don't feel comfortable.

If an anesthesiologist has reservations, the time to voice them is obviously before the case begins.

DOCUMENTATION

Good documentation, including legible and complete anesthesia records, can significantly improve the chances of defending a malpractice claim. A panel of experts reviewing cosmetic surgery malpractice cases, where an anesthesiologist was a named defendant, found only one out of eight had adequate documentation of an informed consent for anesthesia.[2] Whenever possible, the information regarding the planned anesthetic should be provided by the anesthesiologist, not the surgeon. A single sentence related to anesthesia buried in a surgical consent may not offer sufficient protection to an anesthesiologist if an adverse event occurs.[2] One or two sentences regarding the informed consent, written by the anesthesiologist, can go a long way toward making a malpractice claim defensible.

The informed consent need not be extensive, but it should at least mention the type of anesthesia planned (sedation, general, or regional) and the most common and severe injuries possible. A sample informed consent for a general anesthetic might simply read: "Risks explained including possible sore throat, dental injury, pneumonia, and death. Questions answered. Patient concurs." No patient entering surgery wants to hear about possible death. This can, however, be phrased in a reassuring light: "Anesthesia is becoming safer all the time. Death related to surgery is extremely uncommon these days, but I need to mention this as a rare complication of anesthesia."

That advisory is important from a malpractice standpoint because patients who have consented to the remote possibility of death will have a hard time arguing that they never would have had anesthesia had they known a dental crown could be loosened.[3]

It is also a good idea, when consenting patients for sedation or regional blocks, to mention that general anesthesia is a remote possibility should the chosen alternative prove unsatisfactory. The patient should clearly understand what type of anesthesia is anticipated and whether there are any decisions to be made. If there were reasonable alternatives and you failed to mention that fact in advance (or document that such a discussion took place), it could become an issue in the event of litigation. Although informed consent is rarely the main reason why patients file lawsuits against anesthesiologists, it may become a secondary issue when complications related to the anesthesia or surgery occur.

Sometimes patients may not completely understand what monitored anesthesia care (MAC) or intravenous sedation is.

They may have a mindset that they will be completely unconscious during the procedure and then become frightened or angry if they are aware during the surgery being performed. A substantial number of malpractice claims for awareness do occur in patients having planned intravenous sedation or regional blocks where general anesthesia was never anticipated. In these cases, patient expectations and understanding are key. Listen carefully to patients' concerns and wishes preoperatively. If a patient is adamant about not wanting to see or hear anything at all during surgery, this needs to be addressed early on. Either the patient can be led to understand and agree to the reasons for sedation, or consideration needs to be given to changing the plan to a general anesthetic.

There is sometimes a tendency, when procedures are performed in small offices, to do things less formally. Charting standards for anesthesia, however, are universal. Always adhere to all specialty standards and guidelines regarding the documentation of vital signs, oximeter, and end-tidal CO_2 readings, where appropriate, no matter how simple or short a procedure might be. In hospitals, charts are often reviewed for completeness by medical records or medical staff committees. This may never occur in some offices. No chart will be more thoroughly reviewed, however, than one involved in a malpractice action, no matter where the surgical care it describes took place.

A fifty-eight-year-old overweight man had a facelift performed in a plastic surgery office operating room under general anesthesia. In the recovery room, he required several doses of intravenous morphine. Subsequently, he was noted to have shallow, labored respirations and was given naloxone and transferred to a hospital for overnight admission. The remainder of his course was uneventful, but he filed suit, claiming injuries and emotional distress. Review of the records found no mention of informed consent for anesthesia and no recorded vital signs for the entire two-hour recovery room stay. Although the surgeon, anesthesiologist, and nurses all testified that the patient was continuously on a pulse oximeter in the recovery area, and that blood pressure and pulse were checked automatically at intervals, it was felt this case would be very hard to defend as to standard of care owing to the lack of appropriate documentation.

Anesthesiologists need to be proactive in charting *every* case as if it could be the one involved in a malpractice action because, of course, this cannot be known with certainty in advance. In medical malpractice handling, "If you didn't write it down, it didn't happen." Although that may seem harsh, it can be necessary if a physician's routine is not documented anywhere in the medical record. Because many other things are documented, the implication may be that if you forgot to chart it, maybe you also forgot to do it or check it, no matter what "it" turns out to be.

MONITORING

Anesthesiologists performing plastic procedures should use all standard monitors including blood pressure, EKG, pulse oximeter, and end-tidal CO_2 (for general anesthetics).

Vital signs should be recorded at regular intervals on the anesthesia record. When anesthesia records are not meticulous as to monitoring, it can make claims difficult to defend, even when the problem is seemingly unrelated. Sloppy anesthesia records may imply sloppy anesthesia technique to a jury who will have little other tangible evidence to view at trial.

It is also, of course, important *who* is doing the monitoring. It is not uncommon for surgeons to provide their own sedation for cases or to medically direct nurses or ancillary personnel to administer drugs for them. Although it is

certainly preferable to have dedicated anesthesia providers present, if such is not the case, it is highly recommended that someone *other* than the surgeon be designated to watch the patient and the monitors while the operation is taking place. There have been a number of disastrous outcomes that occurred when everyone's attention was focused on the operation and not on the patient.

Whenever anesthesia is provided in an office, someone present should be skilled in emergency airway management and Advanced Cardiac Life Support (ACLS) protocols.

Anesthesiologists should keep their Code skills up to date and be aware of current ACLS guidelines. The author once attended a weekend ACLS course where another anesthesiologist excused his failure to correctly manage a simulated Code situation by stating, "I only work in plastic surgery offices. I'll never need this." As malpractice cases will attest, plastic surgery offices are certainly not exempt from cardiac arrests, and anesthesiologists working in them will be expected to handle emergencies as any skilled physician would.

A thirty-two-year-old man presented for a cosmetic eye procedure. A nurse administered intravenous midazolam and fentanyl for pain and agitation at the surgeon's direction. A pulse oximeter was the only monitor used, but as the patient was moving frequently, it was either silenced or removed. At the conclusion of the one-hour procedure, the drapes were removed and the patient was noted to be profoundly cyanotic. All attempts at resuscitation were unsuccessful.

Although hypoxemia is not unique to plastic surgery settings, a special warning is warranted regarding the silencing of monitor alarms.

Many anesthesia "disaster" claims occur because the pulse oximeter alarm is silenced and the anesthesiologist's attention is temporarily diverted.

Often these happen in the seemingly most innocuous of circumstances, such as sedation cases with supposedly awake patients or in long, otherwise uneventful surgeries where anesthesiologists might be tempted to let their guard down, leaving the head of the bed or engaging in activities such as talking on the phone or reading. In these circumstances, the audible alarms on the monitors are the patients' safety nets, and disabling them for other than extremely brief episodes (i.e., Bovie interference) is ill advised. **There is simply *no defense* for failing to use the monitors or failing to use them correctly.**[4]

A similar scenario was the likely cause of the demise of Olivia Goldsmith, author of *The First Wives' Club*, who in January 2004 was scheduled for a rhytidectomy at the Manhattan Eye and Ear Hospital. Information obtained from the New York Department of Health, through the Freedom of Information Act, is strongly suggestive. However, because of the medicolegal ramifications of the case, the complete story will not likely emerge (*vide supra*).

It is also strongly encouraged that appropriate monitors be available both during the procedure and during the recovery period—especially the capability for pulse oximetry. Patients are variably awake after anesthesia and can have unexpected reactions to postoperative pain medication.

If another case has begun in the operating room using the sole set of available monitors, what will be left for a patient in recovery who needs them? Every office surgery site should have protocols for monitoring patients in recovery, and the anesthesiologist should be aware of them and able to have input regarding their appropriateness. The anesthesiologist is responsible for a patient until they have safely recovered from the effects of anesthesia, and therefore should be notified if any vital signs are considered abnormal.

It is, of course, not the monitors that are watching the patient. It is the person watching (and listening to) the monitors. There have been malpractice claims filed where patients were left to recover alone in rooms far away from all medical and office personnel, who failed to hear the monitors alarming. Obviously, if no one can hear the alarms on monitors, they are essentially of no use at all. Anesthesiologists should know who will be present with their patients for the entirety of their recovery periods and feel comfortable that they have the ability both to detect and react appropriately to any and all alarms.

INTRAOPERATIVE MANAGEMENT

Emergency Planning

As has been mentioned, the handling of emergencies in office operating rooms can be more difficult than in a hospital OR. Help may be far away, so the need for it must be anticipated. Paramedics might need to be summoned or the patient transferred by other means to an emergency room or intensive care area before it is too late. Part of this involves the anesthesiologist's recognizing and acting

on the fact that things may be getting out of hand. Situations that might appropriately be handled with a "wait-and-see" attitude in a hospital might require different handling in a remote office location. If breathing treatments or inhalers are not available in an office, then even moderate wheezing that could exacerbate might be a cause for alarm and reason to consider transferring the patient or aborting the case.

*A thirty-five-year-old female presented to an office OR for abdominal and thigh liposuction with monitored anesthesia care. The surgeon injected a mixture of bupivicaine, lidocaine, and epinephrine. Her pulse and heart rate increased substantially, and the surgeon complained because of increased bleeding, so the anesthesiologist injected hydralazine **and** a beta-blocker. The blood pressure and pulse rate started to fall precipitously and did not respond to atropine and fluids. The blood pressure was no longer obtainable by monitor. The anesthesiologist searched the drawers of the medication cart and could find no injectable ephedrine, neosynephrine, or epinephrine. The locked emergency cart for the facility contained airway equipment, but no drugs. The paramedics were called and responded approximately ten minutes later. Administering epinephrine intravenously, they stabilized the patient and transferred her to an emergency room, but she was eventually declared brain dead and removed from the ventilator.*

In offices, there may be no person designated to stock anesthesia equipment and drugs. The anesthesiologist should personally ensure that all emergency drugs and equipment are available and up-to-date. Emergency airway devices, such as laryngeal mask airways (LMAs), should be present as well as appropriately sized endotracheal tubes and laryngoscopes. Drugs should be checked at intervals to remove outdated vials and replenish used items. It is advisable to develop a checklist for emergency medications such as those stocked in hospital operating rooms. Although rarely used in offices, they can make the difference in avoiding catastrophic consequences owing to delays in the arrival of urgently needed emergency supplies.

An anesthesiologist may have worked with the same surgeon in the same office for years. Together, they will likely have developed a routine and a rapport that allows them to anticipate problems and be prepared with solutions. Sometimes, however, anesthesiologists are called at the last minute and asked to work at sites with which they are totally unfamiliar. Time should always be allotted to become familiar with the anesthesia equipment, OR procedures, and supply system of any new facility. An emergency situation will not be the best time to realize you don't know where needed items are kept.

Anesthesiologists should be aware of the availability and location of emergency supplies, including ACLS drugs and equipment, and where the nearest defibrillator is. If dantrolene were required for an unanticipated malignant hyperthermic reaction, would you know where to get it? Although it's not likely these things will be needed on any given case, playing the odds works only until it doesn't. Anesthesiologists are always expected to be prepared for the worst. Even though rare occurrences, complications such as pneumothorax and pulmonary embolism can and do occur with plastic surgery procedures. The anesthesiologist needs to be both alert to the symptoms and signs of such unusual problems and be immediately prepared to treat them according to accepted guidelines.

A twenty-three-year-old woman presented for bilateral reduction mammoplasty. The surgery proceeded uneventfully. At the end of the case, the surgeon performed bilateral intercostals nerve blocks with 0.25% bupivicaine for postoperative pain control. The vital signs became unstable, with falling blood pressure and oxygen saturation. Suspecting a reaction to the local anesthetic, the anesthesiologist administered ephedrine and epinephrine. The patient remained intubated and on the ventilator. When she failed to stabilize, the paramedics were summoned. On arrival they noted poor breath sounds bilaterally. A needle was placed in a left intrathoracic space with an immediate outflow of air. The patient was ultimately diagnosed with bilateral tension pneumorthoraces.

As is the case with any unusual complication, if the possibility is never considered, it is unlikely it will be treated appropriately. When a patient becomes unstable and fails to respond to standard treatments, it is always a good idea to mentally run through a differential diagnosis of possible causes and rule out the worst-case scenarios clinically rather than simply treating the most likely cause. Uncommon complications happen uncommonly, but that doesn't mean they won't happen to you! The index of suspicion for pneumothorax should also be raised *any* time needles are used around the chest cavity, especially for intercostal blocks. A spontaneous pneumothorax, unrelated to injections around the chest, is far harder to suspect. It is more

likely for the second scenario to play out in a patient with preexisting COPD.

Although statistical studies may not currently be available, it does seem from reviews of medical malpractice claims that the outcomes for patients who arrest in remote sites such as offices and surgery centers are not as good as those for patients in the operating rooms of fully staffed hospitals. Even the fastest paramedics, it seems, cannot always get there in time to resuscitate patients and avoid serious anoxic brain injuries. Anesthesiologists, therefore, need to make sure they have all the supplies available that they might require to stabilize their own patients in the event of serious complications.

Fluid Management

Accurate assessments of fluid intake and output can be a problem in longer surgical cases. Large-volume liposuction (i.e., >5,000 cc) may involve considerable fluid shifts that may make intraoperative management difficult. The California Medical Board discourages >5,000 cc liposuction in the office-based setting. Florida has also limited office-based liposuction to 4,000 cc. The use of compression garments tends to obliterate the "third space" created by the removal of fat deposits.

Efforts should be made to make sure the patient's urine output remains in a reasonable range (at least 60 cc·hour^{-1}) as measured by a Foley catheter for longer surgeries. Some thought should be given, when administering many liters of crystalloid, as to whether the patient actually may need blood or blood products. Just because it isn't available in the office doesn't mean a patient doesn't need it. Aborting a surgical case or transferring a patient is never an easy or pleasant process for the anesthesiologist, but when malpractice claims are reviewed by experts using 20/20 hindsight, it may be determined that that was the only appropriate decision considering the circumstances.

The necessity of giving many liters of intravenous crystalloid in order to stabilize a patient's vital signs or keep up urine output may be a sign to the anesthesiologist that things are getting out of hand. Malpractice cases reviewed where intravenous intake is in the 10-liter-and-up range in an office setting often have end results that might have been avoided had consideration been given to obtaining laboratory work or transfusing blood. One wonders, in reviewing such cases, if there was a discussion between the surgeon and anesthesiologist as to how the case was going and how much more surgery was anticipated.

Blood loss can be quite difficult to determine in procedures such as liposuction, where blood is mixed primarily with other fluids. Clearly, errors can be made on both sides. Too much intravenous crystalloid causes a dilutional anemia and fluid overloaded state, Circulating clotting factors will be similarly diluted whereas too little leads to hypovolemia with hypotension and low urine output.

Anesthesiologists may be accustomed to using laboratory work, such as blood counts and electrolyte studies or monitored central venous pressures to guide them, but these may not always be available or feasible in every office setting. If extensive fluid shifts are expected or possible, the availability of chemistry and hematology labs and the ability to do invasive monitoring might be considerations in deciding where best to do a specific case.

A fifty-two-year-old previously healthy woman had large-volume liposuction, a facelift, and breast implants performed in a plastic surgery office under general anesthesia. Blood pressure initially was 130/85, but several hours into the case, it began to run 80–100 mm Hg systolic. This responded to intravenous fluid boluses of normal saline. After nine hours of surgery, the anesthesiologist had given 12 liters of fluid and the patient's urine output totaled 500 cc. She was extubated at the end of the case, but in recovery, her respirations became progressively more labored. Auscultation revealed bilateral rales and wheezes. She was given intravenous furosemide, but was eventually transferred by paramedics to a medical center, where she was treated for pulmonary edema.

When procedures exceed the time and blood loss originally estimated, it is crucial for the anesthesiologist to discuss with the surgeon whether the case should proceed. Multiple procedure cases can be stopped before new procedures are begun, and the patient can return on another day. It can be difficult to defend claims where the surgery was allowed to proceed under circumstances that should have caused the anesthesiologist concern.

LIPOSUCTION

Since its introduction into the United States, liposuction has advanced from a procedure for minor body contouring to one with the ability to recontour multiple body

areas, with large volumes of fat aspirated.[5] Whenever liposuction is performed, an anesthesiologist should be aware of the extent of the procedure, including how much local anesthesia is being used and how much volume is estimated to be aspirated, and should work with the surgeon to determine a safe limit for the patient (see Chapter 8). Some facilities have their own policies as to what the upper limits for acceptable liposuction volumes are considered to be. Even if no such guidelines exist, anesthesiologists should be aware of what the standards in the community are and what specialty societies currently recommend.

The American Society of Plastic Surgeons (ASPS) issued practice advisories on liposuction in 2003 and 2004. Although it is important to remember that specialty societies do not establish the medical-legal standard of care, many physicians have chosen to adhere to their guidelines. One recommendations states, "Regardless of the anesthetic route, large volume liposuction (>5,000 cc total aspirate) should be performed in an acute care hospital or in a facility that is either accredited or licensed. This generous loophole leaves open the possibility that >5,000 ccs of aspiration could be performed in an AAAASF accredited office facility. Liposuction volumes exceeding 5,000 cc have been associated with higher morbidity and mortality. Postoperative vital signs and urinary output should be monitored overnight in an appropriate facility by qualified and competent staff who are familiar with perioperative care of the liposuction patient."[6,7] Although there is nothing magical about the 5,000-cc number, what appears clear is that the complication rate rises as the volume of fat aspirated increases and possibly as the number of anatomical sites aspirated increases as well.[6,7]

A fifty-eight-year-old man had surgery in an office operating room that included liposuction of 7,500 cc, a facelift, and abdominoplasty. The patient's blood pressure was running between 120 and 130 systolic, but after four hours, systolic pressures were in the 80s to 90s with a pulse rate of 110. The anesthesiologist gave volume, which raised the blood pressure and lowered the pulse rate. By the end of the seven-hour case, the patient had received 11 liters of normal saline. Blood loss was estimated at 1,500 cc. In the recovery area, the patient remained hypotensive and appeared pale and dusky. He was transferred to an emergency room, where his hemoglobin and hematocrit were measured at 5 g/dL and 15%. He went on to have a very stormy hospital course.

Whenever the tumescent liposuction technique is utilized, intake and output measurements should be made of the fluid injected by the surgeon. Because a large proportion of the residual fluid will become intravascular, this should be taken into account in estimating intravenous fluid requirements. Patients with large volumes of residual fluid from the wetting solution are at risk for fluid overload and should be observed for an extended period of time with consideration given to prophylactic diuretic treatment.[6,7]

The anesthesiologist should additionally be aware of the total dose of local anesthetic given by the surgeon and be alert to potential signs of toxicity. Whereas lidocaine used in wetting solutions for liposuction is variably absorbed, it can still result in toxic blood levels. The ASPS suggests limiting lidocaine dose to levels of 35 mg $\cdot$ kg^{-1}, with the admonition that this level may not be safe in patients with low protein and other medical conditions.[6,7] It has also been recommended that epinephrine doses not exceed 0.07 mg $\cdot$ kg^{-1}, although apparently doses as high as 10 mg $\cdot$ kg^{-1} have been safely used.[6,7] (See Chapter 8).

There is a safety concern when multiple surgical procedures are combined, such as in the case described previously. The ASPS practice advisory recommends that large-volume liposuction not be combined with certain other procedures, such as abdominoplasty, because of the incidence of serious complications noted.[6,7]

Communication between the surgeon and anesthesiologist is, therefore, crucial. It is important that the anesthesiologist be included in the planning process and be fully aware of the length and extent of the surgical procedure contemplated. It is always a judgment call to decide when a surgery is simply becoming "too much" for any given patient, but the correct decision will likely be obvious to a malpractice-claims reviewer using 20/20 hindsight.

Multiple or lengthy procedures may better be divided and accomplished in separate operations.

Patients usually prefer to "get it all over with in one session." When the "one session" approach is explained as a potential safety issue, it is much more easily accepted. Obviously, the time for an anesthesiologist to voice concerns is ideally *before* the procedure gets underway. Once the surgery has begun, the anesthesiologist can keep the surgeon apprised of how much has been aspirated—especially when the volumes become large. *It is never too late to stop a procedure if the anesthesiologist has real con-*

cerns about the patient's well-being. A defense attorney or jury member may someday ask, "Why didn't you say something to the surgeon if you were concerned?" There is rarely a good answer to that question. Either you weren't concerned when you should have been or you failed to speak up about it.

OPERATING ROOM FIRES

Intraoperative fires are not unique to plastic surgery. However, it is particularly devastating to a patient who has come in for a cosmetic procedure to end up with a disfiguring burn. When procedures are performed on the face under sedation, there is a necessary proximity of the operative site to supplemental oxygen provided by nasal cannula or facemask that makes this a time of particular risk.

The three ingredients necessary to combustion are (1) an increased oxygen environment, (2) a flammable substance, and (3) a heat source. Judging by numerous malpractice cases, an oxygen pool around the face, a paper drape, and a surgical cautery device are more than sufficient to satisfy these requirements.

A sixty-three-year-old man developed second- and third-degree burns on his face when a cautery device ignited the nasal cannula and drapes during a blepharoplasty. The patient was given propofol during the injection of local anesthesia, but at the time of the fire was completely awake. He was receiving oxygen 4L flow continuously through the nasal cannula. The charted oxygen-4 saturations were all 100%. The patient sued because of the physical complications of the burn and also alleged psychological trauma from having witnessed the flames.

Always an issue in malpractice claims involving burns is whether the surgeon and anesthesiologist discussed discontinuing the oxygen while a cautery or laser device was in use. Avoiding fires on facial cases might involve little more than an acknowledgment that combustion is a risk and that the surgeon agrees to inform the anesthesiologist before a heat source is used so that the oxygen can be temporarily turned off. When burns occur, the anesthesiologist is often asked *why* the oxygen was in use at the time. "Because I always use it on awake sedation cases" is not a very compelling response to that question. If the recorded oxygen saturation was near 100% at the time, it could be argued that the patient did not really require supplemental oxygen at that moment and could easily have tolerated a short period without it.

If the reason for providing supplemental oxygen is patient comfort because of stuffiness under the drapes, consideration should be given to switching to compressed air—which comprises only 21% oxygen, lessening the risk of fire. If a patient does require an enriched oxygen environment because of partial airway obstruction or desaturation without it, an argument may be made by plaintiffs' attorneys or experts that the anesthetic could have been more safely managed utilizing intubation or a laryngeal mask airway (LMA) to provide higher oxygen concentrations in an enclosed system, rather than insufflating increased flows of oxygen near the operative site.

Avoid using the drapes as a tent to enrich the entire area with oxygen. This essentially creates an oxygen balloon that may be ignited by sparks, causing the drapes to engulf in flames as if a bomb had been detonated. Any oxygen delivered through a cannula or mask tends to naturally pool under the drapes and may remain there for some time after the flow meter has been turned off.

Additional risk management suggestions for preventing burns include using moist sponges and towels to drape off the surgical field, keeping the electrocautery device in a holster when not in use, and avoiding foot pedal controls that might accidentally be deployed by stepping on them. Flammable agents such as alcohol or tincture-based products should be avoided as skin-preparation agents. Petroleum-based eye ointments should be used with caution in eye surgeries as they are potentially flammable.[8] If fires do occur, all drapes and flammables should be immediately removed.

Oxygen and nitrous oxide should be immediately discontinued until the fire is extinguished. Use sterile water, if possible, to douse the fire. It is strongly suggested that all operating room areas have a fire extinguisher and that the anesthesiologist be aware of its location and how to use it. Ongoing care involves management of the burn and a frank discussion with the patient and family. An accurate record of all events surrounding the incident should be kept—preferably in the patient's medical record.[8]

Fires around the face may be largely preventable. Malpractice cases involving OR fires are often indefensible and can result in substantial losses. The most critical element in preventing these claims does seem to be good communication among the OR team and an awareness that such an event is always a potential risk.

THE RECOVERY PERIOD

Judging by malpractice claims, the recovery period may be one of the most dangerous for plastic surgery patients. Part of this likely has to do with the variable monitoring standards used in offices and surgery centers compared with hospitals' postanesthesia recovery areas. As has been stated, claims have been seen for patients left to recover alone in remote areas, far away from any medical personnel. Because the anesthesiologist remains responsible for the patient until safely recovered from the anesthetic, any mishaps during this period may incur substantial liability for the anesthesiologist as well. An anesthesiologist planning to perform anesthesia for a plastic surgery procedure should be aware of all recovery-room policies and should feel comfortable that the following have been satisfactorily addressed.

Location

The location of the recovery room should be central enough to be easily accessible to all personnel who might be required. It should be close enough to the operating room to safely transport patients who are still under the effects of anesthesia. Recovery areas should be located so as to assure that someone would hear audible alarms or a patient calling for assistance. Otherwise, an assigned nurse should be continuously present. The danger is that seemingly awake patients arriving in the recovery room might be considered "finished" in the minds of the nurses who have other duties to attend to. As anesthesiologists are well aware, the level of consciousness of any patient can vary widely depending on the amount of stimulation and the addition of any postoperative pain medication. Patients must be frequently reassessed in this critical period.

A fifty-six-year-old woman had a three-hour facelift performed under general anesthesia. She was transported to the office operating room's recovery area, which was a converted room on the opposite side of the office from the OR. The plastic surgeon later explained that "Patients liked it there because it was quiet and private." She received 50 micrograms of fentanyl intravenously for pain, which was repeated thirty minutes later. She stated she was comfortable and was awake and conversant.

The nurse left the area to help get the operating room ready for the next patient. When she returned to check on the recovering patient about fifteen minutes later, she found her cyanotic and in full respiratory arrest. The woman was still attached to a pulse oximeter that was alarming, but it could not be heard by anyone in the operating room area. Although a secretarial station was located directly across from the room, the staff who normally worked there were out on lunch break during this episode.

Cases like this one are often indefensible because they represent a simple failure to monitor at-risk patients effectively. Anesthesiologists may also be named in claims such as these because they have allowed their patients to recover in areas they should have known were understaffed or unsafe. If patients are "fast-tracked" and recovered in the operating room until ready to stay in the waiting room or discharge area, the anesthesiologist needs to be present until the patient is sufficiently awake, and then the patient can be supervised by qualified personnel.

Recovery Room Staffing

At least as important a factor as where the recovery room is located is *who* will be responsible for monitoring the patient there. Typically, the anesthesiologist is available until the patient is stable, and then a nurse or someone else capable of medically evaluating the patient watches the vital signs and monitors the patient's needs for additional medication. In short-staffed facilities, it is important that whoever is assigned to the recovery room does not have competing responsibilities likely to draw attention away from a recovering patient.

It can be an invitation to error if the person watching the patient has little or no medical training. Not every patient will be able to communicate that they are in trouble and someone must be alert for subtle signs before things progress to an emergency situation. More than one claim has involved nonmedical personnel mistaking a recovering patient's being quiet for stability, while failing to recognize oversedation and respiratory insufficiency until it was too late.

Recovery-room personnel ought to have clear guidelines from the surgeon and anesthesiologist as to exactly when the physicians should be notified (i.e., when vital signs fall outside of specifically set parameters). Anesthesiologists should avoid writing pain-medication orders with wide limits that leave dosing decisions largely up to some-

one else. Anesthesiologists might feel comfortable doing this in hospital recovery rooms, where they are familiar with highly skilled recovery-room nurses. However, unfamiliar staff at another facility might handle those orders very differently. For example, ordering morphine sulfate 2–4 mg intravenously every five minutes as needed for pain could result in large doses being given to a patient over a relatively short interval. If the anesthesiologist writes the orders, he could find himself held at least partially responsible for the results—even if he were no longer in attendance.

It is safest to be as specific as possible with postoperative orders, giving the recovery-room nurses some idea of when patients should be medicated and specifying pain scores and respiratory rates for which medication should be held. It is best to anticipate where problems could develop and to take steps to prevent them before they occur.

A continuously present office staff member, who was not an RN, recovered a twenty-three-year-old breast-augmentation patient. The only monitor used was an EKG. When the patient became bradycardic, the monitoring personnel assumed it was due to the fact that the patient was sleeping soundly. It was only when frequent PVCs and bizarre complexes appeared that the surgeon was summoned and a Code was called. The patient developed anoxic brain damage.

Monitoring

Monitoring in the recovery area is at least as important as monitoring in the operating room—if not more so. The anesthesiologist may not be in continuous attendance and may need to rely on the monitors and alarms to notify other personnel of a potential problem. Recovery areas should have a full complement of monitors, including at least EKG, pulse oximeter, and blood-pressure monitoring capabilities. There should be a separate set of monitors for the recovery area if there is a possibility that a procedure might simultaneously be done elsewhere in the facility that would require the same monitors.

A forty-eight-year-old woman presented for breast augmentation and liposuction, which was performed uneventfully under general anesthesia. She spent between one and one-and-a-half hours in recovery and was medicated twice during that period with intravenous meperidine for pain. As she was standing up to get dressed in preparation for going home, she suddenly stated that she felt faint and collapsed on the floor, unarousable. Although there were single readings recorded for oxygen saturation, blood pressure, and pulse on her arrival in recovery, and a short EKG strip, those monitors were on a wheeled cart that had been returned to the operating room by the anesthesiologist when he began another general anesthetic. There were no physicians available and no other functional monitors in the facility with which to even assess the patient. The paramedics were summoned and on arrival found the patient to be in ventricular fibrillation. It was impossible to determine what the etiology of the syncope had been since the patient was completely unmonitored at the time.

From a malpractice-defense standpoint, probably the single most important monitor is the pulse oximeter. Should a patient develop problems, documentation that the oxygen saturation was always monitored and in a satisfactory range or that any desaturations were promptly noticed and corrected can go a long way toward proving that the medical care provided was standard of care. It is crucial to pick up hypoxia as soon as it occurs and imperative that it be treated appropriately and promptly.

Airway equipment should be readily available in the recovery room, including supplemental oxygen. Someone with airway-management skills needs to be available while a patient is still recovering from an anesthetic. From a medicolegal standpoint, charting is as important in recovery as it is in the OR. Blood pressure, pulse, and oxygen-saturation levels should be charted on the recovery-room record at least every fifteen minutes. Physicians should be notified of any instability and written parameters should exist for what is considered outside of normal limits. Any medications should be charted with accurate times and dosages administered. As risk managers admonish, "It isn't what you do; it's what you chart that counts!" Some complications may be unavoidable risks of anesthesia, but the failure to pick them up promptly and treat them aggressively is often a major problem leading to litigation.

Reviewers of medical malpractice claims that contain issues regarding plastic surgery and recovery have recommended that a physician remain in the facility and be readily available during the full recovery period until the last patient has been discharged.[2] This may be either the anesthesiologist or the surgeon. However, an anesthesiologist should verify that the surgeon will remain before personally leaving the area. It is further advised that whenever a patient is placed under anesthesia, someone with advanced life support (ACLS) training will be available on-site. Complications still can and do occur in recovery, and someone who is capable of handling them must be present.

PATIENT DISCHARGE

Unlike other surgical specialties, plastic-surgery malpractice claims frequently involve issues regarding patients' discharge plans after the procedure. This may concern the timing of discharge or the decision of where to send the patient. Cosmetic-surgery patients may be admitted to a hospital, discharged home, sent to outside facilities with skilled nursing available, or to "hotels" with little medical capabilities. Clearly, each of these facilities is appropriate for some patients, but the determination of which is best for any given patient is a decision that should be made after considering the patient's preference, the surgeon's postoperative concerns, and the anesthesiologist's evaluation of the patient's medical status.

Some anesthesiologists simply defer this decision to others, assuming it is outside of their customary responsibilities. From a liability standpoint, though, if it is deemed that a patient ultimately suffered from residual anesthetic effects or from inadequately monitored electrolyte or blood-count abnormalities, a resulting lawsuit might well include the anesthesiologist in addition to the surgeon. When a patient has had extensive blood loss or fluid shifts intraoperatively and laboratory work has not yet been obtained, it would be prudent to discharge that patient to a facility capable of obtaining laboratory studies and monitoring vital signs to ensure that values remain in an acceptable range. If the patient is continuing to bleed postoperatively, this may also require postdischarge monitoring, even if the patient was quite stable throughout the recovery period.

A sixty-two-year-old woman with hypertension and a smoking history had a bilateral blepharoplasty and browlift with abdominal and thigh liposuction performed in an office operating room late in the afternoon. The blood loss was estimated at 500 cc. This was replaced with 3,500 cc. of intravenous crystalloid over the six-hour case. The patient's vital signs were stable in the recovery room. After two doses of intramuscular opioids for pain, she was discharged after one-and-a-half hours in recovery in the care of a nurse, who routinely watched patients overnight in a spare room of her own home.

On arrival at her home, the nurse noted the patient was quite drowsy and dosing on and off. Several hours later, she complained of a feeling that she could not catch her breath. The surgeon was contacted by phone and he suggested loosening the bandages around her face. This was done, and the patient again fell asleep. When the nurse returned to check on her several hours later, she had no spontaneous respirations. Paramedics were called, but she could not be resuscitated.

One concern in the malpractice claim that resulted from this case was the decision to discharge this patient to a private home in the light of the fact that she had had extensive surgery involving fluid shifts, she was elderly, and she had underlying risk factors. Although a nurse was present, there was no ability to check blood pressure or oxygen saturation. Another issue was the nurse's and surgeon's responsibility for acting conservatively when the patient complained of shortness of breath and possible difficulty breathing.

As is the case with the recovery room, it matters not only what capabilities a postdischarge facility has but also *who* will be monitoring the patient while there. Although plastic-surgery hotels may have skilled nursing available, they may not necessarily be assigned to every patient. If an anesthesiologist feels that someone with medical training should be checking on a patient after discharge, this should actively be communicated to the surgeon. Too many malpractice cases involve lay caregivers admitting after an adverse outcome that a patient complained of shortness of breath or dizziness or that they appeared pale or confused, but that they were unsure of how significant that was or what they should do about it.

Clearly, many patients can be safely recovered at home or at hotels if they are given good discharge instructions and if there is a family member or caregiver available who understands the potentially troublesome symptoms and signs for which they should be on the alert. It would certainly be worthwhile for anesthesiologists to be aware of the discharge instructions that are given to their own patients. Patients should be instructed whom to call in the event of questions and to dial 911 or proceed to an emergency room for potentially life-threatening concerns.

If there are conditions specific to an individual patient (e.g., an asthmatic history, insulin-controlled diabetes), the anesthesiologist should make sure that the patient has been instructed on how best to handle this after discharge and knows whom to call with questions or concerns—whether the surgeon, anesthesiologist, or primary care practitioner. If patients have been instructed to resume insulin or use inhalers, this should ideally be communicated in writing—and explained both to the patients and to the individuals accompanying them home. Patients may not completely understand or remember what is told to them in the immediate postop period because of the residual effects of sedative anesthetic agents. All discharge instructions should be documented in the medical record as well.

Factors that may be important in deciding where a particular patient will go after discharge include the surgical procedure performed, the patient's condition during and after the surgery, and the preoperative medical conditions. Physicians should not be reluctant to change discharge plans if one of these variables changes. It is not uncommon for surgical procedures to run longer than planned or for patients to remain more somnolent in recovery than was expected.

One condition that has received increased attention in the anesthesiology literature in recent years is obstructive sleep apnea. Patients with sleep apnea are at risk not only during the operative period but postoperatively as well, especially if they are being given parenteral opioids.[9] Many patients with sleep apnea do not obtain formal sleep studies and have not been diagnosed at the time they present for surgery. The majority of them do not present with the classic Pickwickian appearance of obese males with short thick necks. Many of them have no obvious physical presentations—but they do have physiologically more compliant or narrowed upper airways.

Even if patients are completely unaware they have this condition, they may still be at substantial risk for serious postoperative apneic periods and even death. In order to identify individuals at risk, patients must be asked specifically whether their sleeping partners have ever advised them of loud snoring or whether they suffer from excessive daytime somnolence that interferes with daily life functions. Patients who answer affirmatively to these questions should be advised about the possibility of sleep apnea and treated similarly to those who carry that diagnosis.[9]

When patients with sleep apnea are given postoperative pain medication, consideration should be given to whether pulse oximeter monitoring is appropriate during this period to detect hypoxic apneic episodes. Pulse oximeter monitoring can be accomplished safely in a variety of settings—the critical factors being the presence of a monitor to identify hypoxic episodes and a person capable of responding to the alarms and taking appropriate action. Patients who normally wear continuous positive pressure airway devices (CPAP) at night should be advised to wear them in the postoperative period if at all possible.

Reviews of malpractice claims indicate that when patients have tight abdominoplasty incision closures, they may also be at risk from adverse respiratory events, even if they have no apparent underlying predisposing factors. Although this does not seem to be well described in the anesthesia literature, some plastic surgeons indicate they are aware that increased abdominal pressure can make the work of breathing more difficult. Having to overcome this pressure during inspiration may make respirations shallower than normal, and patients might be at risk, similar to sleep apnea patients, from opioid pain medications and during sleep. If patients have tightly closed abdominoplasties, if they complain at all of feeling short of breath, or if they require substantial doses of parenteral pain medication, consideration should be given to postoperative monitoring with pulse oximetry or placement in a facility where they will be closely observed overnight.

When patients are sent to unmonitored facilities after discharge, special attention should be given to the timing of discharge. The emphasis in recent years has been on "fast-tracking," as newer shorter-acting anesthetic agents make recovery times quicker, and as more complex cases are being done under sedation or monitored anesthesia care (MAC). Still, every facility should have standardized discharge criteria in place that includes evaluations of consciousness, oxygen saturation, circulation, respiration, and activity level. Problems in any one of these areas should be promptly addressed and rectified prior to sending a patient home. A patient with a preoperative oxygen saturation of 99% on room air and a postoperative reading of 92% should not simply be sent home because they meet minimal criteria for saturation. There should be some evaluation of what the problem is (e.g., underlying bronchospastic disease, fluid overload, negative pressure pulmonary edema, splinting, aspiration pneumonia, apneic episodes). Consideration should strongly be given to whether such a patient needs further recovery time, transfer to an acute care facility, or supplemental oxygen

overnight. That is a medical determination best made by a physician.

The timing of the last medications given should also be taken into consideration when determining a patient's readiness for discharge. A patient may be wide awake, conversant, breathing well, and well saturated, but if they have received (opioid) pain medication within the last half hour, all could change within a short period of time. Patients may also have allergic reactions to medication, and sufficient time should be allotted for those effects to become apparent before release from the facility.

A fifty-seven-year-old man underwent an abdominoplasty with liposuction in a plastic surgeon's office. He arrived in the recovery room in the early afternoon. One hour later, he was medicated with 75 mg of meperidine intramuscularly. Twenty minutes after that, he was described in the nursing notes as ready for discharge, and he left the office in the presence of the surgeon and anesthesiologist.

The patient's wife phoned the surgeon shortly thereafter. She stated that whereas he was initially awake and alert, he soon fell asleep and was snoring loudly in the car. On arrival home, he was too sleepy to walk. The surgeon told her to leave the man lying down until he was more awake. A short time later, the wife noted he was not breathing. The patient was taken to an emergency room, but he was declared dead on arrival. An autopsy listed the cause of death as "respiratory arrest in the recovery phase of general anesthesia."

Although there are no concrete guidelines for how long a patient should be observed in recovery after general anesthesia, one hour is certainly within reason, and the patient described did exceed that time in postoperative recovery. The problem arose in the interval of only fifteen minutes between the dose of intramuscular meperidine and the discharge home. Fifteen minutes was barely time for the drug to act and certainly not the point of maximal effect. Reviewers felt an interval of one hour after the last intramuscular opioid would have been more reasonable. Reviewers also suggested that giving the drug intravenously instead of intramuscularly would have had the advantages of acting sooner and clearing faster from the patient's system.

Not infrequently, it is the anesthesiologist who is ordering medication in recovery. Although anesthesiologists may not even be present in the office when patients are discharged, they may find themselves liable for the decisions of others to discharge patients home while still under the effects of anesthetics or postoperative medications. It would, therefore, be wise for anesthesiologists to be aware of and have input into the discharge policies of all facilities where they will be anesthetizing patients.

WHAT TO DO IF YOU ARE SUED

Being sued is a fact of life for most anesthesiologists with busy practices. Although anesthesiology currently has one of the lowest frequencies for lawsuits among all medical specialties, the average anesthesiologist is still sued approximately once every eight years. The good news is that the vast majority of those lawsuits are successfully defended, with between 80–90% of them closing without any payments being made to patients.

Don't Panic

The stress of a lawsuit may leave an anesthesiologist feeling isolated and alone. Unlike physicians in many other specialties, anesthesiologists do not usually have consistent and loyal patient bases. They may have only transient relationships with the other physicians with whom they work. Often it may seem like one is only as good as your last case. Anesthesiologists sued for the first time frequently report feelings of depression or dread or feel like their career is in jeopardy. Familiarization with the legal process and the knowledge that many other anesthesiologists have successfully trod this same pathway can help alleviate that anxiety. The malpractice process can be long and drawn out, with many months elapsing between interviews with claims representatives, meetings with attorneys, and depositions. However, anesthesiologists need to remember that life goes on.

Although sufficient attention should be devoted to the legal process to ensure its proper functioning, this should not substantially impact the performance of job functions or one's personal life. It is simply one more thing an anesthesiologist must deal with in an often overburdened schedule. It may well take years for a legal case to slog toward completion, with mounds of paperwork generated in the process, but this should not be the central focus of life. The vast majority of one's anesthesia peers have likely been through similar processes, although it is not a subject often publicly discussed. It may well be, as one physician put it, "the cost of doing business for the business we are in."

Don't Discuss It

Although it is tempting to review the facts and details of a case with friends and colleagues, technically all discussions about a claim are legally discoverable by the plaintiff's attorney, with the exception of the formal peer-review process and discussions with one's own attorney and malpractice company claims representative. It is not uncommon for the patient's attorney to ask in a deposition, "With whom, if anyone, did you discuss this case?" An affirmative answer provides an opportunity to subpoena any individuals who might be able to furnish information regarding your mindset or conclusions about the anesthesia care. An unexpected patient death can be the stimulus for posttraumatic stages disorder (PTSD) for the involved anesthesiologist. Do not hesitate to seek psychiatric help. Your therapist's conversation with you is nondisconversable.

Clearly, there will be discussions with the patient and family. Refusing to discuss the case with them at all only gives the impression one is hiding something or is afraid. Although physicians are encouraged to be honest and open with patients and their significant others regarding complications or untoward outcomes, it is important to avoid placing blame or admitting one feels at fault. Patients have a right to know the basic facts regarding what has happened, and they additionally want to feel that their physicians care. "I am very sorry this happened" is an empathetic show of support. However, "I really wish now that we had handled this differently" may be an invitation to litigation. Patients' families often have amazing recall for what was told to them immediately after complications occur. Care should be paid to what is said in the heat of the moment.

Get the Facts Down

Write a detailed narrative of the facts as they occurred from your perspective and keep it at home or separate from the patient's medical record. This is for the anesthesiologist and his defense team to have access to all pertinent information, and it should be documented while it is still fresh in one's mind. This can serve as a starting point for explaining the case to an attorney and claims representative. Obtain copies of the pertinent medical records if possible. Once a case enters litigation, medical records may be sequestered and it can be months or even years before they are subpoenaed.

One important caution here: DO NOT ALTER THE MEDICAL RECORD *after* the fact. Although it might be tempting to make the records more perfect or clearer, records alterations are frequently discovered as such and will only impugn one's credibility and honesty. If something is not correct or important information has been omitted from the patient's chart, it is permissible to add an addendum, clearly labeled as such, and dated at the actual time it was written. Remember that medical records may have already been copied by the time one goes back and reviews them and that it is important that all copies be the same, or alternately that there be a very credible explanation for why that is not so.

The medical record is not the place to plead the case. What is charted should be pertinent information regarding the care of the patient. A patient's chart is not the place to explain in detail why something occurred or why there was no one at fault. Stick to the facts. There will be plenty of time for explanations during the legal process. Placing self-serving notes in the record in an attempt to convince potential plaintiffs attorneys of one's innocence may give the impression that one is more concerned about one's own welfare than the patient's.

Plaintiff's attorneys may simply review charts to see if there is anything that seems negligent. One physician attempting to blame someone else is simply a red flag. Basically, this ensures that each physician will make the case against the other, and the only one who will likely win will be the patient. Juries often conclude in such circumstances that someone must be at fault if they are both blaming each other, so why not give the patient the money? It is always important to avoid public "finger pointing." If one honestly believes that a nurse or surgeon is at fault, there will be opportunities to explain this to one's attorney, who will know best how to handle that information.

It is also helpful if time can be spent researching the pertinent medical literature. If there is information available that might be relevant to one's case, the anesthesiologist can furnish and explain this to his defense team. This may include online searches of medical journals for conditions similar to those experienced by the patient or reviews of relevant medical society guidelines and standards. If there is information available, it is always preferable to know this in advance and to be prepared to address it rather than having it be a surprise to the anesthesiologist by the plaintiff's attorney experts. The anesthesiologist's attorney will designate an expert on his behalf who will likely independently search the literature and help establish the standard of care.

Spend Time on Activities You Enjoy

Stress, overwork, and sleep deprivation can have only negative effects on an anesthesiologist's mental state and job function. After being sued, it is more important than ever to have healthy outlets for recreation and stress release. Run, ski, do yoga, meditate, or find something that helps one get one's mind onto something more positive. As many anesthesiologists who have successfully navigated the malpractice litigation process will attest, "This too shall pass."[10]

REFERENCES

1. Personal communication, Mark Gorney, M.D. The Doctors Company, www.thedoctors.com.
2. Bristow J, Charles D, Gorney M, et al.: Plastic Surgery and Anesthesia: A Claims and Risk Reduction Workshop, *The Doctors Company Risk Management Advisory*, 2000. www.thedoctors.com/risk/specialty/plasticsurgery/J4221.asp.
3. Lofsky, AS: Guidelines for Risk Management in Anesthesiology, *The Doctors Company Risk Management Advisory*, 1998. www.thedoctors.com/risk/specialty/anesthesiology/J3221.asp.
4. Lofsky, AS: Alarms Save Lives, *The Doctors Company Risk Management Bulletin*, 2001. www.thedoctors.com/risk/bulletins/alarms.asp.
5. American Society of Plastic Surgeons: *Practice Advisory on Liposuction: Executive Summary*, 2003. www.plasticsurgery.org/loader.cfm?url//commonspot/security/getfile.cfm&PageID/765.
6. Iverson, RE, Lynch DJ, and ASPS Committee on Patient Safety: Practice Advisory on Liposuction. *Plast Reconstr Surg* 113:1478,2004.
7. Friedberg BL: Inaccuracies and omissions with the report of The ASPS Committee on Patient Safety Practice Advisory on Liposuction. *Plast Reconstr Surg* 117:2142,2005.
8. Gorney M, Lofsky AS, Charles, DM: Playing with Fire, *The Doctors Company Risk Management Advisory*, 2002. www.thedoctors.com/risk/bulletins/fireinor.asp.
9. Lofsky AS: Sleep Apnea and Narcotic Postoperative Pain Medication: A Morbidity and Mortality Risk, *The Doctors Company Risk Management Bulletin*, 2001.www.thedoctors.com/risk/bulletins/sleepapnea.asp.
10. Lofsky AS: You Are Not Alone: On Being Sued, *The Doctors Advocate*, 4th Quarter, 2000. www.thedoctors.com.

APPENDIX A

A Guide to Perioperative Nutrition

David Rahm, M.D.

According to the author, nutritional supplementation in the period before and after surgery can have a significant impact on surgical outcome by reducing bruising, swelling, and inflammation; promoting wound healing; enhancing immunity; and reducing oxidation generated by surgery and anesthetic agents. However, supplements must be administered judiciously; some popular herbal products are contraindicated before and after surgery. Insufficient nutrition impairs wound healing and leaves surgical patients more susceptible to perioperative complications. By addressing nutritional status and providing focused guidance on nutritional supplementation, the aesthetic surgeon can positively influence surgical outcome.

OBESITY, AGING, AND NUTRITION

The risk of death from comorbid conditions increases exponentially as weight increases.[1-3] Patients who are poorly nourished, obese, and, especially, diabetic are particularly prone to surgery-related complications, including wound infection and poor healing. Most Americans consume diets too high in calories and deficient in essential nutrients. More than 70% of American adults do not even get two thirds of the recommended daily allowance (RDA) for one or more nutrients; consumption of fruits and vegetables is notably poor.[4-8] American meals, loaded with packaged, processed, nutrient-poor foods, contribute to marginal deficiencies that result in a shortage of micronutrients and antioxidants that are particularly important to surgical patients undergoing anesthesia, trauma, and wound healing. Older patients are more susceptible to wound-healing problems because of the interactions of body systems, environmental stresses, and disease. Although they have the capacity to heal well, older patients have a slower recovery rate. Aging also pro-

duces dysregulation of the immune system resulting from changes in cell-mediated immunity. Deficits in micronutrients such as zinc, selenium, and vitamin B6 (common in older adults) have a negative influence on immune response. Because aging and malnutrition exert cumulative influences on immune response, many older people have poor cell-mediated immune response and are therefore at increased risk of infection. The appropriate use of nutritional supplements can be particularly helpful in improving immune response in aging surgical patients with protein, energy, and micronutrient deficits.

HERBAL MEDICINES, PHARMACEUTICALS, AND ANESTHESIA

With the greater availability of nutritional supplements, many Americans use herbal preparations for the management of specific symptoms and to combat changes associated with aging. For example, men use saw palmetto to treat benign prostatic hyperplasia, and women use *dong quai* to relieve menopausal symptoms. Many herbal users do not understand the interaction of herbal medicines with pharmaceuticals or anesthesia, and so surgeons must pay careful attention to the use of these products by their patients. A smaller proportion of Americans use supplements to maintain good health. The authors of a study published recently in the *Journal of the American Medical Association*[9,10] concluded that all adults should take a daily multivitamin. This recommendation is based on research demonstrating that a multivitamin may help prevent chronic disorders such as heart disease, some cancers, and osteoporosis. For aesthetic surgeons, knowing which nutrients to include and which to exclude is the basis of perioperative supplementation.

SUPPLEMENTS TO AVOID DURING THE PERIOPERATIVE PERIOD

For several years, discussion about which nutritional supplements are contraindicated during the perioperative period has been widespread.[11–14] Although many familiar supplement and botanical therapies are valuable, their use around the time of surgery can be problematic. The five most popular herbal products in the United States, Ginkgo biloba, St. John's wort, ginseng, garlic, and echinacea,[15,16] can all have negative side effects during this time. Adverse reactions that may be caused by supplements include prolonged bleeding, interference with anesthesia, cardiovascular disturbances, and interactions with pharmaceuticals. It is recommended by the American Society of Anesthesiologists that supplements producing these effects be avoided for at least two weeks before surgery and for at least one week after.[17] Table A-1 lists popular supplements that should be discontinued during the perioperative period.

SUPPLEMENTS RECOMMENDED FOR USE DURING THE PERIOPERATIVE PERIOD

Many herbs and nutraceuticals are potentially useful during the perioperative period. Aesthetic surgeons can incorporate nutritional guidance and supplementation into patient-care regimens to mitigate complications and optimize outcomes. Simple, short-term guidance on nutritional therapies can also be effective in enhancing patient satisfaction. Recent statistics indicate that the likelihood that a surgical patient will present with poor dietary habits is quite high.[4–8] Although a surgeon cannot change a patient's eating habits and lifestyle choices in the limited time between consultation and surgery, a focused approach to nutrition is practical. It is important for patients to know that caloric restriction is not recommended during the perioperative period. Patients frequently believe that the inactivity of recovery will cause weight gain. However, the trauma of surgery and the subsequent wound-healing process increase metabolic requirements by 10% to 100%.[18] Cutting calories during the perioperative period can therefore impair wound healing; the reduction or elimination of beneficial nutritional supplements during the perioperative period can deprive the body of vital nutrients when they are most needed. Patients who normally take supplements may experience diminished outcomes if they are instructed to discontinue all supplements rather than to eliminate only those that are contraindicated. I recommend that surgical patients augment the diet during the perioperative period with nutritional supplements. Although there is no universal agreement regarding supplements and dosages in the perioperative period, Table A-2 shows nutrients that are useful for individuals undergoing aesthetic surgery; this listing is based on the best available data and recent expert recommendations. Perioperative supplementation can have a significant and measurable effect on surgical outcome by favorably affecting four primary mechanisms: reduction of oxidation generated by surgery and anesthetic agents; enhancement of immunity; reduction of bruising, swelling, and inflammation; and promotion of wound healing.

OXIDATION AND ANTIOXIDANTS

Many anesthetic agents are a considerable source of cellular oxidation, causing formation of reactive oxygen species or free radicals, which in turn cause tissue damage and affect wound healing. Excessive free radicals have many harmful effects, including suppression of immune function, disruption of normal cell activity, increased lipid peroxidation, and abnormal cross-linking of protein molecules resulting in tissue stiffness. Beneficial antioxidants can deactivate unstable free-radical molecules resulting from surgery, thereby playing an important role in the prevention of further damage. The administration of specific nutrients and compounds before surgery can help protect patients against the more common forms of injury and oxidation induced by anesthesia and surgery.[19] The presence of these antioxidants in the cell can either prevent free-radical formation or minimize damage by interrupting an oxidizing chain reaction. The body also produces its own antioxidant defenses, including several enzymes such as catalase, superoxide dismutase, and glutathione peroxidase; all three can also be taken in supplement form. However, it is usually simpler for patients to take supplements that enhance the activity of these naturally produced enzymes than to take the enzyme supplements directly. Vitamins and minerals, such as carotenoids, vitamins A and C, selenium, and bioflavonoids, act as antioxidants. Because antioxidant systems and requirements in various body organs differ, a combination of these substances

Table A-1. Supplements contraindicated during the perioperative period

Supplement	Use	Adverse effects
Bilberry (*Vaccinium myrtillus*)	Visual acuity; antioxidant	Antiplatelet activity, inhibition of clot formation
Dong quai (*Angelica sinensis*)	Relief of menopausal disorders, menstrual cramps	May potentiate anticoagulant medications
Echinacea (*Echinacea angustifolia*)	Immune-system stimulant	Can cause hepatoxicity; contraindicated with hepatoxic drugs (e.g., anabolic steroids, methotrexate)
*Ephedra (*Ma huang*)	CNS stimulant, appetite suppressant, antiasthmatic, nasal decongestant, bronchodilator	Hypertension, tachycardia, cardiomyopathy dysrhythmia, myocardial infarction
Feverfew (*Tanacetum parthenium*)	Migraine preventive; used to relieve allergy symptoms	May affect clotting components; contraindicated with warfarin and other anticoagulants
Fish oil	Contains omega-3 derivatives DHA and EPA; used to treat hypercholesterolemia and increased triglyceride levels	EPA and DHA inhibit platelet adhesion and aggregation; excessive doses can inhibit wound healing
Garlic (*Allium sativum*)	Antispasmodic, antiseptic, antiviral, antihypertensive; used to treat hypercholesterolemia	Contraindicated with warfarin and other anticoagulants, NSAIDs, aspirin
Ginger (*Zingiber officinale*)	Antiemetic, antispasmodic	Risk of prolonged clotting time; contraindicated with warfarin and other anticoagulants, NSAIDs, aspirin
Ginkgo (*Ginkgo biloba*)	Antioxidant; enhances cerebral blood flow, alleviates vertigo and tinnitus	Inhibition of platelet activity factor; contraindicated with warfarin and other anticoagulants, NSAIDs, aspirin
Ginseng (*Panax gingseng, P. quinquefolium*)	Improves physical and cognitive performance; antioxidant	May interact with cardiac and hypoglycemic agents; contraindicated with warfarin or other anticoagulants, NSAIDs, aspirin
Goldenseal (*Hydrastis canadensis*)	Mild laxative; reduces inflammation	May worsen swelling and high blood pressure
Hawthorne (*Crataegus laevigata*)	Used for ischemic heart disease, hypertension, angina, and chronic congestive heart disease	Potentiates actions of digitalis and other cardiac glycosides
Kava kava (*Piper methysticum*)	Sedative, analgesic, muscle relaxant, anxiolytic	May potentiate CNS effects of barbiturates, antidepressants, antipsychotics and general anesthesia
Licorice (*Glycyrrhiza g/abra*)	Used to treat gastric and duodenal ulcers, gastritis, and bronchitis	May cause high blood pressure, hypokalemia, and edema
Melatonin	Used for jet lag, insomnia, and seasonal affective disorder	May potentiate CNS effects of barbiturates and general anesthetics
Red clover (*Trifolium pretense*]	Used to relieve symptoms of menopause	May potentiate existing anticoagulant medications
St. John's wort (*Hypericum perforation*)	Antidepressant for mild to moderate depression	Contraindicated with other MAOIs or SSRIs; photosensitivity; multiple drug interactions

Table A-1. (Continued)

Supplement	Use	Adverse effects
Valerian (*Valeriana officinalis*)	Sleep aid, mild sedative	Contraindicated with sedatives and anxiolytics
Vitamin E	Antioxidant; used in treatment of cardiovascular disease	Anticlotting activity may prolong bleeding time
Yohimbe (*Corynanthe yohimbe*)	Aphrodisiac, sexual stimulant	Hypertension; tachycardia; increases potency of anesthetic agents

CNS = Central nervous system; *DHA* = docosahexaenoic acid; *EPA* = eicosapentaenoic acid; *MAOI* = monoamine oxidase inhibitor; *NSAID* = nonsteroidal anti-inflammatory drug; *SSRI* = selective serotonin-reuptake inhibitor.

may provide the best protection against free-radical damage. The current evidence does not favor the use of large (megadoses) of individual nutrients. Administration of smaller, more measured doses of a broad spectrum of several supplements is recommended for antioxidant protection. With surgery, decreases in blood and tissue levels of several nutrients have been documented. At the same time, surgery and anesthesia can increase antioxidant requirements. For example, a decrease in the plasma concentration of vitamin C during the postoperative period, frequently affecting patients and associated with organ failure, has been postulated to be caused by increased

Table A-2. Supplements recommended for use in the perioperative period

Supplement/nutrient	Mechanism of action	Dosage range
Vitamin A (*carotenoid or retinol palmitate*)	Antioxidant; required for new cell growth and maintenance and repair of epithelial tissue	15,000–25,000 IU/d (carotenoid/palmitate blend) limit use to 4 wk
Vitamin C (*ascorbic acid*)	Antioxidant; necessary for tissue growth and repair; primary role in formation of collagen	500–750 mg daily (divided doses)
B vitamins	"Anti-stress" group of water-soluble vitamins; necessary for multiple metabolic pathways	Best taken as B-100 complex: thiamine (B_1) riboflavin (B_2), niacin (B_3), pyridoxine (B_6), biotin, pantothenic acid, folic acid, cobalamin (B_{12}), choline, inositol
Zinc	Antioxidant; essential for protein synthesis and collage formation	15–21 mg/d
Selenium	Antioxidant; inhibits oxidation of fats, protects vitamin E	150–210 mcg/d
Copper	Required for cross-linking of collagen and elastin; required for formation of hemoglobin, red blood cells, and bone	1.5–2 mg/d
Arnica montana	Administered in homeopathic remedy for bruising and swelling	
Bromelain	Proteolytic enzyme; used to minimize inflammation and soft-tissue injury	1,500 mg/d, 2,000–3,000 MCU/d
Flavonoids (*quercetin* and *citrus bioflavonoids*)	Antioxidant, anti-inflammatory; function with vitamin C to prevent bruising and support immune function	600–1,500 mg/d

MCU = Milk clotting units

radical-scavenging activity in response to surgical trauma.[20] Nutrient deficiency may be exacerbated because patients typically fast before and after surgery. For the many patients who take antioxidant supplements regularly and may build up an increased requirement, a shortage of these nutrients is particularly detrimental.

IMMUNITY

Marginal nutritional status and aging are associated with alterations in cellular physiology and immune function, both important factors for the surgical patient. Anesthesia, stress, and pain may also substantially alter the immune system, with potential affects on postoperative function. Nearly all nutrients play a crucial role in maintaining optimal immune response; deficient or excessive intake can negatively affect immune status and pathogen susceptibility. Because nutrient status contributes to immunocompetence, the lack of certain nutrients can suppress immune functions that are fundamental to host protection. Excessive caloric intake and obesity can also influence immune mechanisms. Obesity can promote diabetes, which can significantly alter the immune state. In addition, immunity becomes weaker with aging, and this trend is enhanced by poor nutrition. Zinc is particularly important to the immune system, playing a vital role in more than 300 enzymes that facilitate chemical reactions needed for immune function. Zinc is required for development and activation of T-lymphocytes, and even a moderate deficiency can adversely affect the immune system.[21] Zinc deficiency can be manifested in increased susceptibility to a variety of pathogens through many pathways, ranging from the barrier of the skin to gene regulation within lymphocytes.[22] Zinc affects these key immunologic mediators because of its role in basic cell functions such as DNA replication, RNA transcription, cell division, and cell activation. Small doses of zinc supplements can increase T-lymphocyte levels and have the potential to decrease the incidence of postsurgical infection and its associated complications. Vitamin A also helps regulate the immune system.[23,24] Studies in animal models and cell lines show that vitamin A and related retinoids play a major role in immunity, including lymphopoiesis, cytokine expression, antibody production, and the function of nearly all white blood cells. In particular, natural killer cells, macrophages, and lymphocytes are activated by vitamin A. Vitamin A has been documented to boost immune responses in the elderly, people with marginal nutrition, and patients undergoing surgery.

BRUISING, SWELLING, AND INFLAMMATION

An innovative approach used in aesthetic surgery to reduce inflammation, swelling, and bruising is to provide tissue levels of selective anti-inflammatory agents before the induction of anesthesia and surgery. With injury caused by surgery comes the release of vasoactive substances and pain-inducing chemicals. This proinflammatory process can be attenuated by botanical compounds such as bromelain, an enzyme derived from pineapple stem. Bromelain supplementation before and after surgery has been shown to reduce swelling, bruising, healing time, and pain. Bromelain's effectiveness as a selective anti-inflammatory agent has been demonstrated in several published double-blind studies. It is most commonly used to treat inflammation and soft-tissue injuries, and it has been shown to speed healing from bruises and hematomas.[25] Bromelain treatment after blunt injury to the musculoskeletal system results in reductions in swelling, pain (at rest and during movement), and tenderness.[26] Presurgical administration of bromelain can accelerate visible signs of healing.[27,28] Bromelain has low toxicity in the recommended dosage ranges, and in human clinical trials it has been generally well tolerated and free of side effects. Recently, aesthetic surgeons have become familiar with the benefits of bromelain in the treatment of inflammation and resorption of hematomas. A second herbal remedy that has been touted widely for use in plastic surgery is Arnica montana, which is administered in a homeopathic dilution and has the potential to reduce pain and swelling and to improve healing of soft-tissue injuries. Many aesthetic surgeons have recommended this compound, but, like all homeopathic remedies, arnica is the subject of considerable debate in conventional medical circles. The available evidence from clinical trials indicates that homeopathic arnica's toxicity is negligible and that arnica is safe for use in the perioperative period.[29] However, cosmetic surgeons should be cautious. In a small percentage of patients who take excessive doses of arnica before surgery, bleeding and bruising during surgery may be increased. It is probably wise to advise patients to refrain from taking arnica during the preoperative period. Until homeopathy is better understood, it would be wise to keep an open mind with regard to arnica and to maintain communication with patients who use it.

WOUND HEALING

Wound healing is an orderly progression including inflammation, epithelialization, angiogenesis, and the accumulation of cells necessary to heal the tissue. Like many other bodily functions, wound healing is often straightforward and successful. However, a patient in poor health may not heal so easily. From a nutritional standpoint, raw materials are required for the formation of new tissues and blood vessels. This complex activity can be severely hampered by a diet lacking in essential nutrients. Several of the nutrients listed in Table A-2 can affect wound healing. Vitamin C is a key requirement for proper wound healing. Adequate levels of vitamin C are necessary for function of the enzyme protocollagen hydroxylase, which produces collagen, the primary constituent of granulation tissue. The importance of vitamin C in the wound-healing process has long been recognized. It is evident from clinical experience and reported studies that wound healing requires more vitamin C than diet alone can easily provide.[30] The need for daily replenishment through supplements is increased because vitamin C is water-soluble — any excess is excreted rather than stored. Ophthalmologists routinely administer vitamin C to patients undergoing corneal transplantation, in which optimal wound healing is critical. The relative safety and effectiveness of vitamin A in surgical patients is well documented.[31] Vitamin A's significant wound-healing activity is related to the use of corticosteroids before surgery. Anti-inflammatory corticosteroids significantly impair wound healing by interfering with inflammation, fibroblast proliferation, collagen metabolism, and reepithelialization. These actions are mediated by the antagonism of various growth factors and cytokines. Vitamin A restores the inflammatory response and promotes epithelialization and the synthesis of collagen and ground substances.[16] As noted in Table A-2, a typical recommended daily dose is 25,000 IU for no longer than four weeks total perioperatively. Reported incidences of vitamin A toxicity are relatively rare, averaging fewer than ten cases per year from 1976 to 1987. The overconsumption of vitamin A supplements, occurring after ingestion of 500,000 IU or

>100X the RDA), typically produce symptoms that are reversible.[32] The use of vitamin A does require some caution: It should not be used by pregnant women and should be used only for short periods in women who may become pregnant. The importance of perioperative nutrition is growing with the increased likelihood that surgical patients will have age- and obesity-related problems. It is important for surgeons to make patients aware of supplements that are known to cause perioperative problems and to recommend supplements that boost patient nutrition in the critical period surrounding surgery.

REFERENCES

1. Eckel RH, Krauss RM: American Heart Association call to action: Obesity as a major risk factor for coronary heart disease. *Circulation* 97:2099,1998.
2. Allison DB, Fontaine KR, Manson JE, et al.: Annual deaths attributable to obesity in the United States. *JAMA* 282:1530,1999.
3. Calle EE, Thun MJ, Petrelli JM, et al.: Body mass index and mortality in a prospective cohort of US adults. *N Engl J Med* 341:1097,1999.
4. Block G: Dietary guidelines and the results of food consumption surveys. *Am J Clin Nutr* 53:356S,1999.
5. Kant AK, Schatzkin A: Consumption of energy-dense, nutrient-poor foods by the US population: Effect on nutrient profiles. *J Am Coll Nutr* 13:285,1994.
6. Breslow RA, Subar AF, Patterson BH, et al.: Trends in food intake. The 1987 and 1992 National Health Interview Surveys. *Nutr Cancer* 28:86,1997.
7. Kant AK, Schatzkin A, Block G, et al.: Food group intake patterns and associated nutrient profiles of the US population. *J Am Diet Assoc* 91:1532,1991.
8. van der Wielen RP, deWild GM, de Groot LC, et al.: Dietary intakes of energy and water-soluble vitamins in different categories of aging. *J Gerontol A Biol Sci Med Sci* 51:B100,1996.
9. Fletcher RH, Fairfield KM: Vitamins for chronic disease prevention in adults: Clinical applications. *JAMA* 287:3127,2002.
10. Fairfield KM, Fletcher RH: Vitamins for chronic disease prevention in adults: Scientific review. *JAMA* 287:3116,2002.
11. O'Hara M, Kiefer D, Farrell K, et al.: A review of 12 commonly used medicinal herbs. *Arch Fam Med* 7:523,1998.
12. Miller LG: Herbal medicinals: Selected clinical considerations focusing on known or potential drug-herb interactions. *Arch Intern Med* 158:2200,1998.
13. Larkin M: Surgery patients at risk for herb-anesthesia interactions. *Lancet* 354:1362,1999.
14. Cupp MJ: Herbal remedies: Adverse effects and drug interactions. *Am Fam Physician* 59:1239,1999.
15. Ernst E: The risk-benefit profile of commonly used herbal therapies: Ginko, St. John's Wort, Gingseng, Echinacea, Saw Palmetto, and Kava. *Ann Intern Med* 136:42,2002.
16. Petry JJ: Surgically significant nutritional supplements. *Plast Reconstr Surg* 97:233,1996.

17. Ang-Lee MK, Moss J, Yuan CS: Herbal medicine and perioperative care. *JAMA* 286:208,2001.

18. White DA, Baxter M: *Hormones and metabolic control*, 2nd ed. London, UK: Edward Arnold 1994.

19. Kelly FJ: Use of antioxidants in the prevention and treatment of disease. *J Int Fed Clin Chem* 10:21,1998.

20. Irvin TT: Vitamin C requirements in postoperative patients. *Int Vitamin Nutr Res Suppl* 23:277,1982.

21. Beck FW, Prasad AS, Kaplan J, et al. Changes in cytokine production and T cell subpopulations in experimentally induced zinc-deficient humans. *Am J Physiol* 272:E1002, 1997.

22. Shankar AH, Prasad AS: Zinc and immune function: The biological basis of altered resistance to infection. *Am J Clin Nutr* 68:447S,1998.

23. Ross AC: Vitamin A and retinoids, in Shils ME, Olson J, Shike M, et al.(eds.), *Modern nutrition in health and disease*, 9th ed. Baltimore, Williams & Wilkins, 1999.

24. Gerster H: Vitamin A functions, dietary requirements and safety in humans. *Int J Vitam Nutr Res* 67:71,1997.

25. Blonstein JL: Control of swelling in boxing injuries. *Practitioner* 203:206,1969.

26. Masson M: Bromelain in blunt injuries of the locomotor system. A study of observed applications in general practice. *Fortschr Med* 113:303,1995.

27. Tassman GC, Zafram JN, Zayan GM: Evaluation of a plant proteolytic enzyme for the control of inflammation and pain. *J Dent Med* 19:73,1964.

28. Tassman GC, Zafram JN, Zayan GM: A double-blind crossover study of a plant proteolytic enzyme in oral surgery. *J Dent Med* 20:51,1965.

29. Lawrence WT: Arnica, Safety and Efficacy Report. *Plast Reconstr Surg* 15:1164,2003.

30. Bartlett MK, Jones FM, Ryan AE: Vitamin C and wound healing: Ascorbic acid content and tensile strength of healing wounds in human beings. *N Engl J Med* 226:474, 1942.

31. Wicke C, Halliday B, Allen D, et al.: Effects of steroids and retinoids on wound healing. *Arch Surg* 135:1265,2000.

32. Bendich A, Langseth L: Safety of vitamin A. *Am J Clin Nutr* 2:358,1989.

APPENDIX B

Reflections on Thirty Years as an Expert Witness

Norig Ellison, M.D.

INTRODUCTION

Threat of malpractice litigation is a fact of life in American Medicine and well recognized. That the threat and its costs vary greatly by both specialty and geography is equally well recognized (e.g., an academic anesthesiologist in Philadelphia pays more than three times what comparable insurance costs in San Francisco). Physicians in California credit the Medical Injury Compensation Reform Act (MICRA) of 1975 for their low premiums and physicians in Pennsylvania attribute high premiums to an inability to convince the state legislature to pass a "MICRA" equivalent. This failure currently has the potential to effect healthcare in Pennsylvania adversely. For example:

1. Premiums for category 5 (highest risk) specialists are more than $200,000 annually.
2. Young physicians trained in high-risk specialties are electing to go elsewhere.
3. Hospitals are closing labor and delivery suites to avoid carrying insurance coverage for same.

On the positive side, in Pennsylvania, anesthesia has moved progressively from category 5 to category 3 over the past twenty years. This move reflects the national improvement in the safety of the anesthetized patient (Fig. B-1).

WHO CAN BE AN EXPERT WITNESS?

Most witnesses in a trial do **not** express an opinion – that is, they only testify to the events which they have "witnessed" or to the facts as they know them. In contrast, expert witnesses are specifically recruited by lawyers on both sides of a case to express their opinions on the issue, especially on medical malpractice cases. Why is this so? The "jury of peers," who will judge the facts, lack the expertise to take the facts as presented to them by the "fact witnesses"

and reach a conclusion. Lawyers on both sides will bring in expert witnesses to educate the jurors on what constitutes "Standard of Care" and if a particular treatment was appropriate. In fact, in a medical malpractice case, the jury's decision often will depend on which side's expert witnesses are the most credible.[1]

As a defense expert witness, I have had frequent opportunity to review the statements of plaintiff's expert witnesses. Often as I compare my analysis to that of the plaintiff's expert witness, I marvel how two individuals educated in the same profession and practicing the same specialty can profess such divergent opinions as to standard of care in general or a specific physician's practice in particular after reviewing the same set of documents.

"Peer" is defined as "one of equal standing with another."[2] If a pediatric cardiac anesthesiologist is being sued, does that mean the jurors will be pediatric cardiac anesthesiologists? Absolutely not! In addition to the fact that it would be unlikely to find a sufficient number of them within a given jurisdiction to serve as jurors, physicians would almost certainly be eliminated from consideration by the plaintiff's lawyer because of potential bias toward the defending physician. That helps explain why, as previously mentioned, the jury may lack the expertise to reach a conclusion based on just the facts.

Surely, however, the expert witnesses on both sides would certainly be a pediatric cardiac anesthesiologist. Unfortunately, this is not required. In thirty-seven states, expert witnesses are required only to possess a medical license in their state of residency (Table B-1).

While it may be true that, at one time, there was a "conspiracy of silence" that kept physicians from testifying against other physicians, that day is long gone. Why do physicians testify on behalf of the plaintiff? Some might testify to discourage "bad physicians" from practicing medicine. Another motivating factor is the

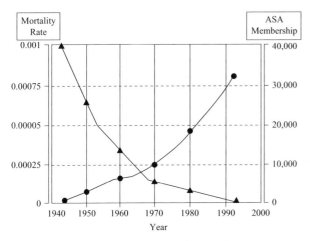

Figure B-1. Anesthesia mortality versus ASA membership. The inverse relationship between mortality and available anesthesiologists is clearly shown by the exponential decrease in mortality being mirrored by an exponential increase in ASA membership. ASA, American Society of Anesthesiologists. From the American Society of Anesthesiologists with permission of the publisher.

financial rewards that can be obtained. Regardless, the AMA Board of Trustees has affirmed that it encourages physicians to recognize their ethical duty as learned professionals to assist in the administration of justice by serving as experts.[3]

Table B-1. States with no expert witness provisions

Alabama	Nebraska
Alaska	Nevada
Arizona	New Hampshire
California	New Jersey
District of Columbia	New Mexico
Georgia	New York
Hawaii	North Carolina
Illinois	North Dakota
Indiana	Oklahoma
Iowa	Oregon
Kansas	Pennsylvania
Kentucky	South Carolina
Louisiana	South Dakota
Maine	Utah
Maryland	Vermont
Massachusetts	Virginia
Michigan	Washington
Minnesota	Wisconsin
Missouri	Wyoming
Montana	

Reprinted from Ellison (1) with permission of the publisher.

Who should be recruited as defense expert witnesses? Partners or close associates would be acquainted with the local standard of care, but the plaintiff's lawyer will quickly bring out the close association and thereby plant the possibility of biased testimony in the juror's mind.

In selecting any expert witness, be it for the plaintiff or the defendant, consideration should be given to such obvious issues as a similar area of practice, certification in the specialty, and experience in the subspecialty (e.g., pain, critical care) if appropriate, and national reputation as evidenced by publications or positions held in national specialty organizations. Less obvious, but equally important, is the impression the witness will make on the jury. A distinctive accent, be it from abroad or just another region of the country, may offend jurors who are parochial. Expert witnesses must also be able to respond quickly to opposing lawyers' attempts to impugn their testimony.

CLOSED CLAIMS PROJECT OF THE AMERICAN SOCIETY OF ANESTHESIOLOGISTS (ASA)

In 1984, the ASA Closed Claims Project began to collect data from closed claim files of (currently thirty-five) cooperating malpractice insurance companies. This data identified the major causes of anesthesia-related patient injury. In this way, ASA can determine where to place emphasis when trying to improve both the care and safety of the anesthetized patient.[4]

While the cooperating insurance companies cover more than 60% of the practicing anesthesiologist in America, the total number of anesthetics administered by these anesthesiologists is unknown—thus, there is no denominator to go with the numerator and an incidence cannot be calculated. However, after twenty years of data collection, it is possible to look at trends over time and the response to interventions. Each year the June issue of the ASA Newsletter features reports from the Professional Liability Committee and these reports reflect both these trends and the responses to interventions. For example:

1. Claims for death and brain damage have decreased, confirming that the severity of anesthesia-related damage has decreased (Fig. B-2).
2. Conversely, the claims for nerve damage have remained constant. In certain susceptible patients, nerve injury may occur in spite of conventionally

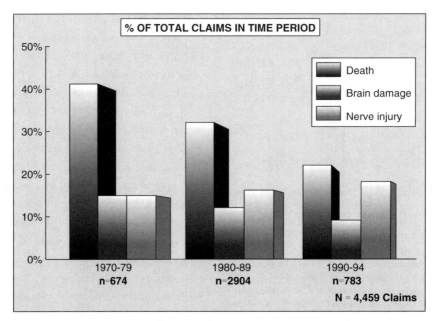

Figure B-2. The incidence of death, brain damage, and nerve injury as a percentage of total claims in a given time period. A significant reduction in the proportion of claims for death and brain damage occurred between 1970–79 and 1990–1994 (p 0.01, _ test). Reproduced with permission from *Anesthesiol* 91:552,1999.

accepted methods of positioning and padding.[5] Therefore, the occurrence, especially of an ulnar neuropathy postoperatively, does not necessarily mean malpractice.

3. Claims for respiratory damaging events have clearly decreased (Fig. B-3). ASA's first practice parameter, Management of the Difficult Airway, was approved in 1992 and revised in 2002 in response to the recognition of this major risk.[6] The decrease reflects favorably on the effect of the parameter. The advent of

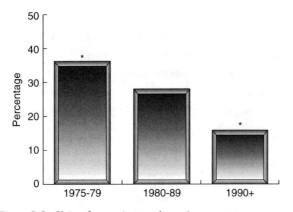

Figure B-3. Claims for respiratory damaging events as a proportion of all claims is the database for each time period. *p < 0.5 for the 1975–90 and 1990+ time periods. Reproduced with permission from *ASA Newsletter* 60:11,1996.

pulse oximetry in the mid 1980s and adoption of capnographic confirmation of tracheal intubation as an ASA standard at that time undoubtedly contributed to this improvement also.

MALPRACTICE INSURANCE CLAIMS

A larger, but more general, source of data regarding malpractice litigation is available from the Physician's Insurance Association of America that summarizes data reported by eighteen physician-owned insurance companies covering all specialties in every region of the country.[7] This data source permits a comparison of anesthesia-related claims to other specialties. For example, in terms of average payout, over $250,000 of all cases between 1985–1997 anesthesia ranked third (Table B-2) and, in terms of average payout of all claims paid, anesthesia ranks eighth (Table B-3).

An analysis of "the most expensive locations" helps explain why anesthesia premiums are what they are. Nearly half the claims (46.6%) originate in the two locations where anesthesiologists primarily work: the operating room and the labor and delivery suite (Fig. B-4).

The most common reason for malpractice claims in general as well as for anesthesia and surgery are listed in Table B-4. In all twenty-four specialties, "no medical

Table B-2. Expert witness requirements by state	
State	Rules
Arkansas	Prohibits testimony from expert witnesses whose compensation depends on outcome of suit. Health care provider shall not be required to give expert opinion testimony against himself or herself except with respect to discovery
Colorado	Expert witness must be licensed physician and substantially familiar with standard of care on date of injury
Connecticut	Expert witness must be licensed physician practicing for five years before date of injury
Delaware	Expert testimony on deviation from applicable standard unless panel found negligence to have occurred and caused injury complained of Expert witness must have knowledge of locality or similar locality in order to testify
	(Locality rule: any Delaware physician in active practice may testify as to standard of care)
Florida	Expert testimony by licensed physician in same practice or practicing for five years before claim filed
Idaho	Expert witness must have knowledge of community standards
Mississippi	Expert witness must be licensed physician
Ohio	Expert testimony limited to licensed physician or surgeon who devotes three-quarters of his or her time to active clinical practice or teaching
Rhode Island	Only those persons whose knowledge, skill, experience or training qualifies them as experts will be permitted to testify
Tennessee	Expert witness must be licensed in Tennessee or contiguous state and practice for one year preceding date of injury
Texas	Expert witness must be practicing physician or training medical residents
West Virginia	Expert witness must be licensed physician and engaged in the same or substantially similar medical field as defendant

Reprinted from Ellison (1) with permission of the publisher.

misadventure" (NMM) was listed among the top three reasons, but only in anesthesia and psychiatry was NMM the top reason. NMM means the physician did nothing wrong but was involved in the patient's care in some way—and on occasion contributed to the payment, obviously sometimes significantly.

A more complete analysis of anesthesia-related claims is provided in Figure B-5. The troika of death, brain damage, and peripheral neuropathy comprises 62% of all claims. In the remaining 38%, another four categories comprising 14% presumably are related to anesthesia procedures: airway trauma, pneumothorax (central line cannulation or high peak conspiratory pressure), headache (post-lumbar puncture), and aspiration.

MALPRACTICE INSURANCE COSTS

A recent survey of forty-six medical liability insurance carriers found the average premium for an anesthesiologist was $20,611, but the range was from $3,458 to $62,400![8]

Part of this range can be explained by history of lawsuits and performance of high-risk procedures such as invasive pain management. The remainder is essentially geographically determined with the highest premiums occurring in Florida, Illinois, Michigan, and Ohio.

Interestingly, when 1985 premiums are adjusted for inflation and compared to the 2004 premiums, the former is 35% higher (Fig. B-6). The aforementioned improvements in patient safety due to the adoption of monitors and practice standards/guidelines have been credited for these savings.

It is paradoxical, and at the same time the administration of anesthesia is becoming safer, malpractice insurance premiums are increasing. Why? Mills has addressed the issue of increasing premiums.[9] While adverse patient outcomes are the underlying factor in establishing rates, the costs associated in both resolving and defending claims have increased between 1994 and 2000, 84% for the former and 39% for the latter. Volatile jury awards have also contributed (Table B-5). Superimposed on these factors have

Table B-3. Which specialties have the biggest payouts?

	% of paid claims $250,000 and over	Average payout
1. Neurology	24	$662,715
2. Pediatrics	26	662,275
3. Anesthesiology	**21**	**639,153**
4. Surgery, Ob/Gyn	26	631,890
5. Radiation therapy	26	626,590
6. Dermatology	12	607,997
7. Pathology	25	603,208
8. Neurosurgery	30	598,850
9. Surgery, *cardiovascular and thoracic*	19	584,722
10. Emergency medicine	16	575,622
11. Cardiology, non-surgical	22	575,123
12. Gynecology	12	574,333
13. Gastroenterology	13	559,336
14. Psychiatry	16	548,217
15. Surgery, general	17	532,389
16. Otorhinolaryngology	19	523,413
17. Internal medicine	19	523,167
18. Radiology	15	503,778
19. FP/GP	14	500,229
20. Surgery, orthopedic	16	490,909
21. Surgery, urologic	14	485,345
22. Ophthalmology	16	466,625
23. Surgery, plastic	8	461,257

For claims that lead to indemnity payments of at least $250,000, some specialists take a harder hit than others. As a group, Ob/Gyns wind up with the biggest total payout. Data are from 1985–1997.

been insurance-industry–related factors. Between 1994 and 2000, there was significant competition within the malpractice insurance industry, resulting in a reluctance to increase premiums despite increased losses. This resulted in several large companies becoming insolvent and others, including St. Paul, which was the largest malprac-

tice insurer, leaving the malpractice market completely. Both the loss of competition with the decrease in insurers and a decrease in investment income, the latter a national factor totally unrelated to the malpractice issue, have further contributed to the premium increase (Table B-6).

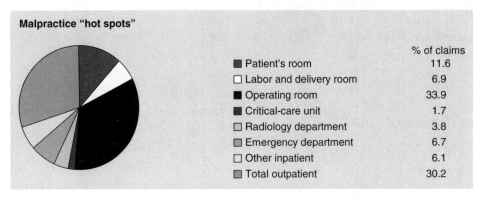

Figure B-4. Malpractice "hot spots." Reproduced with permission from *Medical Economics*, August 24, 1998, p 118.

Table B-4. How 23 specialties compare in number of claims

	Claims	% closed with payout	Average payout
Surgery, Ob/Gyn	22,217	36.43	$216,392
Internal medicine	20,319	27.36	153,028
FP/GP	17,372	37.42	122,172
Surgery, general	16,812	36.06	143,415
Surgery, orthopedic	15,729	30.07	130,563
Radiology	8,162	29.96	127,466
Surgery, plastic	6,105	29.47	83,379
Anesthesiology	**5,940**	**36.65**	**176,544**
Pediatrics	4,783	29.61	226,818
Ophthalmology	4,516	30.29	133,252
Surgery, cardiovascular and thoracic	4,159	24.01	164,727
Surgery, urologic	3,849	30.32	122,087
Neurosurgery	3,798	28.74	235,738
Otorhinolaryngology	2,530	32.20	151,282
Emergency medicine	2,217	28.37	140,038
Neurology	2,194	20.48	215,358
Cardiology	1,978	18.85	182,453
Dermatology (non-surgical)	1,874	32.17	103,285
Gynecology	1,812	32.76	109,333
Psychiatry	1,557	22.86	136,021
Radiation therapy	1,297	22.66	208,879
Gastroenterology	1,105	21.88	127,315
Pathology (non-surgical)	1,006	30.72	204,955

Overall, 89.5 percent of the claims recorded by the PIAA from 1985 through 1997 have been closed. In the nearly 32 percent of cases that resulted in an indemnity payout, the average paid was $154,910.

The figures in this table give only a general idea of how specialties compare. The number of claims is not weighted according to the number of physicians in each specialty. Reprinted from Preston (7).

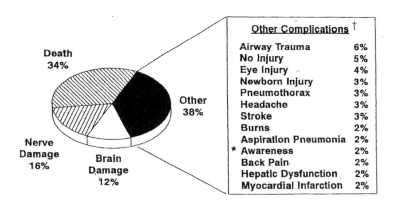

Most common complications in the ASA Closed Claims Project database. Some claims involve multiple complications. †Figures have been rounded.

Figure B-5. Most common complications in the ASA Closed Claims Project database. Some claims involve multiple complications. Figures have been rounded. Reproduced with permission from *ASA Newsletter* 60:15, 1996.

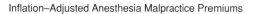

Inflation–Adjusted Anesthesia Malpractice Premiums

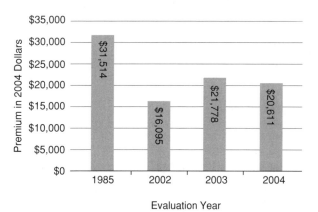

Figure B-6. Inflation-adjusted anesthesia malpractice premiums. Mean premiums for liability insurance. For anesthesiologists in the United States adjusted for inflation in 2004 dollars using the U.S. Consumer Price Index. Adjusted premiums during 2002–04 were still more than 30% below these in 1985. Reproduced with permission *ASA Newsletter* 68:6,2004.

Table B-6. Factors that Influence malpractice premium rates

Medical	Quality of care
	Nature and severity of injury
	Defensibility
	Documentation
Legal	Volatility of jury award
	Level of tort reform
	Limits of coverage
	Increasing defense costs
Economic	Validity of rate level
	Competition entering and exiting malpractice market
	Increases and decreases in investment income

Reprinted from Mills (9) with permission of the *American Society of Anesthesiologists*

Table B-5. What specialists are sued for

	Average payout
All Fields	
Improper performance	$134,360
No medical misadventure	139,411
Errors in diagnosis	169,037
Failure to supervise or monitor case	189,461
Medication errors	114,192
Surgery, general	
Improper performance	$144,419
No medical misadventure	135,377
Errors in diagnosis	180,318
Failure to supervise or monitor case	160,570
Performed when not indicated or when contraindicated	136,931
Anesthesiology (top five causes)	
No medical misadventure	$168,107
Improper performance	118,074
Intubation problems	228,514
Problems monitoring patient during surgery	270,224
Tooth injuries	8,333
Internal medicine (top five causes)	
Errors in diagnosis	$178,189
No medical misadventure	123,117
Improper performance	123,910
Failure to supervise or monitor case	160,944
Medication errors	108,418

PREVENTIVE MEDICINE

The term "defensive medicine" has been used to describe one's practice of ordering unnecessary tests to protect against lawsuits. Here the term "preventive medicine" is used to describe steps that are taken to avoid preventable errors. To prevent **patient mix-up or wrong side/site surgery**, three steps are recommended:

1. Both the anesthesiologist and the circulating nurse independently or jointly confirm the patient's name and the planned procedure with the patient on arrival in the operating room.
2. Prior to induction, the surgeon or his designee mark the operative site.
3. After the induction and prior to the incision, a "TIMEOUT" is called where the surgeon, anesthesiologist, and nurse jointly identify the patient and agree on the procedure. Recording the timeout on the anesthesia record is encouraged.

Documentation legibly and contemporaneously of the administration of anesthesia is essential. If a second sheet is needed before the time graph is filled up, going on to a second sheet is preferred to a cramped inadequately documented record. Equally important is a careful documentation of what may be done in the PACU or ICU. The Anesthesia Patient Safety Foundation advocates electronic records to address both the legibility and timing issue.

The increasing use of electronic instruments in the OR hastened the demise of ether and cyclopropane as anesthetic agents, thus eliminating the risk of explosion from these agents. Today, **intra-operative fires** most commonly involve head and neck procedures with the surgical instrument, either electrocautery or laser, as the ignition source. Use of supplemental oxygen will increase this risk. Communication and coordination between surgeon and anesthesiologist are essential to prevent this risk.

Burns due to inappropriate attempts to warm patients—either with heated bags or unauthorized use of thermal blankets/hot air sources—are other clearly preventable injuries.

EXPERT WITNESS CASE REVIEW

Long before a malpractice case comes to trial, expert witnesses will be recruited by both the plaintiffs' and defendants' lawyers. Indeed, if the former's expert concludes that there is no evidence of malpractice, that may be the end of the case. **Unfortunately, plaintiff's lawyers always seem able to find an anesthesiologist who is willing to say anything to anybody for a price.**

Indeed, a major problem regarding expert witness testimony has been dealing with these "professional witnesses" who appear willing to testify anywhere, anytime, to anything. Defense counsel for many years cautioned about taking any action against these individuals for fear of being accused of witness tampering. The American Academy of Neurosurgeons (AANS) deserves credit for standing up and challenging irresponsible witnesses who develop new theories of causation unsupported by scientific evidence to explain how/why a physician committed malpractice. The AANS expelled a member who was considered to have offered irresponsible testimony. This case went all the way to the U.S. Supreme Court, which affirmed the right of a professional society to police its members.

In 2004, the ASA House of Delegates approved a mechanism for reviewing testimony of expert witnesses in closed cases and, if appropriate, recommending sanctions. These may include either suspension or expulsion of members who are found to have provided irresponsible testimony. One problem is that the anesthesia professional witness

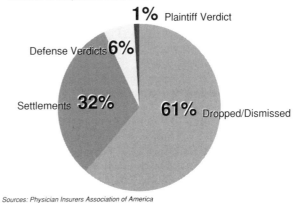

Outcome of Malpractice Case Closed in 2001

Sources: Physician Insurers Association of America

Figure B-7. Outcome of malpractice cases closed in 2001. Reproduced with permission from *Physician Practice* 13:32,2003.

may not belong to the ASA. In these cases, at least the testimony offered can be labeled irresponsible and in future cases, this fact can be introduced to attack the credibility of the professional expert witness.

FINAL REFLECTIONS

The good news is that only 7% of malpractice cases go to trial and 85% of those return a verdict for the defense (Fig. B-7). The bad news is that 32% of cases are settled, invariably with a payment that may be substantial. However, in many cases, a small payment is made "to make the case go away," the thought being that the expense of a trial would be greater than a small payment.

Nevertheless, the current system is broken. Many patients are compensated who have not been injured. The "no medical misadventure" discussed previously attests to this.

Patients who are injured may not be compensated due to failure to file claims or inadequate legal representation. Do I know of any such cases? No, but the statement has been repeated so many times that I suspect somewhere, sometime there may have been a patient who was not compensated.

A new system of medical injury compensation is needed. Alternatives include binding arbitration by impartial panels, no-fault insurance, specialized health courts such as currently exist in the areas of taxes, worker's compensation, and labor issues.

REFERENCES

1. Ellison N: Role of the Expert Witness in Malpractice Litiga-tion. *Problems in Anesthesia* 13:515, 2004.

2. Merriam-Webster's Dictionary, 10th ed. Springfield, MA, Merriam-Webster Inc., 1993.

3. Reardon TR, et al.: Expert witness testimony. AMA Board of Trustees Report 5-A-98, June 1998 Handbook of AMA House of Delegates.

4. Cheney FW: The ASA closed claims project. *Anesthesiol* 91:552,1999.

5. Cheney FW: Perioperative ulnar nerve injury—A contin-uing medical and liability problem. *ASA Newsletter*. Park Ridge, IL, American Society of Anesthesiologists 62:10, 1998.

6. Caplan RA, Benumof JL, Berry FA, et al.: Practice guidelines for management of the difficult airway. *Anesthesiol* 2003; 98:1269–1277.

7. Preston JH: Malpractice danger zones. *Medical Economics* August 24, 1998, p 106.

8. Domino KB: Availability and cost of professional liability insurance. *ASA Newsletter*. Park Ridge, IL, American Society of Anesthesiologists 60:5,2004.

9. Mills EC: Why are my malpractice insurance rates increasing? *ASA Newsletter*. Park Ridge, IL, American Society of Anes-thesiologists 66:13,2002.

10. Administrative procedure for expert witness testimony. *ASA 2004 House of Delegates Handbook*. Park Ridge, IL, American Society of Anesthesiologists, p. 410.

Index

abdominoplasty
  general anesthesia for, 162
  local anesthesia for, 109, 111
  minimally invasive anesthesia® for,
  psychological aspects of, 189
  respiration risks of, 238
accreditation
  for anesthesiologists, 201
  for dentist anesthesiologists, 48
  differing standards for, 212, 218
  issues in, 211
  for office-based anesthesia, 14, 211, 212
  reimbursement and, 223
Accreditation Association for Ambulatory
  Health Care (AAAHC), 211
acetaminophen
  dental procedures and, 55
  in MIA™, 5, 9
  in TIVA, 116, 117
acne treatment, 185
adrenergic alpha-agonists
  dental anesthesia and, 55
  regional anesthesia and, 136
  for TIVA, 115, 116
adrenergic beta-agonists, 17, 118, 119
Advanced Cardiac Life Support (ACLS),
  17, 229
adverse events, 79, 215. *See also*
  complications, perioperative
aging, 184, 241
airway continuum, 120
airway patency management
  algorithm for, 8, 18
  in cosmetic procedures, 121
  in dental procedures, 49, 50–53
  devices for, 18, 120, 121, 122
  interventions for, 12
  legal issues in, 236
Aldrete score, 164
allergy history, patient's, 18
alloplastic body augmentation, 111
alopecia, 186
ambulatory surgery (AS)
  growth of centers for, 171
  vs. office-based surgery, 207

risks associated with, 78, 133
American Academy of Cosmetic Surgery
  (AACS), 183
American Association for Accreditation of
  Ambulatory Surgery Facilities
  (AAAASF), Inc., 11, 211, 212
American Board of Anesthesiology
  (ABA), Inc., 48
American Dental Association (ADA), 47
American Dental Board of Anesthesiology
  (ADBA), 48
American Osteopathic Association
  (AOA), 211
American Society for Aesthetic Plastic
  Surgery (ASAPS), 77
American Society for Dermatologic
  Surgery (ASDS), 77, 183
American Society of Anesthesiologists
  (ASA)
  clinical levels of sedation by, 13
  Closed Claims Project of, 249, 253
  membership/specialties of, 48
  mortality vs. membership in, 249
  office-based guidelines by, 157
  physical status classifications by, 172
American Society of Plastic and
  Reconstructive Surgeons (ASPRS), 79
American Society of Plastic Surgeons
  (ASPS)
  accreditation and, 201
  DVT task force by, 166
  liposuction statistics by, 77
  plastic surgery statistics by, 183
American Society of Regional Anesthesia
  (ASRA) and Pain Medicine, 134
analgesia, adequate
  BIS monitoring and, 3
  inferences regarding, 8, 45
  levels of, 11
  patient movement and, 3, 8, 42
analgesia, preemptive
  clonidine and, 9
  dissociative effect for, 44, 46
  essential concepts of, 43
  ketamine and, 5

in MIA™, 12, 42–45
non-opioid (NOPA), 42
postoperative nausea/pain and, 4
analgesics. *See* non-opioid analgesics;
  opioid analgesics
anatomy. *See* sensory anatomy
androgenetic alopecia (AGA), 186
anesthesia
  goals of, 132
  history of, 86
  primary components of, 37
anesthesia practitioner, 218
anesthesiologist
  attitude of, 20, 43
  due diligence by, 200
  education by, 19, 21–22, 44
  as final gatekeeper, 226, 228
  medical care by, 172
  MIA™ and, 45
  vs. nurse anesthetist, 217
  questions to ask, 56
anesthetic agents, selecting, 114, 157
anesthetic toxicity, 140, 149
anorexia, 192
antacids, 179
anti-aging procedures, 184
antibiotics, 74
anticoagulants, 134
antidepressants, 74
antiemetic agents
  dental anesthesia and, 56
  prophylactic use of, 19, 59, 178
antifungals, 75
antihypertensives, 74
anti-inflammatory agents. *See*
  non-steroidal anti-inflammatory
  agents (NSAIDs)
Anti-kickback Statute, 201
antioxidants, 242
antiseizure agents, 75
anxiety, 177
anxiolysis,
aspiration, 49, 162
aspiration pneumonitis, 178
assessment. *See* pre-anesthetic assessment

257